D1715103

Medicine in Chicago | 1850–1950

Thomas Neville Bonner

Medicine in Chicago | 1850–1950

*A Chapter in the Social and Scientific
Development of a City*

SECOND EDITION

With a Foreword by
Robert C. Hamilton, M.D.

University of Illinois Press
Urbana and Chicago

Material added to second edition © 1991 by the Board of Trustees of the University of Illinois
Originally published in 1957 by the American History Research Center, Inc.
Manufactured in the United States of America
C 5 4 3 2 1

This book is printed on acid-free paper.

Library of Congress Cataloging-in-Publication Data

Bonner, Thomas Neville.
    Medicine in Chicago, 1850–1950 : a chapter in the social and
scientific development of a city / Thomas Neville Bonner.—2nd ed.
      p. cm.
    Includes bibliographical references.
    Includes index.
    ISBN 0-252-01760-9 (cl. : alk. paper)
    1. Medicine—Illinois—Chicago—History.   I. Title.
    [DNLM: 1. History of Medicine—Chicago.   WZ 70 A13 B7m]
R210.C4B6   1991
610'.9773'11—dc20
DNLM/DLC
for Library of Congress   90-11121
                                                  CIP

Contents

Illustrations follow p. 68

Foreword to the Second Edition

Those who cannot remember the past are condemned to repeat it.

George Santayana

Peoples and governments have never learned anything from history, or acted on principles derived from it.

Georg W. F. Hegel

The preface to the original edition of this book entirely justifies its raison d'être. That people have a knowledge of history does not guarantee that they will not let it be repeated; it is hoped, however, that knowledge of previous actions and their consequences may have a positive effect upon our contemporary decision makers, both within and without the medical profession. In the material at hand, it is possible to trace the onset and increasing importance of these outside, though intimately intertwined, governmental and consumer influences.

Thomas Bonner asked several questions in his original preface that should also be answered today: Is the high cost of medical care due solely to the technological and personnel expansion required for treatment? Does this high cost influence the relations between the public, government, and the medical profession? Today the answers are certainly affirmative. The most important current question is can a knowledge of history in the context of present-day medical and socioeconomic conditions be used to make the best long-range decisions for all entities involved? Today the eleemosynary institution and attitude are almost as archaic as the word itself. Medical care is no longer a privilege; it is a right. Life and death, from conception to old age and/or infirmity, including the physician's influence thereon, have been redefined and regulated.

Social and political attitudes of physicians change, perhaps in cyclical fashion. The chapter "Social and Political Attitudes of Chicago Physicians" is included in the main body of this volume for the first time. It was not a part of the original publication because, it is said, the material was too sensitive. Today, however, it is possible, from the vantage point of years, to see parallels and to draw conclusions. The role of medicine and health (or the lack thereof) in the development of civilization cannot be questioned, thus this history applies to many disciplines. Everyone concerned with any aspect of medical care may learn from and be guided by the triumphs and mistakes recorded in this history of *Medicine in Chicago.*

ROBERT C. HAMILTON, M.D.

President, Chicago Medical Society, 1981–82

Preface to the Second Edition

The world of medicine has changed dramatically since the first edition of this book. Much of the research and writing was done more than four decades ago when organized medicine was locked in a fierce struggle with reformers over methods of payment for health care. Voluntary health insurance plans were then new and not yet fully developed; organized labor had not yet made bargaining over health benefits a principal concern of collective bargaining; Medicare and Medicaid were far in the future; and the governmental and corporate stake in medicine was at a low level. The research for the book was undertaken under a generous fellowship provided by the Chicago Medical Society in 1949–50. By the time of the book's publication, seven years later, the manuscript had been the subject of rising controversy, interminable delays, legal challenges, and efforts to stop publication. It is a measure of the sea change in political and social attitudes that the viewpoint of the book and the use of materials that were stoutly resisted then have become commonplace in institutional histories today. The battles that raged over health insurance thirty-five years ago are now largely stilled as the social context of American medicine has shifted to embrace new and wider dimensions. The present crisis of the city's hospital system, on the other hand, could scarcely have been anticipated three decades ago. The recent closing of Provident Hospital and the ending of Cook County Hospital's emergency service would have seemed incomprehensible when this book was being written. As the present edition is being prepared, the city apprehensively awaits the report of an unprecedented summit conference of state, county, and city officials on the future of the health care system of the metropolis.

A chapter of the original manuscript that was omitted to satisfy medical critics of the 1950s has been restored in this edition. The new chapter 12 on the social and political attitudes of Chicago physicians will scarcely be found controversial amidst today's writings on health care. I am grateful to the *Journal of the History of Medicine and Allied*

Sciences for permission to reprint this material, which first appeared in 1953. In addition to this chapter, a note on recent bibliographical sources for Chicago's medical history has been appended to the Bibliography. The assistance of Patricia Spain Ward, medical historian at the University of Illinois at Chicago, has been most helpful in appraising new historical materials and medical developments since 1957.

When Richard Shryock wrote the Foreword to this book in 1957, he expressed the hope that other cities and states would have "future, comparable histories" of their medical experience. By and large, with notable exceptions, this has not happened. Medical historians continue to show little interest in the kind of detailed, institutional history that will alone provide the building blocks for the history of American medical development. In the case of Chicago, suprisingly little has been written in recent decades that would substantially modify the historical judgments expressed in this book.

On rereading the following pages, I am glad to see how they anticipate some of the more recent interests among historians of medicine. The sections on socio-medical problems, political intervention in medicine, class differences in health conditions, and gender and race issues in medical care and training, while spare by 1990 standards, were unusual among studies of that period. I am especially grateful to Ray Allen Billington, my teacher and mentor, and to Richard H. Shryock for awakening my interest in the social aspects of medical development.

From the perspective of more than thirty years, of course, some topics should have been given more space, while others might easily have been given less attention. Clearly, the sections on the health of women and blacks, and on female and black physicians, would now be expanded. Chicago's leadership in the founding of birth control clinics seems more important now than it did in 1957. In that connection, the work of Herman Bundesen in this field appears less impressive than three decades ago. The early success of the public bath movement in Chicago, in which women played a prominent part, somehow escaped my earlier attention. And among the medical "firsts" in the city, the pioneer work of Bernard Fantus in opening a blood bank in 1937, should have been given some prominence.

The present edition is largely unchanged except for chapter 12, the Note on the Bibliography, and a new set of illustrations. It still seeks to record and explain the medical history of a city in the century that ended in 1950. I hope that it can continue to serve a new generation of students of American medicine.

Foreword

Of all the fields usually termed natural sciences, none exerts a more obvious and direct influence upon mankind than does medicine. Most sciences, of course, have important social implications, but rarely are these of such intimate concern to individuals—to all individuals, sooner or later—as is medical science. Presumably for this reason, few sciences have been so influenced in turn by their social milieu as has medicine. So constant and complex are the interactions between medicine and society, indeed, that the field has sometimes been called a social as well as a natural science. Yet one would hardly attain this perspective in reading most of the older histories of medicine, which gave nearly all attention to personalities and to the ideas and methods associated therewith.

Dr. Bonner presents some interesting personalities in the present study, but he does much more than this in providing what is essentially a social history of medicine—an account of how this field evolved and with what results in a major American city. Developments within medical science, as such, are recalled in so far as is necessary in order to explain their impacts upon society; but major attention is given to the interrelations between the medical profession, medical institutions, and the community at large. The result is, in a sense, an "external" history of medicine, in contrast to the traditional "internal" history of medical men and their ideas. The one supplements the other, in making possible a more comprehensive picture of the significance of medicine in our social and cultural experience.

Dr. Bonner's focus on the social history of medicine presumably reflects the interests of the general, as distinct from the strictly medical historian. So, also, does his very thorough use of social data taken from newspapers, institutional records, and the like. But he by no means neglects professional sources, and one of the most arresting aspects of his study is the account of the activities of the medical societies. He does not hesitate to interpret these in the light of his own viewpoints.

Because of the peculiarly human implications of medicine, as well as in consequence of a readable style, Dr. Bonner's work should prove of interest to laymen as well as to physicians. It should also appeal to those concerned with the history of Chicago. No other American city has received so thorough an analysis of its medical experience. No doubt, the Chicago record was typical in some respects of that of all large centers, but it is to be hoped that we shall have future, comparable histories of other cities and also of some of the states. Studies of this nature would be of value to all social historians, and would meanwhile provide the elements essential to any general history of medicine in the United States.

RICHARD H. SHRYOCK,
The Johns Hopkins University

Preface

The medical history of Chicago is important if only because it forms an important chapter in the growth of a great city. The same forces that thrust Chicago to the forefront in matters of trade and commerce also operated to bring her fame in the medical world. The crucial location of the city at the juncture of two great water systems of the continent brought doctors as well as merchants to the frontier village; the later industrialization and urbanization of the area promoted the growth of hospitals as well as factories, demanded specialization in medicine as well as in industry; the accumulation of wealth was used to subsidize medical as well as technical research. By 1893, when a surprised world first viewed Chicago's commercial and industrial achievements at the Columbian Exposition, her fame as a medical center was known throughout the Middle West. In the twentieth century the city has attracted a unique combination of industrial, transportation, and business enterprise to the southwestern tip of Lake Michigan; similarly, she has few peers in point of medical schools, hospitals, and research institutions.

But there are other reasons why an examination of Chicago medicine should prove fruitful. By intensive study of the growth of a single city, some larger hypotheses regarding medical development may be tested. Is it true, for example, that the high cost of medical care may be traced to the technical improvements and expansion of personnel attendant upon the introduction of modern medical procedures? When did the cost of medical care become a factor affecting the relations between the public and the medical profession in Chicago? Does Chicago experience bear out the suggestion that there is intimate relation between disease and social conditions? Why have medical men tended to ally themselves with the conservative groups in the community? What forces have shaped the political and social outlook of Chicago physicians? What part has the medical profession played in attacking those social problems which lie on the borderline between medical and civic responsibility? These are a few of the questions that suggest themselves.

A study of Chicago medicine should also provide an opportunity for assessing the importance of regional factors in shaping imported scientific thought and institutions. Chicago was a frontier town during much of the nineteenth century and she preserved certain frontier characteristics long after the last Conestoga wagon had disappeared. How did immigrant doctors from the more settled and comfortable East adapt to life in the West? Do medical journals reveal important differences between medical thought in the East and the West? Did new ideas from Europe and the East penetrate rapidly into the West? How did Chicago receive anesthesia? antisepsis? the germ theory? Are there evidences of sectional feeling in the writings of nineteenth-century physicians? It is hoped that the reader will find satisfactory answers to at least some of these questions in the following pages.

THOMAS NEVILLE BONNER

Acknowledgements

This book was made possible in large measure by the Chicago Medical Society, which provided a generous fellowship during 1949–1950 for carrying on the necessary research. The Society also permitted me complete freedom in the examination of the minutes of its meetings and other materials in its files. The author wishes especially to acknowledge the help and counsel of Dr. James P. Simonds and the other members of his Committee on Medical History for their suggestions and comments. The generous, helpful, and enlightened attitude of the Society in supporting this project in its initial stages is a strong testimonial to the integrity and objectivity of the Chicago physician's interest in the medical past.

The libraries of Chicago were uniformly helpful in the search for materials. The help of the staffs of the following libraries is gratefully acknowledged: Chicago Public Library, Newberry Library, Church Library of Northwestern University Medical School, Billings Medical Library of the University of Chicago, Quine Library of the University of Illinois School of Medicine, Chicago Historical Society Library, Harper Library of the University of Chicago, Deering Library of Northwestern University, American College of Surgeons Library, Rush Medical School Library, and John Crerar Library. Special thanks is due the staff of the Crerar Library and especially its efficient and kindly medical reference librarian, Miss Ella Salmonsen.

The advice of a number of colleagues in the historical profession was cheerfully given and gratefully received. Professor Ray A. Billington, of Northwestern University, made numerous valuable suggestions at an early stage in the writing and was always sympathetic in counseling me on problems that arose in connection with the manuscript. Professor Richard H. Shryock, director of the Institute of the History of Medicine of the Johns Hopkins University, was kind enough to read the manuscript despite a busy schedule.

My debt to the American History Research Center of the State

Historical Society of Wisconsin is very great indeed. Not only did the Center agree to undertake the publication of the book, but it also persuaded Miss Gayle Thornbrough of the Indiana Historical Bureau to do the necessary editing of the manuscript. Special thanks are due, too, to Forrest McDonald and George Waller, present and former directors of the Center respectively, and to Clifford Lord, director of the State Historical Society of Wisconsin.

Medicine in Chicago | 1850 – 1950

Chapter I

Prologue to 1850:

Medicine in Early Chicago

Philip Maxwell was the last of the Fort Dearborn surgeons. He came to that lonely outpost in 1833, just three years before the fort was swallowed up in the rapidly expanding community of Chicago. A man of Falstaffian girth and temperament, Maxwell brought an infectious enthusiasm, as well as the usual strongbox of primitive medicaments, to his task of guarding the health of the Dearborn garrison. His hale manner and boisterous good humor won him many friends in the Chicago area, while his surgical skill gained him the respect of his professional brethren. As a pioneer doctor in the Northwest his medical experiences were not dissimilar to those of his predecessors; he treated the usual frontier ailments of malaria, typhoid fever, and digestive malaise. When Fort Dearborn was finally evacuated in 1836, Maxwell transferred his colorful activities to the civilian community which had grown up in the shade of the palisades. He thus became one of Chicago's earliest physicians and for the next two decades he practiced medicine intermittently in the young city.[1]

Colorful and interesting though they were, Maxwell and the earlier surgeons at Dearborn exercised little direct influence on the medical development of Chicago. Maxwell was a link between the old and the new. His period of service at the fort coincided with the city's first burst of growth and prosperity. The village which had been incorporated with only three hundred and fifty souls the year that Maxwell arrived could four years later count almost four thousand new inhabitants in the frame shacks and busy stores which lined Chicago's first streets. Like his predecessors, Maxwell had some professional as well as social contact with life outside the Dearborn stockade, but most of his time was spent in treating sick soldiers. Young Chicago was for a brief time dependent on the medical serv-

3

ices of the surgeons at the fort, but as soon as her population had grown sufficiently to warrant full-time physicians, a corps of immigrant doctors arrived to meet the need.[2]

During Maxwell's tenure at the fort the Chicago area was the scene of intense speculation in land. Much of the jobbers' attention was centered on the Illinois and Michigan Canal. Authorized by Congress in 1827, this ribbon of water was to play an important role in peopling the prairie country west of Chicago. Maxwell himself was involved in some of the speculation. In the summer of 1830, lots in Chicago were offered at auction, and the vision of the town as entrepôt for much of the produce of the great Northwest whetted the appetites of the bargainers. Not until the first wave of immigration in the spring of 1833, however, did a real boom develop and it held its pitch until the panic year of 1837.[3] Harriet Martineau, pertinacious and observant British traveler, recorded her vivid impressions of the scene during these hectic years: [4]

I never saw a busier place than Chicago was at the time of our arrival. The streets were crowded with land speculators, hurrying from one sale to another. A negro, dressed up in scarlet . . . announced the times of sale. At every street corner where he stopped, the crowed [sic] flocked round him; and it seemed as if some prevalent mania infected the whole people. . . . As the gentlemen of our party walked the streets, store-keepers hailed them from their doors, with offers of farms, and all manner of land-lots, advising them to speculate before the price of land rose higher.

But the price of land, alas, was to rise no higher. Real estate values were already patently inflated with the breath of future promise and bore no discernible relation to actual conditions in Chicago. The streets marked off in the auction of 1830 were at the time of the panic still indistinguishable in the mud. No drainage had yet been developed in the area; a heavy rain was enough to turn the young town into a swampy morass and the surrounding countryside into a shallow lake.[5] And though the Indian menace could not be considered serious after the Black Hawk War, the boisterous, racist-minded settlers still regarded the remaining red men as a nuisance, as well as a barrier to continued expansion.[6]

Transportation, too, was a serious barrier to be hurdled before Chicago's development could give substance to the airy speculation of the realtors. Despite the boost given commerce and immigration by the opening of the Erie Canal, the approaches to the city were beset with obstacles of all kinds.[7] Roads and paths across the prairie were turned to rivers of mud by a continued rainfall. Travel was hazardous at best and commercial contacts were difficult to maintain. Not until 1842 was the first serious effort at road building brought to completion, but even then stagecoach or private travel was considered an experience to be endured "only at the behest of grim necessity."[8]

The depressive influence of the Panic of 1837 was felt for several years in Chicago. The wave of immigration fell to a ripple; the census of 1840 showed an increase of only three hundred persons over 1837. Business stagnated; some merchants and professional men followed the settlers up the Green Bay road into Wisconsin or took the Ottawa road to the Southwest. Beginning in the early 1840's a sharp upturn in Chicago's fortunes was discernible. Export statistics for the years 1841–1842 revealed a remarkable transformation in the nature of the city's commerce, one that heralded the mighty economic expansion that was to follow. The number of bushels of grain shipped east by water jumped from 212 in 1841 to 586,907 in 1842! It was apparent that the farmer-immigrants who had gone to Wisconsin, Minnesota, and northern Illinois were now producing foodstuffs beyond the power of local communities to consume them. They needed an outlet to the populous East for their surpluses and they were choosing the northern route through Chicago. The opening of the Illinois and Michigan Canal in 1848 joined together the water systems of the Great Lakes and the Mississippi and assured a prosperous future for the Lake Michigan city as the great funnel through which the lion's share of East-West commerce would pass.[9]

But despite the importance of the Michigan Canal, Chicago had to develop more satisfactory roads if she was to make the most of her location. As a correspondent had remarked earlier in a daily newspaper, Chicago's harbor was important, but "if the people cannot reach it for commercial purposes from the back country . . . you lose so much of the advantages which would accrue . . . from having the first harbor on the Lake."[10] The city's answer to the problem was the construction of wooden roads. These plank roads, as they were called, brought excellent results, and Chicagoans were delighted with them. Their success was sufficiently notable to cause merchants to oppose early attempts to bring the railroad to Chicago on the grounds that, as a retail center, the city was dependent on farmers who came to trade. If the settler could ship his produce by rail, the merchants reasoned, he would not come to Chicago and the city's retail trade would be dead. But continued growth, coupled with a change-over from retailing to wholesaling on the part of the larger houses, brought a change in the attitude of civic leaders. By 1855 Chicago found itself one of the leading railroad centers in the United States.[11]

Living in Chicago during these early years was a trying experience. Building a frontier community entailed a strenuous, exciting, and occasionally dangerous existence. While the early settlers had to contend with potentially hostile Indians, later immigrants faced the less heroic, if no less real, danger from primitive sanitary arrangements, bad food, infected drinking water, and lack of medical care. The crowded, unventilated structures which provided shelter exacted further tolls on the frontiersman's life. One of Chicago's early physicians, Dr. Nathan S. Davis, condemned the city's dwellings roundly in a public lecture in 1850. The houses were built too closely together and lacked ventilation, he charged. Five women and children, according to figures he cited, were sick for every adult male stricken in the city. The explanation, according to Dr. Davis, lay in the freedom of the latter to leave their stuffy, often windowless habitations.[12]

The tempo of life in a new community affected adversely the dietary habits of the settlers. Some poorly cooked meat, a few vegetables, and great quantities of boiled coffee, all hastily consumed, was a normal fare for a busy frontiersman. An Indiana physician protested in 1850 that "it is not at all uncommon, indeed it is very common for nervous and exsanguineous females to consume, during a single meal, two, three, four or six cups of strong coffee, almost boiling hot, and perhaps, entirely unqualified by . . . cream and sugar." [13] Daniel Drake, the great prophet of western medicine, pronounced a more judicious criticism of the western diet: [14]

As the time is indefinitely remote, when the density of our population will limit the supply of animal food, it will long continue to enter inordinately into our diet; and, mingled with a great variety of vegetables, unskillfully cooked, indiscriminately mixed, imperfectly masticated, and rapidly swallowed, will constitute our national feeding. That such fullness and crudeness of diet, through successive generations, must work out peculiarities of constitution, and tendencies to some forms of disease, while it gives protection from others, can scarcely be doubted; but these things have not yet been made subjects of accurate observation.

The diseases which affected the white man in the Illinois country were those which laid settlers low everywhere: malaria, typhoid fever, pneumonia, and a loosely defined group of digestive ailments.[15] Illinois, however, early acquired an unusual distinction for unhealthiness. Governor John Reynolds confessed in his memoirs that during the first years of the nineteenth century Illinois was widely thought to be a "grave yard." [16] Malarial or so-called "miasmatic" fevers wiped out 80 per cent of one Illinois county in the 1820's, while Charles Dickens immortalized the abominable conditions in southern Illinois during the early 1840's in his *Martin Chuzzlewit*. The "American Bottom" area in the southern part of the state was long considered uninhabitable because of the widespread incidence of fevers there.[17]

In Chicago, cholera inspired the greatest dread. Even a rumor of this pestilence was enough to rouse officials into attempting some sanitary reforms and appropriating money for the normally neglected Board of Health. The disease had first broken out in 1832 as a result of contact with Gen. Winfield Scott's troops, who were en route to combat with Black Hawk's Indians; the ensuing epidemic had taken a heavy toll of life.[18] For the next seventeen years Chicago enjoyed relative immunity from the scourge, though the town's physicians became excited on numerous occasions over the rumored approach of the disease.

So pronounced did Chicago's reputation for unhealthiness become that the city's promoters frequently felt called upon to refute the charge. In 1835, for example, when rumors were circulating that cholera had struck the town, the editor of the *Democrat* trumpeted that Chicagoans were "uncommonly healthy," and another newspaper boasted that "Chicago is doubtless the most healthy town of any in the state of Illinois." [19] But while the description of the city as a hotbed of disease was repeatedly and vehemently denied, the impression of unhealthiness persisted. As late as 1854, a visitor was surprised to find Chicago "not as unhealthy as has been supposed." [20]

The city's detractors had just cause for criticism. No sewerage system worthy of the name existed in 1850; garbage and refuse were still being thrown into the Chicago River or allowed to accumulate in filthy alleys; drinking water came either from shallow wells or from the lakeshore. Public-spirited citizens like Dr. Nathan S. Davis worked and pleaded for improvements. In a leading article in the *Weekly Democrat* in 1850, Davis called attention to the urgent need for a serviceable system of sewers. The engineering problem, he stated, was similar to that encountered by certain eastern cities, and could be similarly overcome. He outlined in detail a system of sewerage for the city, thereby displaying that universality so characteristic of the nineteenth-century man of science. Davis' plan was typically dedicated to permanence rather than expediency; he warned that an expanding Chicago would soon be overwhelmed in filth and disease.[21] Nor was the doctor's interest confined to matters of public hygiene. He delivered the same year a series of lectures on personal health care in the young city. The lectures contained much practical, common-sense advice on such subjects as adequate ventilation, infant care, temperate eating, and the use of alcohol.[22]

Davis, it must be said, was not typical of his medical confrères in pioneer Chicago. He was abreast of the newest scientific and sanitary discoveries of Europe. These were important years for medicine, and Davis' life span (1817–1904) embraced the crucial period in the evolution of modern medical science. When he came to Chicago in 1849, Xavier Bichat had already accomplished his significant work on animal tissue and demonstrated that tissues, not organs, were the seat of disease. The distinction, though not fundamental in the light of later events, proved a decisive step in the direction of a localized pathology. The concept of disease invading the solid parts of the body and being there subject to arrest or extirpation implied a revolution in medical theory and practice. In medical school, Davis had been taught that the blood was the carrier as well as the starting point of disease; the way therefore to combat illness was to treat the blood, either through withdrawing it by venesection or purifying it with medicines. Now this classical plan of management of the febrile diseases would have to give way when the full implications of the new pathology were grasped.

Another development in French medical circles which was to have enormous significance for the future was the meaningful application of statistical techniques to clinical data. Pierre Louis was a leader in demonstrating the value of correlating ward and post-mortem records, studying vital statistics for clues to the secrets of disease, and using clinical tests in the diagnosis of illness.[23] The importance of statistical studies was not lost on Dr. Davis, who pioneered locally in the movement for a more complete and more careful compilation of vital statistics.

Modern surgery was also emerging in the first half of the nineteenth century. At the beginning of the century, surgeons still confined themselves to the treatment of fractures, flesh wounds, abscesses, bladder stones, and hernia; but the idea of surgery as a last resort in more serious cases faded with the coming of a localized concept of disease. If illness was conceived as arising in the organs or tissues of the body, then surgery might be employed to cut away the ailing members. The development of anesthesia is usually cited as the key to modern surgery, but it is probable that the humoral theory of disease did more than anything else to hinder surgical development. In Chicago, for example, Daniel Brainard performed a number of painful cosmetic operations before the introduction of anesthesia, but he operated otherwise only after internal treatment was found to have no effect. It was medical theory, not dread of pain, which deterred Brainard from greater surgical exploration. But the fear of pain, it should be added, deterred the patient if it did not deter the surgeon; the use of ether and chloroform brought thousands to the operating table who could not otherwise have been induced to appear.[24]

If medical theory and medical research were pointing the way to modern practice in 1850, there is no evidence that the practicing physician in Europe and America was eager to grasp the latest findings of the laboratory. Medical men were used to theories in 1850—the journals were full of them—and there was no reason to believe that any one of them could embody the whole truth. Doctors, indeed, were unusually skeptical of new theories because of the widespread controversy stirred by the homeopaths with their monistic pathology. Nor were young men prepared by the medical schools to receive the new truths coming out of the laboratories of Paris, and later Germany. The first half of the nineteenth century witnessed an unprecedented increase in American medical colleges. As though from the same mold, there sprang up a number of small, often rural, schools with low standards, brief courses of instruction, and inadequate teaching staffs. They taught nothing of the new theories and discoveries. The country's practitioners were inclined to rebel at attempts to break down older doctrines and methods of treatment. When Oliver Wendell Holmes announced in 1843 his conviction

that puerperal fever was a contagious illness preventable by prophylaxis, his message was received indifferently by his countrymen, and
a leading authority on the subject retorted that puerperal mortality
was not only unavoidable, but was the "justification of Providence, a
judgment instituted to remind us of the sin committed by the mother
of the race." [25]

American medicine, in particular, was prone to ignore pure
theory in the search for effective therapeutical procedures. Nowhere
was this clearer than in the American West of a century ago. Experience was the test of a practitioner's reliability here, and little was
said of knowledge gained from books. Western medical journals
were marked by their intensely practical bent. The meetings of medical societies were frequently taken up with discussion of favorite
remedies or proven dosages. A resolution adopted by the Illinois State
Medical Society at its first meeting in 1850 illustrates this practical
quality of mind: [26] "In consultations, theoretical discussions should
be avoided, as occasioning perplexity and loss of time. For there may
be much diversity of opinion concerning speculative points, with perfect agreement in those modes of practice which are founded, not
on hypothesis, but on experience and observation."

The pioneer practitioner differed in other ways from his more
comfortable, settled counterpart in the East. The scattered population and the loneliness of practice induced a gregariousness in the
early western physician which his eastern colleague did not always
share. Few eastern medical societies could boast the loyalty of a member such as Dr. Van Dusen of western Wisconsin, who drove to
Milwaukee for the meetings of his state's society, occupying two or
three days each way in traveling over the hazardous country roads.[27]
Fortunately, his example was becoming rare by 1850 as barriers to
professional co-operation were gradually broken down. The laying of
better roads, the coming of the railroad, the advent of cheap postage,
and lower printing costs all served to bring the members of the profession closer together.[28]

The isolation of the western physician from his colleagues to
the east served for many years to promote a strong feeling of sectionalism on medical matters. Western medical schools, western journals, and western medical societies were acclaimed as superior to
anything the East could produce, and the slightest hint of criticism
from the seaboard brought a storm of disapproval and rebuttal.
When the American Medical Association met in St. Louis in 1854,

the *North-western Medical and Surgical Journal* announced its intention of showing easterners that "though west of the mountains, we are not beyond the reach of light. We speak honestly when we say, we believe that no section of the United States is supplied with better practical men . . . possessed of better common sense in the application of therapeutical rules, than in our North West." [29]

Several physicians of note—Drake, Dudley, McDowell—were produced under these isolated, primitive conditions. Few medical historians have been able to ignore Drake's great geo-medical treatise on disease in the valley of the Mississippi. Traveling the length and breadth of the great valley, questioning, reading, observing, and writing, he accumulated data for two volumes of source material on the relation between the topography, climate, and peoples of the region, and the diseases which attacked them. No environmentalist has investigated the nonconstitutional factors in disease on so broad a basis; no sociologist has grasped more firmly the correlation between social habits and health. Like his colleagues west of the Alleghenies, Drake believed that western physicians had more in common with one another than with doctors beyond the mountains. His advice to readers of the first medical journal in the West was typical: "those who have original matter to communicate, should consent to publish it in the interior, where they live and to which it relates, instead of sending it to the periodical presses of the sea board." [30] His great work excited the admiration of western medical men and at least one western reviewer thrilled with pride at the "appearance of *an Original Medical Book.*" [31]

The typical western practitioner of the period before 1850 still employed bleeding, emetics, and purging as the three mainstays in his armamentarium. Normally a physician was required to treat only a limited variety of diseases and his chief problem at the bedside was to decide upon the proper proportion in which to administer the dreaded trio. In addition to the favored calomel, the medicines most frequently given were quinine, jalap, and occasionally opium.[32] The prescription book used at Fort Dearborn in the 1830's contains such cryptic notations as "Bled"; "Blister"; "Calomel xx gr."; "Poultice of bread and milk"; and "Bleed and Blister." The favorite combination of Dr. Maxwell, the last Dearborn surgeon, was twenty grains of calomel and twenty grains of rhubarb. A typical patient at the Dearborn Hospital underwent the following experience on successive days: [33]

Monday	Tuesday	Wednesday	Thursday	Friday
calomel gr xxx & rhu xv	rest	calomel gr xx jalap gr xx	rest	duty

These remedies, administered in heroic doses, often had a violent effect on the unfortunate patients. Loss of teeth from calomel dosing, for example, was common in the West. Large quantities of mercury given during a malaria epidemic sometimes produced mercury poisoning.[34] And yet, despite their harsh medicines and their bleeding, physicians usually found themselves helpless in the face of epidemic fevers.[35]

This helplessness of regular physicians, coupled with popular distaste for bleeding and vile medicines, goes far to explain the success enjoyed by large groups of irregular practitioners, especially in the West. According to one count, there were seventeen different kinds of "doctors" practicing medicine in the Middle West before 1850.[36] Some of them—homeopathic, eclectic, botanic—continued their profitable existence into the twentieth century; others, such as the uroscopian, hydropathic, vitapathic, physio-medical, and hygeo-therapeutic varieties, enjoyed only faddist popularity. Virtually all of these groups, however, had one thing in common: rigorous abstinence from the use of lancet, mercury, and calomel. A typical botanic physician in Chicago advertised that he "was educated in accordance with the principles of the Old School, but practices upon a system materially different. He substitutes vegetable agents in the treatment of diseases in place of the mineral preparations, so deleterious to the human system." [37] A not uncommon shingle advertisement in these early years was: Dr. John Doe: No Calomel.

In addition to the irregulars, the nineteenth-century physician had to compete with folk medicine, a well-developed set of superstitions and half-truths which carried far greater influence than in our own skeptical age. The amateur healer, according to one legend, could cure a baby's bedwetting by baking a fried-mouse pie; or he could rub off a baby's birthmark by stroking it with the hand of a corpse. Whooping cough would succumb to a bag of live ground-bugs hung around the neck or, if this were not convenient, the victim might "eat the cast-off skin of a snake or eggs obtained from a person whose name had not been changed by marriage." [38]

With the spread of cheap newspapers came another rival of the regular doctor, the patent medicine.[39] The advertising columns of

Prologue to 1850: Medicine in Early Chicago 13

the daily newspaper were the most effective medium for selling patent remedies, though the colorful medicine show continued to attract purchasers for small-scale distributors. In Chicago, not only were vendors of these bottled panaceas successful during the pioneer years, but regular physicians engaged in their manufacture or gave testimonials to their efficacy. Dr. Egan's Sarsaparilla Panacea, for example, which was heralded as the "most perfect restorative ever yet discovered for debilitated constitutions and diseases of the skin and bones," not only enjoyed the publicity attendant upon having the name of the respected Dr. William B. Egan stamped on its label, but was endorsed by some of the city's best-known regulars, the outstanding homeopath, and a judge of the Supreme Court.[40] The pioneer doctor, Edmund S. Kimberly, ran a drugstore during the 1830's which served as an agency for a number of patent medicine firms.[41] Nor were drugstores the only local agents for patent medicines at this time. The early bookstores were heavy competitors, some holding exclusive franchises to sell certain remedies.[42]

Despite the large number of quacks and irregular practitioners in Illinois during the frontier era, there was little disposition to undertake the regulation of medical practice. An "Act for the Establishment of Medical Societies" made it obligatory in 1819 for physicians to police their own profession. The state was divided into four districts with a board of physicians in each to examine candidates for medical licensure. But the law was never enforced, though it was subsequently revised; the amended statute was repealed completely in 1826.[43] For the next half century the practice of medicine was unregulated by public act in Illinois. The experience of the state in this regard, it is fair to say, was quite normal. In the East, as well as in the West, attempts at regulation were defeated by public indifference on the one hand, and by mercenary medical colleges on the other. The latter handed out unearned diplomas and accepted students who lacked any pretense of preliminary education. The sectarian schools were even freer in awarding degrees.[44]

Nor were the regular physicians themselves enthusiastic about licensing the profession. Protection against the irregular practitioner, it was felt, might be bought at too high a price. Public licensure would mean the stifling by the heavy hand of government of individual freedom and the democratic right of free choice. "Much then, as we are scandalized by the wide-spread medical quackery of our time," commented a Chicago medical journal, "we shall do well to adhere to our democratic notions of government—giving the fool full liberty to preach folly, and his hearers abundant permission to trust in him." [45]

Within the profession, however, there existed a genuine desire to elevate the standards of the medical schools, and thus defeat quackery by example if not by law. Dr. Nathan S. Davis, whose importance in the early development of Chicago medicine cannot be overestimated, had early taken the lead in calling for a national convention of medical men to deal with the disgraceful condition of the profession. At an organizational meeting in May, 1846, to which Davis' native state of New York sent over half the number attending, resolutions were adopted asking that the requirements for entering medical school and conferring medical degrees be raised. From these inauspicious beginnings—the schools of Boston and Philadelphia and some of the best-known men in American medicine boycotted the meeting—came the formal organization the following year of the American Medical Association. Though the Association exerted no immediate or striking influence on medical standards, it did provide a forum for the airing of new ideas and its actions did carry a certain moral sanction which represented a step forward in the fight for medical reform.[46]

Conditions in Chicago were no better and no worse than elsewhere. A number of irregular practitioners flocked to the new community in the 1830's, but they were probably outnumbered at most times by the regular physicians. By 1839 twenty-six doctors, most of them regulars, were listed in the Chicago directory, though not all of them were in practice.[47] The number of practicing physicians did not increase appreciably in the following decade, the directory for 1846 listing twenty-four, but there was apparently no shortage.[48] Daniel Drake, who visited Chicago in the mid-forties, warned doctors against rushing to the boom city; there was, he said, already an abundant supply.[49] The city, moreover, had begun to produce her own physicians after 1843 in the Rush Medical College.

Most of Chicago's pioneer doctors emigrated from the East, especially from New York State.[50] Dr. William Todd and his family followed a typical route in reaching Chicago: they left their home in Burlington, Vermont, in 1837, traveled by boat across Lake Champlain to Whitehall, New York, took a canal boat through the Erie Canal to Buffalo, and then steamed around the lakes to their destination aboard the noted side-wheeler, *James Madison*.[51] The typ-

ical practitioner who came to Chicago in the 1830's was married, usually had children, and came with the hope of improving his lot.
Goaded by poverty to seek to improve his fortunes in the West, the
immigrant physician seldom came intending to follow his profession
in his new home.[52] Agriculture or land speculation often occupied
his attention immediately after his arrival, but sooner or later the
physician felt the call to return to his profession. Frequently he continued to work at farming or real estate, while practicing medicine
in his remaining time. An early practitioner in the Illinois country
later recalled that "Anterior to eighteen hundred and forty, nine-
tenths of all the physicians who had located themselves in this region,
had done so with reference to pursuing agriculture, and with the
avowed intention of abandoning medical practice; most of whom,
either from the necessity of the case, or from finding more truth than
poetry in pounding out rails, resumed their profession, and divided
their attention between farming and medicine." [53]

Even those who practiced medicine from the outset in Chicago
usually found some additional pursuit to supplement the meager income of a pioneer physician. Thus Dr. William B. Egan, a native
of County Kerry, Ireland, who had come to Chicago with federal
troops in the early thirties, found additional sources of income in
real estate and patent medicines.[54] Medical practice was combined
with commercial pharmacy by Edmund Kimberly, who also secured
the election of a business partner to the state legislature to work for
his canal interests.[55] Levi D. Boone, later mayor of Chicago, and
Charles V. Dyer, a prominent antislavery advocate, were partners in
the railroad business as well as in medicine.[56] John T. Temple,
another early comer, divided his time between care of the sick and
operation of a stagecoach line.[57]

Since physicians were often the only men boasting any kind
of liberal education in a new community, they frequently stood high
in civic and social life. In western New York, former home of many
Chicago immigrants, medical men served as judges and town officials, and this was likewise true in the West.[58] It was natural that
Kimberly should have been chosen Chicago's first village clerk and
elected to the town's first board of trustees.[59] William Egan served
as county recorder at one time and as a member of the state legislature at another.[60] Another early resident physician, Joseph C. Goodhue, was active in the organization of the city's first school system.
He signed the petition calling for zoning the township for school

purposes, and later as councilman he strongly backed the bill which established Chicago's public schools. Goodhue was active in other educational and civic ventures. He was, for example, an incorporator of Rush Medical College and a frequent disputant on the lyceum platform. His tragic end illustrates the hazards of practice in early Chicago: he died from a fall into an open well while on a night call in 1847.[61]

The early faculty members of Rush Medical College were active in politics and civic affairs. The president of the college, Daniel Brainard, sought the Democratic nomination for mayor several times, finally receiving it in 1858.[62] Graham N. Fitch, the professor of medicine, was elected to Congress in 1849,[63] and N. S. Davis, his successor at Rush, was much in demand as a campaign orator for the Democrats. The energetic and aggressive professor of obstetrics, Dr. John Evans, was active in national politics and played a significant behind-the-scenes role in the Chicago nomination of Lincoln in 1860; he received as his reward the appointment of territorial governor of Colorado.[64]

Perhaps the most notable of Chicago's pioneer physicians was Daniel Brainard, president of Rush Medical College.[65] This remarkable educator and surgeon had much to do with shaping the distinctive pattern of early Chicago's medical growth. He represents the best type of medical man driven into the West by the twin spurs of ambition and desire for adventure. In 1835 Brainard guided his small Indian pony into Chicago after a long trip from the East. He arrived penniless, and it is said that he was forced to sleep on his knapsack until he could afford a bed. The young surgeon struggled along until in 1838 he performed successfully a difficult amputation of a canal worker's leg in the presence of most of the town's physicians. News of this feat spread rapidly and brought him the patronage of the prairie aristocracy.

Thought by strangers to be cold and reserved, Brainard was in reality serious and dedicated. He was genial and polished, yet a hater of sham and pretension. Fellow doctors thought him bold and cool in the operating room. He was the product of eastern schools and European experience, but he was even more the pioneer. He embodied the frontier characteristics of individualism, courage against nature, originality, manual dexterity, and industry. In the years before anesthesia he operated for abdominal tumor, strangulated hernia, strabismus, and obstruction of the lachrymal duct; he extirpated the submaxillary gland and removed encephaloid tumors from the neck; and he performed plastic operations for ectropion and cicatrix of the chin and sternum.[66] The following operation for malignant tumor was performed by Brainard in less than ten minutes with the patient wholly conscious during the entire process: [67]

The integuments were dissected up so as to form a broad flap and entirely expose the tumor. . . . The lip and ala of the nose were then dissected up, and the incisor tooth next the median line extracted. . . . With a common narrow saw of the amputating case, introduced into the nostril, the alveolar and palatine processes of the superior maxillary bone, and the palate portion of the palate bone, were easily divided, as far back as the soft palate. The nasal process of the maxillary, the connexions of the malar bone to the external angular process of the os frontis, and zygomatic process of the temporal bone, were then divided up with the bone scissors, leaving only a posterior bony attachment. To divide this a chisel about one inch wide was placed in the temporal fossa, and with a couple of blows of the hammer it was entirely loosened. It only remained to divide the soft tissues below the orbit and the vail of the palate, at its attachment to the bone, and the whole mass was removed.

The patient, commented Dr. Brainard with masterful understatement, "was considerably depressed from the shock and loss of blood." [68]

Brainard's contributions to surgery and medical education won him fame which was not confined to Chicago or the West. His papers on the treatment of serpent bites and the healing of un-united fractures brought him the vice-presidency of the American Medical Association.[69] In 1853 he was invited to address the French Academy and apparently won the acclaim of that body. A fellow Chicagoan traveling in Europe reported that "Our townsman, Dr. BRAINARD, has made quite a sensation here in scientific circles, and is treated with marked distinction." [70] Upon his return to Chicago the doctor sought political office, but was defeated for mayor in 1858 in a scurrilous campaign.[71]

Brainard died in 1866. His death closed a remarkable career. He had been an active combatant in the front line against disease. His had been the active role of the pioneer; he had personally participated in the establishment of the first medical school, in the founding of the first hospital; his had been the first original research to come out of the new metropolis of the Northwest. It was somehow fitting that he should fall victim to a cholera onslaught just as he was preparing a scientific paper on that disease. His death, according to one journal, "excited a profound sensation in our community. The day was dark and gloomy; the epidemic was at its height; the ensigns of mourning were overshadowing the public buildings. . . ." [72] Brainard had outlived the city's pioneer era; with his passing one of the last landmarks of Chicago's early medical history was gone.

Chapter II	Medicine and the Expanding City, 1850–1900

By 1850, the year that Dr. Davis first excoriated the city's sanitary habits, Chicago was a strapping young community of thirty thousand inhabitants. Its strategic geographical location was already paying dividends in the form of increased trade and the attraction of newcomers to the city. The story of Chicago in the 1850's is dominated by the steady extension of railroad lines into the lumber, corn, and wheat areas north and west of the city. By 1860 the growing metropolis was uniquely prepared to benefit from the tremendous stimulus to industrial development afforded by the Civil War. Resources, manpower, transportation, and entrepreneurial energy awaited only the spark which was to set off a blaze of activity in the sixties. During the Civil War Chicago became a focus for the country's grain, lumber, and meat packing business, while manufactures accounted for an even larger share of her mounting wealth. In the next two decades population increased fivefold as a swarm of immigrants arrived to work in the stockyards and man the new machines. Proud citizens boasted of their part in building the new agricultural machinery which was appearing on farms all over the West, or the Pullman palace cars which carried busy men of trade on errands across the fertile mid-continent.[1]

The Great Fire which leveled the city in 1871 halted only momentarily the city's phenomenal industrial and commercial expansion; in fact, it proved to be only a salutary sweeping out of the Augean stables before newer and greater projects were inaugurated. Feverish rebuilding by business and industry and a new boom in real estate brought a vigorous renewal of prosperity. Even more significant for the future economy of Chicago was the introduction by Gustavus Swift of the refrigerator car into the meat packing business

19

in 1879. The exploitation of this discovery by local packers ensured the city's overwhelming dominance in this important industry. By 1893, the great year of fulfillment for Chicagoans, the world's eyes were fixed on the sprawling giant at the foot of Lake Michigan. At a nodal point in an industrial civilization, Chicago had pushed with unprecedented rapidity into a front-rank position among the world's great cities.[2]

This rapid and relentless transformation of Chicago from a town into a metropolis brought in its wake a host of problems: long hours of work, low level of wages, employment of women and children under unsanitary conditions, lack of public solicitude for the jobless and the aged, and, above all, the mushrooming of slums and crowded rooming houses. All these held ominous implications for the health and happiness of the swelling army of laborers and technicians. And it is impossible to take any measure of the psychological effect on the workers of the breaking down of the integrated operations performed by older skilled craftsmen into numerous routine jobs to be performed by nameless and easily replaced operators. In 1890 Chicago's commissioner of health reported that peddling, carting, and dressmaking were virtually all that remained of the individualistic, self-contained employments of an earlier day.[3]

At the time Chicago was receiving the world's plaudits at the Columbian Exposition in 1893, it had already outdistanced other cities in the misery and degradation of its citizens. Some progress had been made in reducing the amount of child labor by 1893. The number of children under fifteen employed at full-time jobs fell from about nine thousand in 1884 to fewer than two thousand the year of the Exposition.[4] With respect to sweatshops, however, there was no such record of improvement. These unsanitary hovels, with their deadening fatigue, filth, and disease, were mushrooming in the nineties. A sharp smallpox epidemic occurred in the sweating district in 1894 following the Exposition. But it was the housing situation in Chicago which deserved most censure in the closing years of the century. The United States commissioner of labor reported that sanitary conditions were worse in Chicago than in New York, Philadelphia, or Baltimore. In one small area in Chicago there were 811 sleeping rooms without outside windows; only 2.8 per cent of the families in the slum area had their own bathrooms.[5] The hapless industrial worker, according to a writer in the *Weekly Medical Review,* faced an impossible choice: "The sole recourse usually is to the tenement where, heaped floor above floor, in a tainted atmosphere, or in low fetid hovels, amidst poverty, hunger and dirt, in foulness, want and crime, crowded humanity suffers, and sickens, and perishes; for the landlord here is also the air-lord, the lord of sunlight, lord of all the primary conditions of life and living; and these are doled out for a price, failing which the wretched tenant is turned out to seek a habitation still more miserable." [6]

Working conditions in the new factories and packing houses were reflected in the growing concern of medical authorities over accidents and diseases peculiar to industry. The treatment of traumatic injuries and the rendering of emergency care more and more occupied the attention of the city's physicians. In the early 1880's, a paper on "Packing House Wounds" was read by Dr. William L. Axford before the Chicago Medical Society, warning of the danger from cuts inflicted by contaminated knives in slaughter houses. [7]

Not until 1880 was any inspection of Chicago workshops attempted. The problem had become increasingly acute with the growth of new industries and the expansion of older ones; by 1875 manufactories were providing livelihood for over half the population of the city. [8] In 1880 the Board of Health, which was charged with conducting the first inspection, reported that the six inspectors authorized by the City Council were not sufficient for a thorough investigation. The board emphasized that, so far as it could learn, overcrowding, particularly in the garment and tailoring industries, was the worst evil to be met. [9] Public indifference hampered the work of factory regulation for a number of years. At the close of the century several attempts were made to secure more satisfactory legislation at the state level, but not until 1907 was a Department of Factory Inspection created under Illinois' health supervisory powers. The new department was given wide discretion in the enforcement of laws relating to health, especially those governing sweatshops, child labor, occupational diseases, and safety conditions. [10]

Working conditions of women in the 1880's and thereafter were supervised with greater diligence than those of male workers. The Department of Health investigated a large number of complaints against firms employing women—unnecessary standing, filthy dressing and rest rooms, unsanitary surroundings—with apparently good results. A large number of abuses were corrected, but the new conditions could hardly have occasioned the change which a boastful health department inspector attributed to his work: "The sallow hue of disease has given place to the bloom of youth, and the elastic step of the shop-girl as she treads homeward, merrily chatting, meanwhile, with her companions, is a gratifying change from the sad and oftentimes mournful trudging from a laborious day's labor to a cheerless home." [11]

The rise of slaughtering and packing establishments on the south side of the city created health problems peculiar to those industries. The Board of Health did not concern itself greatly with the meat packing concerns until the early 1870's, when regulations were adopted governing the use of steam-tight tanks in the hope of obviating the unpleasant odor which came from the stockyards. [12] In 1877 Health Commissioner Oscar De Wolf received orders to reform the slaughter houses. He found seventy-four such houses within the police jurisdiction of Chicago, in addition to 292 rendering tanks, only eleven of which had any apparatus to suppress the "pungent, acrid, horribly fetid gasses generated." De Wolf at first sought the co-operation of the packers in his cleanup campaign but this he found analogous to making "the Jaguar . . . ameniable [sic] to the influences of christianity." Several packers were actually taken to court, but in each case the twelve jurors, hastily rounded up in neighborhood saloons, according to the health commissioner, censured De Wolf for interfering with legitimate business. Finally, in 1878, the City Council made the slaughter houses subject to license, which meant that failure to conduct an establishment properly could be punished by revocation of license and closing by the police. [13]

Commissioner Swayne Wickersham succeeded De Wolf in 1889 in the war against the packers. He became particularly interested in the practice of the State Live Stock Board of bringing diseased cattle to Chicago for rendering purposes. He was incensed at the board's policy of allowing private dealers to use the city as a disposal center for infected carcasses. Wickersham secured butchers' testimony and the confession of one member of the Live Stock Board that thousands of cattle with actinomycosis had been shipped to Chicago and there sold for food. The commissioner's complaints forced the board to open a special slaughter house for diseased animals. But only three weeks after the opening of this house, health department officers discovered a ton and a half of infected meat in the basement, cut and ready for market. Wickersham then began to insist that the state law which gave the Live Stock Board its power be amended. [14]

Medicine and the Expanding City, 1850–1900   23

Conditions grew worse rather than better in the early years of the new century. Medical and health workers continued to protest, with no success, the packers' indifference to the public welfare. Small wonder that medical journals and public health officers so strongly endorsed Theodore Roosevelt's investigation of packing conditions in Chicago, after Upton Sinclair had exposed them so sensationally in *The Jungle* (1906). One sympathetic journal urged its readers to "Hold up the hands of Hercules Roosevelt" in his fight against the meat industry.[15]

The effect of slums on the health of industrial workers was in many ways more critical than the impact of actual working conditions and industrial hazards. Responsible medical and health workers had early recognized the relationship of slum life to public health. One of the first realistic descriptions of slum conditions in American cities was published in the report of a committee of the American Medical Association in 1849.[16] But though well-demarcated areas of poverty and poor housing existed in Chicago and other cities before the Civil War, it was not until the 1870's that the tremendous pressure of large-scale immigration produced the dangerous overcrowding characteristic of modern slums.[17] Cottages which had formerly housed single families were now packed with a family in each room. A house-to-house check of Chicago's fourteenth ward in 1881 showed that 18,976 persons were sheltered in 1,107 dwellings; significantly, this ward suffered that same year the highest mortality from infectious diseases. Health Commissioner De Wolf attributed the popularity of saloons to the comfort found there by workers and their older sons, since their dwellings—usually kitchen, living, and sleeping room all in one—did not afford even standing room for a whole family.[18] The census of 1880 revealed the number of tenement dwellers in Chicago to be about equal to the number of foreign-born. Though the correlation was not complete, the commission decried the situation which forced most foreign laborers into the tenements.[19]

No public regulation of housing in Chicago was undertaken until 1880; in fact, despite terrible conditions, there was very little that could be done. The critical need was for more housing which would remove pressure from crowded sections and permit the resumption of normal domestic life; but realtors and contractors were unable to meet the skyrocketing demand for new dwellings and it was, of course, the more lucrative suburban construction for the prosperous middle class which received their first attention. Beginning in 1880 attempts were made to control at least the grosser sanitary abuses associated with tenement life. Complaints received regarding plumbing, sewerage, and garbage disposal were acted upon. Enforcement, however, was far from satisfactory. Chief Tenement Inspector Andrew Young assailed his predecessors in 1889 for failing to carry out the law in all cases. He found numerous fictitious reports, calls for re-examination of new plumbing, and other evidences of fraud and bribery.[20] In 1902 a tenement act designed to control conditions of construction and provide more rigorous inspection of existing buildings was passed, but little additional effort was thrown into its enforcement. Hull House residents discovered in 1903 a number of uncovered privy vaults, supposedly outlawed, which were responsible for a sharp outbreak of typhoid fever in their neighborhood. The health department and its chieftain were censured heavily by the investigators and also by the Chicago Civil Service Commission for their negligence.[21]

There was a real relationship between the city's growth and the prevalence of epidemic disease. The congregation of great numbers of people in cities was a direct cause of the high incidence of communicable illness in the nineteenth century. The intimate character of urban living, particularly in the poorer sections, undoubtedly facilitated the spread of germ-borne disease. As early as 1861 one critic complained of the "Narrow and crooked streets, want of proper sewerage and ventilation, the absence of forethought in providing open spaces for the recreation of the people, the allowance of intramural burials, and of fetid nuisances," all of which had "converted cities into pestilential inclosures." [22] Since the urbanization process took place within a framework of individual effort and hostility to governmental interference, cities grew for the most part without the benefit of overall planning. Adequate provision for pure water and the disposal of wastes, for example, seem today a prime necessity of urban life, yet most cities were slow in providing these services. Although the city dweller was eventually to benefit most from the public health work undertaken after 1890, the early effects of urbanization on health were distinctly unfavorable.[23]

This does not mean that all effective epidemic control awaited the coming of the germ theory. In Chicago, as elsewhere, cleanliness, quarantine, and a pure water supply were long advocated by some medical men as prophylactic safeguards against the common epidemic diseases. The importance of the germ theory in public health work was the rationale which it gave to practices long in use. Vaccination against smallpox, for example, dates back to the eighteenth century as an empirical operation, but not until the twentieth, with its systematic health campaigns and public education measures, was the disease virtually wiped out. Public co-operation and financial support were more readily forthcoming when doctors clearly understood and could explain why certain procedures were necessary.

An examination of Chicago mortality tables reveals the effectiveness of empirical sanitary measures undertaken before 1895. During the period between 1855 and 1895, roughly the years of greatest growth for Chicago, the mortality rate was actually reduced, and no epidemic took a toll comparable to the great cholera and typhoid fever outbreaks of the earlier years. The annual death rate dipped to below twenty per thousand persons on a number of occasions, a figure equalled only once in the years before 1855. Cholera, always the most dreaded of pestilences, made its last important appearance in 1866.[24]

There were, in general, two widely prevalent theories of the way in which diseases like cholera were transmitted before the work of Louis Pasteur and Robert Koch put an end to speculation. An older view, that of the *contagium vivum*, held that malignant microorganisms were responsible for illness. This hypothesis has been traced back to a fourteenth-century pest tract and was in considerable favor until the eighteenth century. But with the increased use of the microscope and the actual discovery of bacteria, the omnipresence of these invisible creatures made it seem highly improbable that they could be responsible both for the infinite variety of human afflictions and for the selection of individual victims. Motivated by an increasingly scientific spirit, medical authorities tended to see the contagionist theory as impossible of proof, as the product of a prescientific mysticism. In its stead they clung to an even finer theory of disease transmission by the atmosphere. This so-called "miasmatic" hypothesis placed curious emphasis on contaminated air and malarial exhalations in wafting disease from one place to another. These anticontagionists, strangely enough, were in ascendance during most of the nineteenth century, and it was Jacob Henle, predecessor of Pasteur, who was hailed as a reactionary and defender of the old order in the medical world.[25] There were also political and social factors involved in the controversy. The doctrine of contagion, with its corollary of governmental regulatory action, met with disfavor from liberal thinkers nourished on the laissez-faire postulates of Adam Smith and John Stuart Mill.[26]

It was not strange, then, that an aggressive, young Chicago physician who sought a quarantine during the city's great cholera epidemic of 1849 should encounter robust opposition. Dr. John Evans, who had only recently come to Chicago to teach at Rush Medical College, had taken part in the frantic preparations to ready the city for the expected invader. When cholera was brought to the city with the immigrant boat *John Drew*, in April, Evans began a study of the first cases. The outbreak was unfortunately reinforced by infected newcomers from the East, and in a single month a thousand persons were stricken and over three hundred died.[27] Evans kept a careful statistical record and came to an important conclusion respecting the disease: "Cholera is subject to no boundaries except those that prevent human intercourse." This conclusion was forced on Evans, who as a man heavily engaged in commercial ventures, was reluctant to see the city's trade hampered by quarantine. He admitted in his report that his findings ran counter to his "prepossession against the doctrine of contagion." [28]

But once convinced that cholera was contagious, Evans unleashed a heavy attack on the miasmatic hypothesis. He invited his readers to consider the naïve logic which underlay this theory: [29]

To explain the spread of cholera by the atmospheric theory, requires us to *suppose* in the first place, that the air is contaminated. . . . Then that this poisoned air travels regardless of the course of the winds.—That small bodies of it may go to great distances in very narrow channels.—That a streak of it crosses the ocean . . . at a single point, and invariably that point a sea-port town.—Then that it will tarry a month at the quarantine within eight miles of New York city. . . .—Then that it will travel the whole length of the navigable waters of the Mississippi and its tributaries without varying to the right or to the left, and that it will hover over ships, steam-boats and caravans as they journey on their way. And finally, that like contagion, it follows individuals in their journeyings to the interior, and where they stop it for a time, hovers immediately around them.

When the epidemic had passed, Evans continued to work for an effective quarantine law, on the national as well as on the local level. He was territorial governor of Colorado when the last great wave of cholera struck the West in 1866.[30] In a petition to Congress he observed that the division of opinion which marked the controversy of 1849 no longer held. Only two facts, he declared, need be cited in support of a national quarantine law: first, that cholera had been seen to spread along lines of communication and, second, that cholera had in fact been held off by quarantine.[31]

Dr. Evans, however, was far ahead of his time. Even Chicago's sanitary superintendent, John H. Rauch, a leader in the national health movement, continued to warn as late as 1869 against the fatal exhalations arising from certain waters; he recommended the planting of trees to absorb "the noxious gases which are generated in every populous city." [32]

Typhoid fever in particular seemed to lend itself to interpretation by Rauch's miasmatic theory. Long after most authorities had accepted the germ theory, typhoid continued to be held up as a disease whose etiology was more clearly explained by the atmospheric hypothesis. It was popularly known as the "filth disease" and with considerable justification, since the number of cases seemed to increase proportionately to the coming of industry and the expansion of cities. Typhoid fever was the disease which was to react most spectacularly to sanitary prophylaxis, especially after the role of bacteria laden water in its pathogenesis had been demonstrated.

The seeming relative absence of typhoid fever during Chicago's early years may be at least partially explained by the sparsity of population and the difficulty of differentiating typhoid from other fevers. With the decline of malaria, the prevalence of which on a large scale often served to obscure the presence of typhoid fever, and improved methods of diagnosis, recognition of typhoid became easier and more certain. Chicago sanitarians found the disease surprisingly amenable to prophylactic measures once a clearer idea of its origin had been gained. The mortality rate for typhoid fever in the city fell from more than seventy per one hundred thousand population during the 1860's to less than six in the decade following 1911, and is virtually nonexistent today.[33]

Malaria, unlike typhoid fever, played an important part in the pioneer period of Chicago medicine, but declined gradually in the second half of the nineteenth century. Few settlers escaped a bout with the "ague" during the years of settlement; Governor Reynolds wrote of it as a "seasoning" which every newcomer must endure.[34] As late as the 1850's malarial fevers still accounted for much of the city's illness—a notably sharp epidemic occurred in 1854—but beginning in the late 1860's the disease appeared only rarely in the reports of the Illinois State Medical Society. By 1890, northern Illinois was free from malaria. A number of factors were responsible for the curious disappearance of malaria from the upper Mississippi Valley before Laveran had discovered its cause and before its method of transmission had been announced. These were land and drainage improvements, the use of quinine, and other factors.[35]

Smallpox was the last eradicated of the quadrivium of infectious diseases which attacked nineteenth-century Chicagoans. The first serious smallpox scare came to the city in 1848. The city marshall was commissioned by a frightened Common Council to call on all physicians and ascertain which of them would be willing to perform free vaccinations. All unprotected citizens were then called upon to submit themselves to vaccination immediately.[36] The disease appeared again in December, 1850, and probably was present each winter thereafter.

Not until 1864, when an alarming increase of cases occurred, was a satisfactory pesthouse constructed, though a smallpox hospital had been in existence for more than a decade. At the same time additional policemen were assigned to assist in health work, which was under the supervision of the Police Department during these years. These measures were taken none too soon. By the end of 1865, over two thousand cases of smallpox had been reported. Hardly had the city recovered from this attack when the confusion and crowded living conditions attendant upon the Great Fire of 1871 brought another epidemic of the disease. During this outbreak house-to-house vaccination was tried for the first time with seemingly good results.[37] An important obstacle to effective control of smallpox was the reluctance of victims to be taken to the pesthouse. Commissioner Oscar De Wolf attempted to meet this problem in 1881 by undertaking the forcible removal of sufferers, but public indignation soon brought a halt to the practice.[38]

The last important epidemic of smallpox came in the aftermath of Chicago's Columbian Exposition. The relative immunity enjoyed by the city for nearly a decade fostered a neglect of vaccination which, coupled with the large influx of strangers at the Exposition, increased the severity of the outbreak. This epidemic was particularly sharp in the sweating district where clothiers and their employees resisted efforts of health department officers to destroy possibly infected garments in their possession. The worker who held a

garment representing his food and shelter for a week did not will-
ingly surrender it for the privilege of destroying germs whose existence he probably doubted anyway. Dr. Bayard Holmes, a humanitarian physician with a strong social conscience, flayed the sweating
system, clothing manufacturers, and the Chicago health commissioner for the parts they played in the spread of this epidemic.[39] His
indictment was supported by the report of the factory inspector of
Illinois.

Along with exposure to infectious diseases, Chicago women
faced grave hazards in childbearing. The mortality from childbed
fever, an ancient killer, rose ominously in the second half of the nineteenth century. The reasons for this seem obvious enough, but escaped the practitioners of that day; the likelihood of puerperal contagion like other disease increased in the crowded city. Most births
took place under unsanitary conditions in small, unclean apartments
in tenement areas. And in the hospitals there was the potentially
greater danger of direct infection from the accoucheur's hand, as both
Oliver W. Holmes and Ignaz Semmelweis had demonstrated.[40] Mortality records in Chicago reveal that during the period from 1856 to
1896 puerperal infection was given as the cause of death of 13 per
cent of all women dying between the ages of twenty and fifty years.[41]
One Chicago doctor rose at a medical society meeting in 1874 to announce that he no longer attended puerperal cases, having "essayed
to treat five cases and buried them all." [42] Despite an occasional
allusion by physicians to cleanliness as a factor in preventing infection, not until the 1880's were professors of obstetrics recommending
fresh air and sunlight, good ventilation, adequate sewerage, and
aseptic obstetrical procedures as prophylactic measures.[43]

The smallest chance for survival, however, was held by infants and children. The ratio of deaths among children under five to
all deaths in Chicago rose considerably in the second half of the
nineteenth century, reaching the almost incredible proportion of
70.7 per cent in 1871.[44] For the period from 1843 to 1872, children
under five accounted for over half of all deaths occurring in the city.
In this respect, the record of Chicago exceeded that of any other
city. It was young children who suffered most from the poverty
and uncleanliness of tenement life. The illiteracy and ignorance of
their parents, who clung to long-discarded practices in infant care
or were unable to follow the instructions of patient internes in clinics
and hospitals, made the situation even more difficult. The propor-

tion of children of immigrant parents who suffered from "summer complaint"—a vague term applied to certain undiagnosed digestive infections—was much higher than among the native-born. A partial explanation lay in the fact that the foreign-born inhabited, for the most part, the undrained sections of the city.[45]

From the medical point of view, the diseases of children were considered simply the diseases of adults in miniature. Pediatrics as a specialty had not yet broken off from obstetrics and gynecology. The special hazards of infant life—contaminated milk and water, lack of proper food and clothing—were not recognized by many physicians. Instead they assigned teething, convulsions, or other vague conditions as the causes of sickness and death among children. The six leading causes of death among children under five in 1872, according to a Board of Health report, were cholera infantum, convulsions, diarrhea, dysentery, tabes mesenterica, and teething. This last affliction carried in six months 106 infants to their graves! [46] The newborn suffered, too, from ophthalmia neonatorium, a serious eye infection now routinely prevented by the administration of silver nitrate, and from numerous other nonfatal illnesses. Of 312 children born in one Chicago hospital in the 1880's, twenty-one were afflicted with ophthalmia neonatorium, while a number of others were treated for conjunctivitis.[47]

The social factor involved in the high mortality rate among children was clearly seen in the occasional investigations of sanitary conditions undertaken by the Chicago Medical Society. Typical was the explanation of the inaccuracy of child mortality statistics given by the well-known ophthalmologist Edward L. Holmes: [48]

Undoubtedly, numerous deaths have occurred among children of the abject poor, without the knowledge of physicians. I infer this from the fact, that I have several times heard reports of such cases from people who knew the circumstances. I have also in my visits . . . seen children in a dying condition, to whom no medical assistance . . . had been called. The parents of these children, from the difficulty of gaining a support, seemed indifferent to their recovery, and even wished them to die.

These observations by Dr. Holmes were confirmed by a report on conditions in another section of the city.[49]

Whatever the ailment—cholera, teething, or puerperal convulsions—the medical treatment continued to be almost the same.

Illness, as the second half of the century opened, was closely identified with fever and its symptoms, which were regarded as in themselves injurious phenomena. The approach to disease, therefore, was largely antiphlogistic (i.e., counteracting inflammation) and the chief remedies employed were bleeding, mercury, and antimony. During Chicago's cholera epidemic of 1849, for example, the usual plan of treatment was some combination of bloodletting, stimulants, opium, mercury, and tartar emetic.[50] The work of Pierre Louis and his school in Paris, however, followed by the convincing demonstrations by Josef Skoda and Josef Dietl in Vienna, began to undermine faith in the efficacy of bloodletting.[51] By 1862 the *Chicago Medical Journal* could call attention to the "striking discontinuance of the heroic general bloodletting." [52] But so-called local bloodletting, by means of leeches, cups, and incisions, continued in favor for some years, though its advocates spoke now of using it "judiciously" or "in moderation." Force of habit proved so strong in some cases that at least one Chicago practitioner continued to draw blood "more to gratify the whim of his patient than in pursuance of any positive therapeutical indication." [53] The practice had almost entirely disappeared by 1885, except in treating pneumonia patients, despite the boost given it by the venerable Dr. Samuel D. Gross in a widely publicized address in 1875 and occasional pleas from lesser lights for its resumption.[54]

Thus Chicago's tremendous increase in population in the last half of the nineteenth century created many problems pertaining to the health of its inhabitants. These involved chiefly two types of diseases: those that were spread by close association, such as diphtheria and smallpox, the dissemination of which was favored by the overcrowding in poorly ventilated buildings in slum districts; and those that were spread by contaminated food and water, such as cholera and typhoid fever. That the constant smouldering of these diseases in endemic form frequently led to epidemics with staggering death rates was not surprising; as late as the year 1886 there were 5,000 cases of typhoid fever in Chicago. Heroic efforts by doctors helped alleviate suffering in such periods of great epidemics, but the surprising decline in the death rate during the period was due more to gradually improved sanitary conditions and a concatenation of circumstances than to the efforts of the physician. The practice of healing was plagued by a variety of quack methods, but even "regular" medicine had in many respects advanced very little, and neither the bewildered sufferer nor the conscientious physician had any real way of knowing what was quackery and what was not. Doctors labored under numerous handicaps, but their helplessness in the face of disease resulted primarily from the lack of knowledge of the nature of disease and the lack of weapons with which to combat it. It was not until the bacterial causes of infectious diseases were discovered, beginning in the 1870's and 1880's, that the medical profession and public health authorities had a logical and scientific method of controlling these transmissible diseases and of preventing the terrible epidemics of the past. And many more years of waiting were necessary before the discovery of sulfa drugs and antibiotics were to give the doctor the means of controlling bacterial infections in individual patients.

Chapter III

The Birth of Modern

Medical Science, 1850–1900

A rational plan of medical treatment had to follow a more definite knowledge of the etiology of disease. So long as illness was thought to emanate from subtle miasmas, only the brilliant insight of a Jenner or a Semmelweis would occasionally lighten the dark cloud of mystery which hung over the method by which disease was transmitted. The remarkable Frenchman, Louis Pasteur, was the first to rend the cloud in demonstrating the role of bacteria in fermentation. Pasteur's epoch-making work attracted the attention of an English surgeon, Joseph Lister, whose mind leaped to a profound insight: the possibility that the role of bacteria in wound pus might be causative, rather than incidental. This hypothesis led Lister to the development of antiseptic surgery, first by using a layer of carbolic putty and then a carbolic spray to protect fresh wounds from invasion by micro-organisms. In 1876, Robert Koch, last of this remarkable trio who transformed modern medicine, stated his famous postulate that specific bacteria were responsible for specific diseases, a conclusion reached independently by Pasteur. Koch now led the great microbe-hunting procession which in the last two decades of the nineteenth century discovered the germs responsible for tuberculosis, cholera, bubonic plague, diphtheria, typhoid fever, pneumonia, and dozens of other diseases. These new developments inspired a tremendous burst of energy in surgery, provided a new and broader basis for public health work, and opened up a new world of protection against illness through deliberate immunization.[1]

In the United States, the early work of Pasteur and his associates passed almost unnoticed. The significance for medicine of the relationship between micro-organisms and disease, which seems of such momentous importance to a later generation, was lost on the great Frenchman's contemporaries in America. The germ theory, argued an early Chicago commentator, left too much unexplained. The idea that an invariable relationship existed between the mystery of human illness and the subvisual creatures studied by microscopists seemed the product of wishful oversimplification; "the mere fact of the . . . association of microscopic organisms with contagious diseases," concluded the Chicago writer, "is incidental." [2] But the results obtained by Lister's antiseptic surgery, coupled with a few successful attempts at self-inoculation with catarrh, convinced some Chicago medical men, notably Isaac N. Danforth, that the germ hypothesis went far to explain the nature of disease. Danforth apparently accepted the germ theory as early as 1872, though admitting that the "idea of such multitudes of parasitic tenants seems, at first sight, revolting and unendurable." [3] For the great majority of medical men, however, acceptance lay at least a decade in the future.

But if the abstract theory of a germ cause of disease attracted little attention in America, the practical results obtained by Lister's surgical antisepsis did excite the interest of physicians and surgeons. A number of men have been given the credit for introducing antiseptic techniques in Chicago, but the priority of claim goes to Edmund Andrews.[4] Andrews was a versatile scientist and surgeon with a notable Civil War record when he made a trip to London in 1866. There he was greatly impressed by Lister's methods. Returning to Chicago, he tested Lister's carbolic spray on operative cases in the wards of Mercy Hospital.[5] He found it effective in reducing wound infection and postoperative mortality, but discarded the spray as clumsy and unnecessary. For it he substituted carbolated water in cleansing the wound, followed by carbolated oil and collodion in dressing it. An explanation of his modification of Lister's technique was published in 1869.[6]

But not until 1878 was antisepsis made part of the routine at the famous Cook County Hospital in Chicago, and not until 1882 were most of the city's hospitals following some form of Listerism in their operative procedures. Nor were all surgeons as quick to adopt antisepsis as Andrews had been. A discussion on surgical infection by Illinois doctors in 1870 found a large number skeptical, if not hostile, to the use of carbolic acid in treating wounds. Even the most famous surgeon in Chicago in the 1870's, Moses Gunn, who had come from Michigan to replace Brainard in the chair of surgery at Rush, clung to the doctrine of "laudable pus" in gauging the success of operations. After his conversion to antisepsis, Gunn still insisted that suppuration was not an unmixed evil. It was, he said, "a dangerous thorn, from which occasionally, at least, a fragrant flower was plucked." [7]

With respect to the trial and acceptance of antiseptic surgery, Chicago, and notably Dr. Andrews, were abreast of the American profession. A noted British surgeon visiting the United States in 1874 observed that antisepsis was rarely employed and two years later Lister himself found almost no one using his technique when he toured the country. Robert Weir, surgeon to the New York and Roosevelt hospitals, wrote in 1877 that only since Lister's appearance at the Medical Congress in Philadelphia had antisepsis attracted much attention in the United States. He added that aside from an article in a New Orleans journal, he knew little or nothing of results obtained from using the antiseptic method in this country.[8]

The gradual growth of asepsis began even before antisepsis had been universally accepted. The British surgeon mentioned above remarked that antisepsis was needed less in American hospitals because they were relatively clean and sanitary. "Cleanliness," he noted, "is the best and most efficient antiseptic." [9] The one great obstacle to the adoption of asepsis was the widely held belief that the bacteria which frequented the air of the operating room could infect wounds. With the demonstration that it was the hands and clothing of the operator and his attendants which brought the pathogenic organisms, the development of asepsis was speeded. The great Chicago surgeon-pathologist, Christian Fenger, showed by exposing gelatin plates for long periods that the air of operating rooms was virtually free from responsibility for infection. The disinfection of instruments and the use of gloves in Chicago followed in the 1890's. Fenger himself was the first to use rubber gloves in the city, after discarding silk and cotton as unsuitable.[10]

During the 1870's interest in the germ theory had lain dormant in America. But the announcement in 1882 that Robert Koch had discovered the bacillus of tuberculosis inspired a marked change. The isolation of the tuberculosis germ, unlike earlier developments in bacteriology, fired the enthusiasm of medical men. The "white plague," as it was called, was the leading cause of death at the time and interest in the subject was always intense. Many who had looked askance at Pasteur's work found cause for excitement in the results of Koch's patient search. A number of physicians refused at first to accept the truth of the discovery, believing that Koch's explanation failed to account for those social and constitutional factors which they had observed to be associated with the coming of tuberculosis.[11]

The news from Germany caused hundreds of Americans, including many Chicagoans, to flock to the laboratories of Koch, Behring, and Pasteur. The Chicago Medical Society was the scene of the keenest excitement during these years as young doctors fresh from Europe exhibited Koch's cholera bacillus or his much-discussed bacillus of tuberculosis; at one meeting, William T. Belfield showed lantern slides of many of the new micro-organisms. The youthful Frank Billings returned from Vienna and proudly explained the new urine tests, instruments, and microscopic slides which he had brought back to Chicago. The obstetrician Charles W. Earle described the method of keeping premature infants alive which he had seen in Paris, and he told his listeners of the progress of Pasteur's work on hydrophobia.[12] Young surgeons like Franklin Martin and John B. Murphy did not consider their education complete until they had spent a year or two in Europe.

Two professors in Chicago medical schools were among the first in America to make systematic studies of the whole range of bacteriological investigations and report their conclusions in writing. William T. Belfield, a lecturer on pathology at Rush Medical College, was requested to give the Cartwright Lectures at New York's College of Physicians and Surgeons in 1883 on the subject of the relationship of bacteria to disease. These pioneer lectures were published and provide one of the earliest American sources of information on bacteriology. Belfield accepted all the implications of the germ theory and attacked the skeptics who doubted Koch's tuberculosis germ: "I would call your attention to the fact that Koch's assertion embodies not a theory, but simply an ocular demonstration. If a man is seen to plunge a knife into the heart of another the killing is a fact, not a theory; if Koch saw tuberculosis invariably follow the introduction of isolated bacilli, the relation of cause and effect is a *fact, not a theory.*" [13]

The other pioneer was Henry Gradle of the Chicago Medical College. Gradle gave in 1883 a series of eight lectures on "Bacteria and the Germ Theory of Disease." Like Belfield's, his book showed familiarity with the latest researches and attracted wide attention. The work was translated into a number of other languages, including Japanese.[14]

The first laboratory work of any significance in Chicago was accomplished by Dr. Bayard Holmes in the washroom of the Cook County Hospital. Holmes was a graduate of a homeopathic medical college and as such was suspect to other internes who ridiculed his makeshift laboratory as "an extension of the high potency fad which their professors of medicine had caricatured in the annual lecture against homeopathy." [15] Holmes's work, it should be remembered, was accomplished at a time when Chicago boasted no public medical library and when laboratory materials were extremely difficult to come by. The young scientist had to wait months for the delivery of a few ounces of agar-agar from abroad, since none was obtainable in the United States. But Holmes, nevertheless, teamed with Christian Fenger to perform important pioneer work in experimental asepsis.[16] In 1888 he was called upon to give the first course in bacteriology at the Chicago Medical College. Chicago's other important school at this time, Rush Medical College, was slower in introducing bacteriology but tried to make up for this in 1896 by persuading Edwin Klebs, famed German investigator of typhoid fever and diphtheria, to take the chair.[17]

If the germ theory found rapid favor among younger medical men, there were many older doctors who found acceptance difficult. Although they might approve of antisepsis for its practical results, older men found difficult adjustment to a world in which disease was thought to result from the accidental, undirected attacks of numberless microscopic organisms. The experience of William Allen Pusey with his father was typical: [18]

Like most men of his generation he never came fully to grasp the significance of bacteria in disease. . . . When I began to study medicine and began to talk bacteriology to him, he was greatly interested, and for the remaining years of his life it was a common topic of conversation and correspondence between us. He accepted its importance in surgery promptly, but, in spite of real effort on his part, he found it hard to see the new point of view in disease.

It was the venerable Nathan Smith Davis of Chicago who rallied the forces of opposition to the new ideas. Davis had come to teach at Rush Medical College in 1849 after a farm boyhood in Chenango County, New York, and a medical education climaxed by two years at the country medical school at Fairfield, New York. His had been the energy behind the push for a national medical asso-

ciation, and in Chicago he had helped found Mercy Hospital, the
Chicago Medical School, the Chicago Medical Society, and dozens
of other civic and medical enterprises. No medical man, and few men
in the whole city, commanded the respect accorded Dr. Davis. His
kindness and helpfulness beneath a gruff exterior won him a large
number of devoted friends, particularly among his students. His ora-
torical ability and his wide knowledge of medical lore created a vivid
impression which was reinforced by the shaggy hair, erect carriage,
and the swallow-tail coat which he wore to the day of his death. It
is not strange, therefore, that Davis' opposition to the newer trends
in medicine should kindle a spark of resistance in fainter hearts; it
is unfortunate, but probably inevitable, that Davis' fight should have
been so largely misunderstood by his contemporaries.[19]

Davis' quarrel with the bacteriologists began almost immediately. In 1876 he attacked with vigor the idea of specificity in disease. If specific toxins or specific bacteria were responsible for specific
diseases, he scoffed, then practitioners must differentiate at the bedside between dysentery, which was thought to be specific, and colitis,
which was not. "Yet in general symptoms and morbid anatomy,"
argued Davis, "they are the same." [20] Only coincidence, he continued,
was responsible for the discovery of certain well-marked germs in the
bodies of patients suffering from particular diseases. If the bacteria
hunters would search for their pet germs in persons not afflicted with
a special disease, he declared, they would find them there as well.
Davis was not the only man to find the phenomenon of natural immunity a stumbling block.

The similarity between the development of Davis' thought
and that of the noted contemporary German sanitarian, Max von
Pettenkofer, was too striking to be altogether coincidental. Like Pettenkofer, Davis insisted that typhoid fever, whatever its germ cause,
was primarily explainable in terms of filth and lack of sanitary pre-
caution. Like him, too, Davis placed heavy reliability on his own
observations of social and soil factors involved in the genesis of
typhoid. He followed Pettenkofer in citing the case of isolated villages where the disease had broken out *de novo* with no apparent
contact with the outside world. Both men, finally, recognized the
role of constitutional factors—of the *vis medicatrix naturae*—in predisposing the body to attacks of disease.[21]

Whatever their contemporaries thought, Davis and men of
like view performed a notable service in opposing the extremes to

which the enthusiasm of the early bacteriologists was carrying them. In urging men to hold fast to that which had been proven true, Davis was in the van rather than the rear guard of medical thought. In denying the ultrascientific trend in medicine, which was to reveal its limitations in the twentieth century, he deserves the praise, rather than the censure, of modern medicine. Although he came eventually to accept the germ theory of disease, and even the doctrine of specificity, Davis continued to warn of the folly in concentrating on bacteriology as the only avenue of approach to the secrets of human illness.[22] Davis' influence probably held many back from joining the hunt for the specific bacterial causes of cancer, heart disease, and other noninfectious afflictions. In the 1890's, not only was the microbic origin of cancer generally believed, but many thought that the specific parasite had been found.[23] Davis pointed also to the setback in the management of tuberculosis victims occasioned by the discovery of the responsible bacillus. Since its discovery, medical men had concentrated on a means of destroying the bacillus, while neglecting the accumulated knowledge of predisposing influences and prophylactic safeguards.[24] The year before his death in 1904, the octogenarian Davis was still stressing to his colleagues the "predisposing causes of disease . . . temporarily neglected on account of the zealous search for specific causes and specific remedies." [25]

Davis thus anticipated the twentieth-century reaction to the extravagant excesses of the microbe hunters in applying the doctrines of specificity and solidism to all pathological conditions. His rich experience and healthy skepticism preserved him from the prevalent belief that the etiology of all disease was about to be solved for all time. He pleaded for the study of medical history to teach students that the blocks of medical knowledge, put together so carefully throughout the ages, could not be pulled down by a single discovery, or even by a series of them.

The shift in medical attention from therapeutics to etiology, from cures to causes, explains in large part the rapid growth of homeopathy and other medical sects in late nineteenth-century Chicago. Just as large segments of the public had earlier deserted the regulars because of their fondness for calomel and bleeding, so now did people forsake them for the homeopaths whose intricate and carefully prepared *materia medica* inspired at least the promise of hope. The therapeutic nihilism of the regulars frightened a generation schooled in the virtues of drugs and medicines. Of what value was the positive identification of illness by means of microbes if physicians threw up their hands in helplessness when asked for remedies? There had been only forty-nine homeopathic practitioners in Chicago in 1870; a decade later there were 112, and by the turn of the century the number had climbed to about five hundred.²⁶ Since the popularity of the homeopaths was tied so closely to their empirical belief in the efficacy of drugs, they tended quite understandably to resist the germ theory even more forcefully than the regulars. The pathogenic role of bacteria was burlesqued throughout the 1880's and 1890's in homeopathic journals; even the new diphtheria antitoxin was summarily rejected in favor of their own remedies.²⁷ Other sects joined the homeopaths in their attack on the germ theory; eclectics, chiropractors, and osteopaths outdid each other in denouncing the doctrines of Koch and Pasteur. As late as 1923 a leading osteopath seized upon the renewed interest of doctors in constitutional factors in disease to announce a trend toward the non-bacterial explanation of the osteopaths.²⁸

The story of homeopathy in the West begins with the conversion of Dr. David S. Smith to the principles of Hahnemann. A graduate of the Jefferson Medical College in Philadelphia in 1836, Smith had practiced regular medicine until 1843 when his eldest daughter, seriously ill, responded only to the medicines and the like-cures-like principle of the homeopaths. Smith became an enthusiastic convert and carried the banner of homeopathy throughout the West, winning the support of such influential Chicagoans as J. Young Scammon, John Wentworth, and William B. Ogden. Chicago was already a center for irregular medical practitioners, and now became a focus of homeopathy, not only in the West, but in the country as a whole. By 1905, Chicago schools had sent out more homeopathic graduates than any other city, including Philadelphia, the American home of homeopathy.²⁹

Smith, meanwhile, put to good use his considerable talents as an organizer and educator. He played an important role in founding the first hospital, the first medical society, and the first medical school devoted to Hahnemann's teachings in Chicago. The charter for the Hahnemann Medical College of Chicago was drawn up by Smith in the law offices of Abraham Lincoln in Springfield.³⁰

The inevitable battle between homeopath and regular in Chicago was precipitated by Nathan Smith Davis, then secretary of Rush Medical College. Davis refused peremptorily in 1850 to admit a homeopath into his school. The homeopaths exploited the matter as an invasion of the sacred right of each man to his own opinion, while Davis defended his action on the ground that no one should be allowed to trifle with human life.[31] The press of the city, together with many of its more influential residents, tended to side with the homeopaths. Having witnessed the rise and fall of a number of medical theories, the public thought Davis' pronouncement a little too *ex-cathedra* in the existing fluid state of science. "Homeopathy," warned the *Gem of the Prairie*, "is something that can not be ignored nor sneered out of existence." [32] It is curious that although autopsical and statistical means of checking the claims of the homeopaths existed by 1850, the regulars consistently refused to test their own results against those of their competitors. Perhaps they feared that despite the inanity of homeopathy, the mortality lists from their own bleeding and dosing would be even longer.

The controversy was heightened by the action of city officials in 1857 in admitting a petition from 183 prominent citizens for a separate homeopathic division of the new City Hospital. The subsequent appointment of two medical boards, one homeopathic and one "allopathic," was answered by the prompt refusal of Davis and others to serve in such an organization. In a letter to the *Chicago Times* Davis explained that his conscience would not permit him to take the position; but another paper censured him for his "peculiar notions" of morality. To the suggestion that it might be wise to serve in view of popular feeling on the subject, Davis replied that the perpetuation of popular errors was dangerous. The ignorant poor, Davis argued, would be given no choice under the City Council's plan—those without preference would be arbitrarily assigned to one section or the other—and this, he claimed, was submission to the erroneous idea that one system of medical practice was as good as another.[33] The controversy abated temporarily when the perplexed City Council decided against staffing the institution immediately. The Civil War prolonged the indecision; when the hospital was finally opened in 1865, only regular physicians were in attendance. Further petitions and arguments resulted in 1881 in the authorization of a separate staff of homeopaths who were given the care of one fifth of all patients. In 1889 a similar agreement was reached with the eclectic physicians, a group purporting to select the best from all systems of medicine but in truth relying on botanical remedies. These agreements lasted until the adoption of civil service at the hospital in 1905.[34]

A number of factors operated in the closing decades of the nineteenth century to bridge the chasm of ill will between the homeopaths and the regular profession. Chicago's Great Fire of 1871 brought both groups together in a common fight against the sickness and sanitary dangers which threatened the city. A homeopath wrote that "Our school learned that the other side were not all bigots, with the intolerance of a Torquemada, and they . . . discovered that homeopaths were not born with hoofs and horns." [35] Perhaps more significant in resolving the differences between the rival groups was the gradual broadening of homeopathic education on the one hand, and the dropping of the old heroic remedies of the regulars on the other. The rise of new cults, too, such as osteopathy and chiropractic, tended to promote a closing of ranks against the new heresies. With the admission of homeopaths to the regular schools, beginning in the 1890's, another old sore was healed.

But probably most important in restoring a united profession was the intransigence of the older homeopaths in the face of the new science of bacteriology. In editorial after editorial, the journals controlled by the older, conservative element fought the trend away from the parent doctrine. They excoriated the "Benedict Arnolds . . . who would surrender our birthright for a mess of pottage." [36] Many of the younger men, however, saw in the work of Pasteur and Koch the death sentence for homeopathy and refused to follow their elders in an uphill battle against the germ theory, antitoxins, and serums. By the turn of the century, the decline of interest in Hahnemann's principles was lamented in every journal and medical meeting, and a decade later homeopathy had all but disappeared from Chicago.

With the remarkable developments of the second half of the nineteenth century there had come a revolution in the scientific climate of opinion. A medical world was being constructed in which the older physicians did not feel at home. The bottle-crammed laboratory with its silent men of research was replacing the busy practitioner as the cynosure of attention, while medicine was being broken down into compartmentalized specialties which could be mastered only by concentrated study and experience. The intellectual atmosphere of the 1850's had encouraged medical men to become amateur botanists, geologists, and naturalists, but such diversity of interest was becoming increasingly rare.

The surgeon Edmund Andrews was a fine example of the

older type. He had been a founder of the Chicago Medical College and a pioneer in the use of antisepsis, but he was also an expert in botany, zoology, ornithology, and geology. His was the first scientific explanation of the intermittent eruption of geysers and he made notable studies in philology. With a number of physicians and others interested in natural science, he had helped to found the Chicago Academy of Natural Sciences in 1856; his interest and devotion kept the society alive in the lean years following the Great Fire.[37] By the addition of oxygen to nitrous oxide he made prolonged anesthesia safe, a contribution of the first importance to surgery. Andrews has been compared with Billroth, Albrecht von Haller, and von Helmholtz in the catholicity of his interests and accomplishments.[38]

But by 1900 the atmosphere in scientific circles was quite different. Daring young surgeons who spoke and knew only surgery now held the center of the stage. After apprenticeship in the clinics and hospitals of Europe, they returned with unbounded confidence to make their marks in their fast-growing art. Unexplored cavities of the human body were entered for the first time, better techniques for ancient operations were devised, and all manner of surgical appliances appeared to lighten the work of the operator.

Chicago surgeons and doctors alike had come a long way from the "heroic" period of Chicago medicine a half century earlier. The city had changed from a struggling commercial outpost to the throbbing center of a dynamic midwestern economy, doctoring of the desperately ill to a highly skilled profession. Most of all, the doctors themselves had changed. The wealthy city specialist of 1900, confining his practice to certain diseases in a downtown office, would have seemed useless to his pioneer colleagues of the 1840's. Medicine had grown more scientific, more daring, and consequently more respected, but also, it seemed, more impersonal and esoteric. In effecting this transformation, no force was more important than the medical school, giving the rudiments of technical training and turning out "educated medical gentlemen."

Chapter IV	Medical Schools in Chicago,
	1850–1900

The acceleration of medical discovery in the second half of the nineteenth century created serious problems for those concerned with the training of young men for careers in medicine. Medical schools, with their limited funds and their isolation from the great universities, found adjustment of their curricula to the changing needs of the time difficult; private students, to make the matter worse, often discovered that their preceptors had added little to their store of knowledge since graduation from medical college. The greatest problem in medical education therefore was how to make the new researches and discoveries in medicine a vital part of each student's preparation for professional work.

There was certainly no lack of medical schools. In the fifteen years ending in 1845 the number of colleges devoted to medicine in the United States doubled, and the growth was to continue until the end of the century.[1] The rapid settlement of the West, added to the expanding population of the country as a whole, produced a great need for doctors and facilities for their instruction. But the colleges which sprang into existence to meet this need were ill-suited to the task. Medical schools, for the most part, were staffed by men who considered the education of physicians a business, and a profitable one at that.[2] The entrepreneurs in these ventures were frequently physicians or even instructors in the schools themselves, and the commercial instinct, unfortunately, proved stronger than the professional one in most cases.

The economic motivation which lay behind these institutions was best seen in the sharp competition between schools for students. In their zeal to outrival each other, colleges shortened their curricula, reduced fees, and established easy requirements for degrees.

Preliminary study for medical school was almost unknown. The few standards which had existed in medicine fell before the pressure of competition from new schools, or from the lack of a disinterested board of governors. The idea of a private medical school, separated from any contact with a university or even a college of liberal arts, was English in its origin, but was carried to its illogical extreme in America. The proprietary professional college was in a very real sense a product of the rampant spirit of free enterprise and unrestrained laissez faire which characterized American life in the nineteenth century.[3]

One of the most frequent complaints against medical schools of the last century was their failure to demand a preliminary education. The American Medical Association discovered early in its history that law and theology claimed the allegiance of the better-educated young men, and that the general standard of education in medicine was much lower than in the other professions.[4] The fear of losing students kept admission requirements in medicine at the low level of approximately eight months of "reading medicine" with some local practitioner; this was supposed to supplement the usual four-month lecture course. In practice, however, the duties of a medical apprentice normally prevented him from devoting much time to his studies. No better account of the wearisome rounds of the would-be doctor has been recorded than that of the historian, John Bach McMaster: "He ground the powders, mixed the pills, rode with the doctor on his rounds, held the basin when the patient was bled, helped to adjust plasters, to sew wounds, and ran with vials of medicine from one end of the town to the other. In the moments snatched from duties such as these he swept out the office, cleaned the bottles and jars, wired skeletons, tended the night-bell, and, when a feast was given, stood in the hall to announce the guests."[5]

The number of professors in the pioneer schools was small, varying from five to seven, depending on enrollment. The chairs most often included were those of surgery, medicine, therapeutics, *materia medica*, and obstetrics; the holder of this last chair was usually responsible, too, for teaching the diseases of women and children. Clinical and basic studies were not infrequently combined in one professorship as, for example, anatomy and surgery.[6] Disagreements among the faculty, particularly over division of students' fees, were frequent in these early institutions. In Chicago, the Rush Medical College was warned at the outset that "most of the medical schools of our country have been seriously injured and some entirely prostrated, in consequence of the spirit of rivalry and jealousy indulged in by the professors." [7] The commercial character of the colleges was largely responsible for this feeling of suspicion and distrust. The words of a departing Rush professor in 1849 echoed a common complaint during these years: [8]

I shall finish my course tomorrow and start then or the next day for home. I have notified the other Professors that I *shall not return*. In fact it is a small potato business of which I am most heartily tired. I have been ashamed tó spend my time in this unprofitable manner for two or three years past—but have constantly been in hopes it would improve.

The money is not divided and will not be. In truth I fear me there is "something rotten in Denmark."—The resident faculty make all the money which is made—make no division of funds on hand until we are gone, and then decide to suit themselves. They say they pay debts . . . with the matriculation and graduation fees—but the debts are usually going to themselves.

There were a number of other unwholesome aspects of medical education in these proprietary schools. Traditionally in America the common practice in arranging a two-year curriculum was to require students to study all subjects offered in the school, normally about seven, the first year, and then repeat them the second year. Another shortcoming was a woeful deficiency in facilities for practical training. Many of the schools were located in rural areas with no prospect of clinic or hospital work. Of thirty-three institutions asked to report to the American Medical Association in 1849, only nine indicated that hospital attendance was a requirement for the doctor of medicine degree. A final weakness of the mid-nineteenth-century medical school was the brevity of its courses of instruction. A school term was commonly limited to the winter months to accommodate rural students, usually extending over a period of about sixteen weeks.[9]

In Illinois, during this early period, there was a real shortage of physicians, yet few families could afford the expense of sending a son back to an eastern school. A demand arose, consequently, for local schools where a farmer might send his son for schooling during the slack season. Some of the more ambitious doctors who were already teaching private students began to band together to form centers of medical instruction. These preceptors, as they were called, seldom resided in the towns where the lectures were given, but were forced to snatch a few weeks each year from busy practices to come to the school. The fees and graduation requirements in the embryonic medical colleges showed a large measure of uniformity. The usual charges were ten dollars for each course, a graduation assessment of twenty dollars, and an optional dissection fee of five dollars. Though standards varied slightly from one school to another, all agreed that the recipient of an M. D. degree must be twenty-one years of age, of good moral character, and he must have studied three years with a preceptor and attended two courses of lectures. He must also have submitted an acceptable thesis and paid his fees in advance.[10]

The medical schools of Illinois were not below the national average in the 1840's with regard to length of courses, number of professors, and requirements for graduation. During this decade there existed five medical colleges in or near Chicago, but of these, three had by 1850 closed their doors, one had moved to Iowa, and only Rush Medical College remained.[11]

The founder of Chicago's first medical school was the restless pioneer surgeon, Daniel Brainard. After study at the College of Physicians and Surgeons of the Western District of New York, a small rural institution in Fairfield, Brainard went on to further study in Philadelphia before coming to Chicago.[12] When the young surgeon had been only two years in the western city, he confided to an influential friend his desire to establish a medical college. A charter was obtained from the state legislature in 1837, the first granted to an institution of learning in Illinois.[13] The press applauded Brainard's initiative in giving young men of the West an opportunity to be educated at home.[14] But the financial panic which struck Chicago later in the year brought his plans to an abrupt halt, since he had counted heavily on public support in his venture. For six years the project lay dormant while Brainard studied in France and conducted private classes in anatomy in Chicago.[15] Finally, in December, 1843, the doors of Rush Medical College, named for the famed Dr. Benjamin Rush, were thrown open to a class of twenty-two students.[16]

During the first session of the new school, lectures were held in a rented hall in the Saloon Building on Clark Street, but plans for a college building were inaugurated early. The financing of such a structure proved to be the chief barrier against its realization. Some of Chicago's wealthier men aided with gifts of land and money; one group of businessmen headed by Walter Newberry and William B.

Ogden contributed a lot and five hundred dollars in return for a promise to locate the college on the north side of the river where, it was hoped, the presence of the school would heighten commercial values. The building was erected in the summer of 1844 at a cost of thirty-five hundred dollars, the faculty paying the bulk of the amount after loans and subscriptions were exhausted. The new college was considered quite handsome by the *Chicago Democrat*, which looked on it as "an ornament to the city." The newspaper was lavish, too, in its praise for the work of the college: Rush's success was held up as *bona fide* evidence of Chicago's "capabilities . . . for holding a commanding rank among her sisters of the west in an intellectual and moral, as well as in a commercial point of view." [17]

The faculty which Brainard gathered about him during the early years of the college was remarkable for its youth and ability. Of the fourteen men of professorial rank who taught at Rush in its first sixteen years, twelve were under thirty-six years of age, and four were still in their twenties.[18] James Van Zandt Blaney, distinguished professor of chemistry and pharmacy, was only twenty-three when the college opened, yet his role was second only to Brainard's in settling Rush on a firm foundation. As the founder and editor of the *Illinois Medical and Surgical Journal*, he gave the city doctors their first medical journal. Blaney was a much sought-after lecturer before various civic and social groups in Chicago; scarcely a week passed without some enthusiastic comment from the press concerning one of his lectures at the Mechanics Institute, the Young Men's Association, or the Chicago Female Seminary. Blaney succeeded Brainard in the presidency of Rush on the latter's death in 1866, but poor health forced him to sever his connections with the college in 1871.[19]

Professor William B. Herrick was thirty-one years of age when Brainard offered him the position of lecturer in anatomy at Rush. He had graduated in medicine from Dartmouth in 1836 and had settled in Illinois three years later. So popular was Dr. Herrick with the Rush students that he was made professor of anatomy in 1845 over the objection of several faculty members. In 1846 he was awarded a commission as surgeon in the Mexican War and saw service at Buena Vista. His letters to Blaney's medical journal form an interesting commentary on medical and health conditions among the troops and natives in Mexico. After his return to Rush, Herrick continued to teach courses in anatomy and other subjects until 1857.[20]

Another notable member of the Rush faculty was Austin

Flint, who taught the Institutes and Practice of Medicine. Flint came west to teach at Brainard's school in the middle forties, but returned after a few years to the East, where he became an eminent author and professor in the Bellevue Hospital Medical College in New York.

Not all of Brainard's choices proved as fortunate as these; in at least one case a faculty member was dropped after only one year of service. The contract of Moses Knapp, one of the four professors to welcome the first class at Rush in the winter of 1843, was not renewed at the close of the sixteen-week term. Brainard felt apparently that Knapp's lectures were not well received by his students, and student approval was the only test of fitness for teaching. After his dismissal Knapp spread all manner of false stories about his former colleagues at Rush, causing Blaney to comment privately that all doubts concerning the wisdom of removing him from the faculty were now resolved. Brainard's evaluation of Knapp's character was subsequently confirmed when he was fired from the medical school at La Porte, Indiana, for attempting to seduce a young girl the night after commencement.[21]

One of the major problems facing Rush during the first two years of its existence was how to contact prospective students and persuade them to come to Chicago. Recruiting students was an important part of a faculty member's job in this era, and Brainard was ever on the alert for ambitious and enthusiastic young salesmen for his faculty. In 1844, the president's attention was captured by a dynamic young physician named Evans from Attica, Indiana, who had just gained the approval of tough-minded legislators for a state insane asylum at Indianapolis.

Dr. John Evans was born near Waynesville, Ohio, in 1814. After an adolescence spent in service in his father's store, he resolved to study medicine against his stern parents' wishes. He pleaded with his father that "If it is convenient thow [sic] mayst say whether thee can consent to my wish to study or not, and please do not send me back into the old store to loll on the counter. O, I cannot do it unless I have to, but thy word is sovereign and I hope to be dutiful." [22] The old Quaker relented, and Evans enrolled in the medical department of Cincinnati College, where he graduated in 1838. He settled first in Illinois, and then in Indiana; it was in the latter state that his labors first commanded attention. His work on behalf of a more humane treatment of the insane earned him the praise of Dorothea

Dix; he was also a pioneer in Indiana in the education of deaf mutes.[23]

Evans' ambition could not be held within the bounds of medical practice. His talents found additional outlets in education, real estate, railroading, and politics. In Chicago he invested heavily in land and buildings, and became an early director of the Fort Wayne and Chicago Railroad. As a philanthropist, he played a decisive role in the founding of Northwestern and Denver universities. His political interests by the 1850's were focused on the slavery question; his influence was largely responsible for the Indiana delegation's consistent support of Lincoln at the Republican Convention in 1860. In return for Evans' help, Lincoln offered him successively the territorial governorships of Washington and Nebraska, which he rejected in favor of Colorado. After thirty-six stormy years in Colorado politics, he died in 1897 at the age of eighty-three years.[24]

At Rush, Evans' infectious enthusiasm was an important factor in publicizing the school and attracting new students from all over the Northwest. He seized upon the medical journal founded by Blaney as a fine medium for publicity, writing another professor that "you must see that the character, usefulness and success of our school must depend upon the reputation of its teachers. Then it becomes important for each of us, not only to teach well and profoundly, but to write well and extensively." [25] The aggressive newcomer took the lead in rounding up students for the school. A typical letter to the more reticent Dr. McLean, professor of *materia medica*, read as follows: "Now Doctor I tell you what it is you must be up and doing—We must have 150 students this winter or break a trace and at least 25 of them must come from Michigan [McLean's state]—now if you do not know where they are to be found it is time you were looking them up. I will take 25 & Fitch [another faculty member] 20 from this state [i.e. Indiana] and the other 75 must come from Ills. Wisconsin Iowa and elsewhere." [26]

Like most medical men of his day, Evans considered medical education a sound investment. Not only did students' fees provide an additional source of income, but the general enhancement of professional prestige which went with a college appointment also had a real momentary value. Evans found that Rush Medical College was not dissimilar in financial organization to the usual proprietary school of a century ago. Ownership and control of the college was vested almost entirely in the faculty. Upon rebuilding in 1875, a check of outstanding bonds disclosed that only ten were in nonfaculty hands. These had somehow gotten "embarrassingly" into the hands of lay- men during the confusion attendant upon the Great Fire. The Rush professors, of course, constituted virtually the entire board of trus- tees, although an occasional outsider was invited to serve. This re- lationship continued until the affiliation of Rush with the University of Chicago in 1898, when the old professor-trustees stepped down in favor of a nonfaculty board of directors.[27]

The size of the Rush student body was small in comparison with older institutions, but it continued to grow, passing the one hundred mark in 1849 and reaching one hundred and fifty by 1856.[28] The students came from a wider area as the publicity of Evans and of his co-workers spread across the Middle West. In 1846 forty- four men enrolled from Illinois, fourteen from Indiana, five from Michigan, four from Wisconsin Territory, and three from Ohio and Pennsylvania combined. The following year the faculty was pleased to welcome the first student from New York.[29] By 1848, President Brainard and his colleagues were growing sensitive to the competition of other schools in Illinois and the Northwest. An edi- torial signed by John Evans protesting the opening of new medical colleges at Rock Island and Iowa City appeared in the Rush journal. Evans pointed to the disadvantages of small towns as centers of med- ical education, citing particularly the lack of clinical and anatomical material; he forgot apparently that Chicago had been just as small when Rush was chartered. He criticized, too, the lack of hospital facilities in these places, although Chicago had yet to open her first permanent hospital.[30] These arguments had some validity when ap- plied to conditions in the more settled East, but no one could pre- dict the potentialities of small communities in the growing West, as the example of Chicago herself was proving.

So long as competition between medical schools was keen, Rush found it difficult to raise the level of teaching and require- ments. In the existing state of things, any significant rise in standards was sure to be followed by a general exodus to less strenuous aca- demic surroundings. The only solution, some faculty members be- lieved, was co-operation with other institutions in a national move- ment such as the American Medical Association to raise standards slowly but steadily together. Rush had sent representatives to the first meetings of the Association, and in 1849 John Evans was dis- patched to Boston to attend the third session. While there Evans met Dr. Nathan Smith Davis, founder of the Association, and invited him to accept the chair of physiology and pathology at Rush.[31] Davis' acceptance of this offer had tremendous significance for the future development of medical education in Chicago.

The ideas of Dr. Davis on medical schools and their problems were already well known throughout the country. He had begun his campaign for a national association of physicians primarily to correct some of the weaknesses in America's system of training physicians. At the time of the first meeting of the American Medical Association, he had drawn the fire of Professor Martyn Paine, a well-known New York educator, for his speeches and writings in favor of a longer course of study and a more exacting premedical education. Paine and others saw an aristocratic bias in Davis' proposals, since it was farm boys, attending medical school in the winter season, who would suffer most from the enlarged requirements.[32] Davis' concern, however, was centered on the recipients of medical care; he persevered in his attack on what he thought were the evils of the existing system. Aside from short sessions and inadequate premedical education, he considered the absence of clinical and practical demonstrations, the lack of hospital experience, the large number of lectures each day, and the repetition of courses as the major problems which educators must meet. A score of years earlier, Daniel Drake, famous pioneer in early western medicine, had enumerated an almost identical list of the shortcomings of American medical schools.[33]

The first lecture given by Davis after his arrival in Chicago was on the subject "Free Medical Schools." In this address he told his audience that the cost of a thorough education in medicine barred students from spending as much time as was necessary to truly master their profession. This was fair, he challenged, neither to the physician who must enter practice with inadequate preparation, nor to the community which he served. Davis announced the goal of the Rush faculty as the abolition of all professors' ticket fees; to show the school's good intentions he promised that tickets for three courses would be given forthwith without charge.[34] This action caused other schools to complain of unfair competition; several threatened to report Rush to the American Medical Association. But Davis continued to insist that the way to achieve higher standards was to decrease, not increase, the cost of a medical education, thus making it available to all. The only qualification for study, he believed, should be the native ability of the applicant. To charges of impracticable idealism he replied that his goals were attainable. He demanded, indeed, that they be realized in the near future because of the vital importance of well-trained physicians to the health of every community. "Is it not the physican," Davis queried, "on whom the whole community leans, when pestilence stalks abroad, clothing all ranks in the habiliments of mourning?" [35]

When Davis heard the report of a special committee on medical education at the American Medical Association meeting in 1856, he learned that that group had decided on certain steps toward ending the senseless repetition of courses in medical schools. The committee recommended that eight distinct courses of instruction be set up, with each course divided into two parts. Each student, according to this plan, would take the first half of all eight courses the first year, and complete them in his second year. Davis felt that his own scheme was more simple and practicable. He wanted full instruction given in four basic subjects the first year (anatomy, chemistry, *materia medica*, and physiology), before proceeding to the clinical subjects of surgery, obstetrics, and the practice of medicine the second year. In 1857 the Rush faculty voted unanimously to establish a graded course along the lines outlined by Davis, but President Brainard vetoed the idea because he feared the plan would drive students elsewhere.[36]

When Davis began to insist on grading the Rush curriculum, the faculty split into two groups, culminating in the establishment of a new medical school in 1859. At the head of the two antagonistic groups were Brainard and Davis, men of strong personality and fixed beliefs. While each respected the other's accomplishments, a mutual feeling of suspicion and distrust grew up in the two years following Brainard's veto of the graded course. Early in the spring of 1859, Dr. Hosmer A. Johnson and several other of Davis' supporters were approached by the trustees of the recently organized (and short-lived) Lind University, who were seeking to organize a medical department in connection with their school. Johnson and three other members of the Rush faculty, Professors Rutter, Isham, and Andrews, met in March to consider the proposition. They decided to accept the offer and a committee was appointed to urge Davis and William Byford to join them on the new faculty. When both men agreed, the six Rush professors became the nucleus of the medical faculty of Lind University.[37]

The first course of lectures in the new school was given the following fall in Lind's Block, at the corner of Market and Randolph streets, with a class of thirty-three present.[38] In his inaugural address, President Davis reviewed reforms which he was introducing: a college term extended to five months, fewer lectures per day, the number of professorships increased to thirteen, clinical subjects now endowed with full college chairs, daily clinical experience in hospitals, and a graded course of study divided into junior and senior departments. That the study of anatomy and physiology should precede practical medicine and surgery was as obvious, Davis assured prospective students, as that arithmetic should precede algebra.[39] Although Charles W. Eliot of Harvard is usually given credit for introducing the graded curriculum in America, it was not until 1871, twelve years after Davis' plan was put into operation at Rush, that President Eliot reordered the course of study at the Harvard Medical School and inaugurated the graded system there.[40]

To teach anatomy, Davis was fortunate in securing the services of a French scientist, Titus De Ville, who had commendatory letters from Brown-Sequard and others. De Ville attracted a moderate number of students to his lectures and demonstrations, but was disillusioned by the prospects offered him in Chicago. He resigned his connection with Davis' school after the first year; his account of his disappointment afforded an interesting insight into conditions at the new college: [41]

In the short space of twelve months, I am obliged to return to my native country, for my means will not permit me further to prolong my stay. . . . No one is responsible, it was my own act in coming out here. I thought that this would be a good point to meet with pecuniary success, that the opportunities which I had enjoyed in my profession would be duly appreciated, and remuneration sufficient to meet every moderate requisite immediately attained. I found on my arrival a great commercial depression, no money to be had, and but a few students.

Even if the school's financial standing did not provoke optimism, a swelling enrollment augured better things for the future. Despite the fact that Rush was already well established with a sixteen-week term, and that seemingly there was little call for another medical school, particularly one with higher standards, enrollment at the new college jumped from thirty-three the first year to fifty-four the next and to eighty-one in 1863.[42] After the Civil War, the faculty moved to admit Negro students, a step taken by Rush some years before the conflict.[43]

A serious blow to Davis' financial hopes came with the dissolution of Sylvester Lind's fortune in 1861 and the resulting collapse of the Lind University plans. The Lind trustees had agreed to provide the medical department with a new building at the expiration of a three-year term, but Davis and his faculty saw now the futility of expecting help from this quarter. A building fund entirely from lecture fees was commenced in 1863, but until 1870 the school, renamed the Chicago Medical College, held its classes in rented rooms on State Street.[44]

The Civil War tended to put a temporary quietus on the drive for medical reform. A few months after Appomattox, Davis reorganized further the curriculum of the Chicago Medical College by adding a third year of medical studies. In 1868 the three-year course of six months each was made compulsory for all candidates for the M.D. degree.[45] A nominal affiliation with Northwestern University was reached in 1869, whereby the Chicago Medical College retained its name, yet became a department of the university. Such agreements were not uncommon in this period, being inspired by the mutual gain of university and medical school alike from the arrangement. The medical school earned the privilege of bestowing degrees in the name of the university, an inducement not to be overlooked in the harsh competition for students, while the university benefited from the appearance of expansion given by the affiliation with the medical school.[46]

The split between Brainard and Davis proved to be a permanent one. The withdrawal of six of the most able men from Rush was a hard blow for Brainard to bear, despite his unconvincing declaration that "the means of teaching . . . will be rather increased than lessened, by the effect of this withdrawal." [47] When Davis left Rush, he took with him, too, the clinical facilities of Mercy Hospital, which he had helped to found, forcing Brainard's students to rely on the inadequate resources of the college dispensary and the Marine Hospital. Brainard's opposition to medical reform now deepened into bitterness as he castigated the "incompetent, noisy individuals" who, he said, thrust their reform tirades upon the patience of more level-headed educators. Medical knowledge, he insisted in the pages of the *Chicago Medical Journal*, could not be legislated nor voted onto a higher plane. His own pioneer resourcefulness taught him that individual rather than group action was the remedy for low standards. Each physician by his own industry in practice, teaching, and writing could provide the example which would stimulate progress in medicine. More specifically, he contended that the way to improve teaching was to hire better lecturers rather than revamp the curriculum. Better educated physicians would come from constructing more medical libraries from more students' fees rather than lengthening courses of study.[48]

Brainard made no attempt to lengthen the Rush term in the years following the establishment of Davis' college. He based his opposition to the longer period of study, as had earlier critics of reform projects within the American Medical Association, upon the economic status of his students, maintaining that few had the means of attending school for more than four months. Davis' charge that the country was "full of half-educated physicians" was labeled by Brainard "an unjust attack upon physicians and schools, especially in the West, which irregular practitioners will not fail to turn to account." [49] Nor did the graded course find any favor at Rush. Even after Brainard's death (1866), his colleagues continued for more than a decade to fight its adoption. They argued that dividing the curriculum into two groups of subjects only forced students to cram in the elementary courses given the first year, while encouraging them to neglect these important studies the second year.[50] As for Davis, the Rush organ caricatured him for years as "the Apostle," while his medical school was referred to constantly as "the Reform School." [51]

With President Brainard's passing in 1866, much of the illwill between Rush and her rival began to disappear.[52] The optimistic Davis even drew up a plan for reuniting his college with Rush. According to the terms of his draft, Rush was to increase her term to five months and her professorships to thirteen, while the proprietory relationship of the faculty to the college was to be terminated. Davis did not insist on grading the course of study, though he contemplated an informal division of subjects into elementary and advanced groups.[53] But this proposal for a united medical school was never seriously entertained by the Rush professors and was soon forgotten by faculty and historians alike.

The enrollment at Rush did not suffer from the competition of another medical school in Chicago. The number of students rose steadily from 119 in 1859 to a high mark of 374 the year of Brainard's death, while Davis' school did not matriculate a hundred students in any year before 1865. The Civil War seemed to have no adverse effect on the numbers attending the two schools. Indeed, the need for trained physicians and surgeons in the northern armies was probably responsible for some of the increase in registration during the war years. The only noticeable changes in Chicago's medical schools occasioned by the war were the inauguration of studies in military surgery at Rush, and a few faculty replacements as a result of enlistments.[54]

Both Rush and the Chicago Medical College faced a number of problems common to all medical schools in the second half of the nineteenth century. One of the greatest was the securing of anatomic material for dissection in the college laboratory. The medical school of this period was the victim of a vicious paradox in which it was held responsible, on the one hand, for the training of students in practical anatomy and yet was told, on the other, that the public would not tolerate the dissection of unclaimed bodies. The gallows apparently furnished the only bodies made freely available to the Chicago medical profession in the years before 1850; the earliest recorded dissection in the city was on the body of a criminal executed in 1840.[55] But with the rapid growth in demand for medical education, other sources of supply were, of necessity, sought out and the result was a wave of body snatching throughout the West around the middle of the century. The peak of public indignation was reached at Cincinnati when the body of William Henry Harrison's son was discovered in the dissecting rooms of the Medical College of Ohio. So great was the demand for material in comparison with the meager legal supply, that the procuring and disposing of bodies attained the status of a regular employment, with prices ranging from ten to twenty-five dollars a body.[56]

In Illinois, the zeal of body snatchers was largely responsible for the dissolution of at least two early medical schools. George W. Richards, president of the short-lived college at St. Charles, was shot at and wounded by a member of an enraged mob for shielding a student accused of stealing a corpse from the local churchyard. The college was closed in haste and Richards removed to Rock Island, where he helped organize another medical school.[57] At the Illinois Medical College, which held classes in Jacksonville for five years during the 1840's, the securing of material for dissection was more difficult than elsewhere because of the location. One student recalled that the college catalogue advertisement of "an ample supply

of fresh subjects . . . from abroad" was spurious: "every corpse for
dissection was taken from a barrel, sure, dripping with alcohol. What
I may happen to know about how some bodies got there is neither
to be printed nor written." [58] This school closed its doors in 1848 as
public sentiment reached a level dangerous to the safety of the professors.

In 1857 Rush Medical College found itself in public disfavor
when a student and the city sexton were charged jointly with "resur-
rectionism," as body snatching was jocularly known among the students. In a slashing attack the press branded the robbers as "hyenas"
and "barbarians." Dr. Davis courageously penned a reply to the ac-
cusations, asserting that the procuring of bodies could not be in its
nature criminal if necessary for a physician's education. He announced his intention of seeking a law which would give medical
schools the unclaimed bodies of those dying in hospitals, poor houses,
and other public institutions.[59]

The struggle for such a law proved to be a long one. Another
scandal in 1867, when two Negroes were arrested in possession of
several cadavers intended for the anatomical theater, created further
antagonism toward the profession, but the press, at least, began to
show some realization of the medical educator's predicament. The
Chicago Times, for example, held that "It is both an absurdity and
a tyranny, to hold the Physician accountable for a lack of knowledge,
and, at the same time, to hold him accountable when he endeavors
to supply himself with that knowledge." [60] The repeated outrages
to public feeling culminated in a state anatomical law in 1885 which
provided, in self-protection, for the turning over to a medical institution of any body which would otherwise be buried at public expense.[61]

Another problem which Chicago schools shared with other institutions was the vexing matter of admission requirements. If a student were turned away from one college because his preliminary education was inadequate, he could simply turn to another with every
hope of gaining entrance. The competition for students' fees allowed many men to become physicians who would never have been
permitted entrance to other professional schools. The long-range success of the drive for reform in this regard was clearly linked to the
spreading common school movement of the Jacksonian era, which
had to precede any effective enforcement of higher admission standards in secondary school or college. In the meantime, only joint

action by all the schools in an area seemed to guarantee the enforcement of even a modicum of preparatory studies.

As in most matters pertaining to medical education, it was Dr. N. S. Davis who took the lead in seeking to force action. At a convention of medical educators which met in Cincinnati in 1867, Davis demanded that each matriculant at the colleges represented be required to show some knowledge "of the common English branches of education," including elementary mathematics, the rudiments of natural science, and a sufficient acquaintance with Latin and Greek to comprehend technical terms. But a number of schools refused to co-operate in Davis' plan, including his Chicago rival, Rush Medical College. For a number of years only pious resolutions were adopted at these meetings, expressing hope that the colleges would "endeavor to conform" with Davis' or other reform proposals.[62]

While Davis' school required from the outset that candidates show some knowledge of English, mathematics, and natural science, other Illinois schools waited until 1877, when the state undertook the regulation of medical practice, to raise their requirements. Rush raised her requirements slowly, at first examining prospective students in elementary physical science and arithmetic "to cube root," and then, in 1891, asking all students to prepare themselves in algebra and geometry, rhetoric and logic, Latin and English, and physics. The level of premedical education at Rush remained low nevertheless in comparison with later standards. Dr. James B. Herrick recalled that in his class of 1888 only seven of 135 men entering the school boasted a college diploma of any description.[63]

The problem of college fees was equally troublesome. Since many of the students attending early medical colleges came from struggling farm families, tuition costs were a major factor in choosing a school. As early as 1829, Daniel Drake had protested that the cost of education was a serious hindrance to would-be physicians; he urged needy parents not to place their sons in the study of physic until they had accurately counted all the costs.[64] Fees during the first years at Rush amounted to sixty-five dollars, plus an optional five-dollar dissection charge, and a graduation levy of twenty dollars. But with the coming of N. S. Davis and his "free course" policy in 1849, fees were reduced to about thirty-five dollars. While this amount was frequently a burden on the indigent student's family, boarding was remarkably inexpensive, even for that period. "Good

Boarding," read the second Rush catalogue, "with room, fuel, lights, and attendance, can be obtained in Chicago, at $2.00 per week." [65]

While Rush insisted that all lecture fees be paid in advance, exceptions were frequently made and credit extended to students whose notes were endorsed by responsible persons. Occasionally, a charity student was admitted without payment of fees. The collecting of notes written by students often proved a difficult matter; the disgruntled Austin Flint refused to return to Rush unless the full value of the notes in his possession was assured him. [66]

The lowering of tuition charges at Rush upon Davis' insistence brought a storm of disapproval from other western schools. Davis defended his action as arising from educational principles and not commercial motives. The medical schools connected with the universities of Michigan and Iowa were also experimenting with lower fees at this time, forcing other colleges to slash fees to remain in competition. After Davis broke with the Rush faculty, he began to co-operate with other western schools in attempting to stabilize lecture fees. A plan for a uniform scale of charges was decided upon at a meeting of educators in Louisville in 1869 but abandoned when it was learned that several schools had already issued their annual announcements. Finally, ten years later, an agreement was reached between all the regular medical colleges of Chicago and Cincinnati to hold tuition costs at seventy-five dollars, a figure representing an average rise of 50 per cent over existing charges. [67] With ratification by all the more important schools in the West, one more step in taking medical education out of the category of competitive commodities was completed.

Another question, less urgent but no less agitated, which the medical colleges faced during this period was the training of women in medicine. This problem must be seen against the background of attitudes, beliefs, and prejudices which constituted the average doctor's view of the female sex during the nineteenth century. Women were widely thought to be mentally, as well as physically, inferior to men. Few persons thought it possible for a woman to engage successfully in a business or profession. Most observers, including women themselves, concurred in the judgment expressed by Dr. Alfred Stillé in his presidential address to the American Medical Association: "On the whole, then, we believe that all experience teaches that woman is characterized by a combination of distinctive qualities, of which the most striking are uncertainty of rational judgment, capriciousness of sentiment, fickleness of purpose, and indecision of action, which totally unfit her for professional pursuits." [68]

Not only were women thought to be mentally unsuited for professional study but, in the case of medicine, there were additional reasons why it was felt they should be disbarred. Victorian concepts of modesty and morality made the joining of women with men in listening to physiological discussion and cutting up the human body seem most unladylike. Emily Blackwell, sister to the noted Elizabeth, was denied permission to complete her studies at Rush in 1852 when the Illinois State Medical Society censured the school for its impropriety in admitting a woman.[69] In 1869 women were accepted by the Chicago Medical College at the earnest solicitation of Dr. William H. Byford, a faculty member. But the male students at the college petitioned at the close of the year to have them dropped, charging that certain clinical materials and observations had been omitted by the faculty because of the presence of the young women. This prudishness, of course, was not confined to medical men; indeed, they tended to be far more realistic than the general public in such matters. One can only marvel at the narrowness of the male who offered his body to the Rush Medical College with this stipulation: "I desire that my remains shall be preserved from any *indignities*. . . . And that no female medical students shall work over me." [70]

Some of the leading physicians of Chicago were among the most vociferous opponents of medical education for women. A medical society discussion in 1869 found N. S. Davis upholding the action of the Chicago Medical College in closing its doors to women, though several women members of the society were present at the time. Davis, while he grudgingly approved of separate colleges for female instruction, was strongly opposed to the idea of co-education in the medical school. He fought, too, against the admission of women into the American Medical Association, but it was a Chicago woman, Sarah Hackett Stevenson, who courageously took the first seat ever occupied by a woman in the history of the Association. Dr. Stevenson was a native of Illinois, valedictorian of her class at the new women's medical school in Chicago, and a student of Darwin and Huxley at the famous South Kensington Science School in London.[71]

The Chicago school from which Sarah Stevenson graduated was the Woman's Hospital Medical College, an outgrowth of a hospital established in 1865 by Mary H. Thompson for indigent women and children. While managing this hospital, Miss Thompson applied unsuccessfully to both Chicago medical schools for permission to complete her medical education. Finally, in 1869, she was selected as one of the four women admitted to the Chicago Medical College in its one-year experiment and received her degree from that institution at the close of the year. The other three candidates, however, were left stranded by the decision of the college to admit no more women. A sympathetic member of the college staff, Dr. Byford, proposed to Miss Thompson that a woman's medical college be organized in connection with her hospital. Classes were inaugurated in the hospital building in the fall of 1870, but disaster struck the following year; hospital and college alike were swallowed up in the Great Fire of 1871. The school was removed to a hastily remodeled barn until a new building was erected on Lincoln Street.[72]

Women graduates were admitted to competition with men for interne positions at the Cook County Hospital and Insane Asylum in 1879. A woman who placed second in her examination for the asylum, however, was denied the post with the explanation that the city commissioners could not ratify the appointment of a woman to such a place. In 1881, however, Dr. Mary Bates actually won a place at County Hospital, though considerable difficulty was encountered in securing the approval of the County Board. Her internship passed successfully, her mentor predicting a brilliant career for her.[73]

A changing attitude toward the education of women was reflected in the new and larger building erected by the Woman's Hospital Medical College in 1890 and in the action of Northwestern University, two years later, in making the college a department of the university. The arrangement with Northwestern continued until 1902 when the university decided abruptly to adopt a policy of co-education in medicine. Rush Medical College, in the meanwhile, had affiliated with the co-educational University of Chicago in 1898, which meant that there, too, the old policy of discrimination was dropped. By the close of the century opposition to women in medicine had all but disappeared. The transformation was seen clearly in the editorial pages of the *Medical Standard*, which had fought the idea for many years. Now, the *Standard* retracted, "we must admit that the woman is peculiarly at home in the sick room—both as doctor and patient. Her deftness of hand, her sympathy, her hopefulness, furnish a medicine to the soul which often does more for the patient than anything which the pharmacist can dispense. . . . Yes, we believe in the woman doctor!" [74]

Aside from the regular schools there were, of course, a number of institutions in Chicago devoted to the propagation of various sectarian doctrines. The first homeopathic college, for instance, was opened in 1860, largely through the efforts of the pioneer homeopath, David S. Smith. Despite its inadequate quarters—several rooms over a drugstore on South Clark Street—the Hahnemann Medical College prospered during the Civil War years and added a hospital in 1870. Smith was president of the college and an able faculty, including such noted homeopaths as Reuben Ludlam and George E. Shipman, was engaged to conduct the lectures and demonstrations.[75]

In 1876 a number of the faculty seceded to found a second school devoted to Hahnemann's teachings: the Chicago Homeopathic Medical College. The reason given for the separation was the desire of the withdrawing homeopaths to elevate standards and introduce a broader training in the basic medical studies. Nicholas B. Delamater, who was the man primarily responsible for the introduction of homeopathy into the Cook County Hospital, was the leading spirit in the organization of the new institution. The Homeopathic Medical College enjoyed a robust existence for the next two decades, but with the decline of interest in sectarian medicine around the close of the century, it began to fail; in 1905 the school was recombined with the Hahnemann Medical College.[76]

Other sects had their own schools. The eclectics founded a college on their negative principle of condemning all depleting measures in the treatment of disease. The Bennett College of Eclectic Medicine and Surgery, as it was called, was open to women from the first.[77] Like the homeopathic schools in Chicago, Bennett began to lose its distinctiveness under the pressure of revolutionary medical discoveries; in 1910 the college became one of several which merged to form the medical department of Loyola University. Among the newer medical sects, osteopathy attracted the most attention. A school was opened in Chicago in 1900 to accommodate students interested in mastering the principles of that sect. Known as the American College of Osteopathic Medicine and Surgery, this institution enrolled students from a wide geographic area. After 1913 the college was known as the Chicago College of Osteopathy.[78]

The regular schools, too, were responding to the expansion of medical knowledge in the last quarter of the nineteenth century. Important curricular changes, the building of laboratories, the introduction of bacteriology and other new subjects, and the appearance of a new medical school, all heralded significant growth in the concept of an adequate medical education. The contemporaneous rise of Chicago made that city a natural center for the exploitation of the new developments. By 1896, an enthusiastic partisan trumpeted that "Practitioners now, as well as pupils, come from all sections of the West to pursue special lines of study and investigation. In fact, no city in the country can offer more complete clinical advantages than Chicago, and the faculties of her colleges embrace not a few specialists whose fame is international." [79]

But before medical educators could embark on their programs of expansion, the heavy losses incurred in the Fire of 1871 had to be replaced. The destruction of medical facilities was immense. Rush Medical College was totally destroyed, six hospitals and more than a hundred wholesale and drug stores were burned to the ground, and four medical periodicals, with their offices, account books, and subscription lists were lost to the flames. Over two hundred physicians, including most of the Rush faculty, lost their homes, offices, libraries, and practices. Moses Gunn, professor of surgery at Rush, lost not only his books, office, and instruments, but also a cabinet of anatomical specimens years in the making, as well as the manuscript of a compendious work on surgery. Many of the students living in the vicinity of Rush not only lost everything they owned but lacked the wherewithal to replace it. The Chicago College of Pharmacy, whose library on chemistry and pharmacy was the most complete to be found anywhere in the West, was burned completely.[80] The Woman's Medical College, inaugurated only the year before, suffered the loss of its rooms with all their contents.

The Chicago Medical College, located on the south side of the city, escaped damage and offered the Rush students free attendance until Rush could be rebuilt. The offer was refused; Rush resumed classes four days after the fire in the clinical amphitheater of the Cook County Hospital.[81] A temporary building was erected on the grounds of the Cook County Hospital and a decision was reached to postpone erection of a permanent building until the new county hospital was completed, when the college would build on adjoining land. The advantages of such a location, it was felt, would more than compensate for the destruction of the old college. Not until 1876 did hospital and college move to their new accommodations on the west side.

Despite the setback, Rush continued to attract more students than her rival. While the Chicago Medical College graduated only 45 students in 1881, Rush sent 172, one of the largest classes in the country, into the practice of medicine.[82] A nominal agreement with Lake Forest University, similar to Northwestern's relationship with the Chicago Medical College, was in force between 1875 and 1887 but was dropped in favor of another loose tie, this time with the old Chicago University, in 1887.[83] The Rush faculty had been greatly strengthened since the break with Davis by the addition of James Nevins Hyde, who was becoming widely known in his specialty of dermatology, and Edward L. Holmes, whose fame as an ophthalmologist was not confined to Chicago. Holmes had an unusual background, especially for a medical school professor. As a youth he had associated with the historian John Lathrop Motley, had received his instruction in German from Henry Wadsworth Longfellow, and had spent his summer vacations with the communistic society at Brook Farm, Massachusetts. After graduating from the schools of liberal arts and medicine at Harvard, Holmes studied in Vienna, Paris, and Berlin before coming to Chicago in 1856. The genial eye specialist taught for about forty years at Rush, becoming its president in 1890. He was for almost a generation the leading ophthalmologist of the West. His scholarly character and quiet strength were an inspiration to several generations of Rush students.[84]

The great importance attached to lecturing began to fade somewhat in the 1880's as the newer trends in medicine began to turn attention toward the laboratory and practical demonstrations. The didactic lecture was the chief, almost the only, means of instruction in the early years. It had been the practice at Rush to choose teachers according to their performance in lecturing on topics selected at random, a terrifying procedure for the self-conscious candidate.[85] In 1884, N. S. Davis suggested to his faculty that the usual lectures be supplemented with recitations by students, in order to encourage them "to study more attentively and systematically." [86] Laboratory work played an increasingly important role in the curriculum in the closing decades of the century. At the Chicago Medical College laboratory work in chemistry was begun in 1868, in histology in 1877, in pathology and bacteriology in 1893, and in physiology in 1895.[87]

The first instruction in bacteriology in Chicago was given by

Bayard Holmes at the Chicago Medical College in 1888, though Henry Gradle had done much to popularize the germ theory earlier. Holmes had the co-operation of Adolph Gehrmann, recently returned from intensive study in European clinics, Isaac Abt, a future pediatrician of note, and Daniel Eisendrath.[88] Chicago schools were not unduly slow in thus introducing the new science; a graduate of the Medical Department of the University of Pennsylvania in 1889 recalled that he "never heard a lecture upon a bacteriological subject, made a culture of any kind or was shown a culture of any kind." [89]

The work of William T. Belfield at Rush aroused an early interest there, too, in bacteriology. One student remembered an autopsy he performed in 1883 on a tuberculosis victim and his invitation to his audience to come down into the arena to see under the microscope the new bacillus tuberculosis. But the systematic teaching of bacteriology at Rush was not begun until the 1890's when the college became a center of interest with the appointment of Edwin Klebs to the faculty.[90]

The specialization of medical knowledge was proceeding at such a rapid rate by the end of the century that colleges were forced to create new departments and staff them with practicing specialists who were expected to impart some of their hard-gained experience to the fledgling physicians. During the twenty years following the Great Fire, for example, the Chicago Medical College added departments of gynecology, histology, pediatrics, physical diagnosis, dermatology, laryngology and rhinology, and nervous and mental diseases. Within the next few years, departments of orthopedics, bacteriology, and genito-urinary surgery were appended to the expanding list of subjects taught.[91] It soon became obvious that the term of study must be lengthened if the student were to make more than a passing acquaintance with these new studies. A proposal was made in 1888 that the college year be increased to seven months, but the faculty voted to postpone for one year a decision on the change.[92] Beginning in the fall of 1889, however, all students were required to attend three yearly terms of seven months each to qualify for the M.D. degree.

Another result of the growing interest in medicine was the organization of a new medical school in 1881 to accommodate the larger numbers of young men seeking medical education. A well-known obstetrician, Charles W. Earle, joined an ambitious young surgeon named A. Reeves Jackson in securing a charter for the Col-

lege of Physicians and Surgeons of Chicago. With the noted internist, William E. Quine, the surgeon D. A. K. Steele, and Frank E.
Waxham, who was to achieve fame as the pioneer in intubation for
diphtheria in the West, they became the nucleus of the new faculty.
The graded curriculum was decided upon at the outset and the college gave every promise of competing successfully with the two older
schools.[93]

A further development of the 1880's which reflected mounting concern for the complexity and rapidity of change in medical
practice was the inauguration of post-graduate education in medicine. New York City had begun post-graduate work in 1882 to stop
the wholesale emigration of young doctors to European clinics. Four
years later the Chicago Policlinic commenced instruction in a rented
house on the corner of Chicago and La Salle avenues. The methods
employed at the Policlinic were almost exclusively practical and
clinical. A number of brilliant practitioners and specialists were induced to come and give demonstrations of their particular skills; the
early faculties included such well-known surgeons as Christian Fenger, Nicholas Senn, and Fernand Henrotin, internists Henry B.
Favill and E. Fletcher Ingals, the neurologist Archibald Church, and
the genito-urinary specialist William Belfield. The goal of the school
was to bring the new ideas and theories of the laboratory, together
with the latest improvements in operative procedure, within the
reach of the working physician.[94]

A second graduate institution came into existence in 1888
when Franklin H. Martin, W. F. Coleman, and several other of the
younger teachers at the Policlinic resigned to form the Post-Graduate Medical School and Hospital. Although no reason was given for
the withdrawal, it may be guessed that they felt their work would
find fuller expression in a school not dominated by older and better-
known men. Martin and Coleman were aided by the young internist,
Frank Billings, in organizing the school; they were fortunate in soon
obtaining the services of Bayard Holmes, the Viennese dermatologist Joseph Zeisler, and the brilliant young surgeon, John B. Murphy.[95]

As the century ended, the importance of Chicago as a center
of medical education was assured. The city had already outdistanced
Louisville, Cincinnati, and St. Louis in the number of regular graduates in medicine and no new challenger was expected. In a sample
year, the number of young men from Nebraska who received di-

plomas from Chicago medical schools was five times that of those
who graduated from schools in St. Louis. Not only was the Lake
Michigan city attracting students from all over the Middle West by
1900, but an increasing proportion of her own practitioners were
trained in local schools. As late as 1877, only 36 per cent of physicians practicing in Chicago were graduates of the city's schools, but
a decade later the proportion had risen to 56 per cent.[96] A civic-
minded educator in 1900 could muse that since 1843 Chicago had
produced four regular medical colleges and two post-graduate schools,
had stopped the emigration of western students to eastern medical
schools, and had won a name among centers of medical instruction.
The pioneering optimism of Daniel Brainard had not proved unjus-
tified.

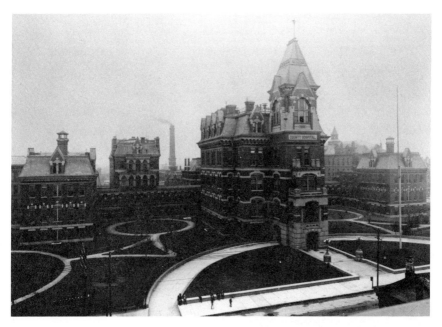

Cook County Hospital, 1905 (Courtesy of the Chicago Historical Society, #ICHi-19012).

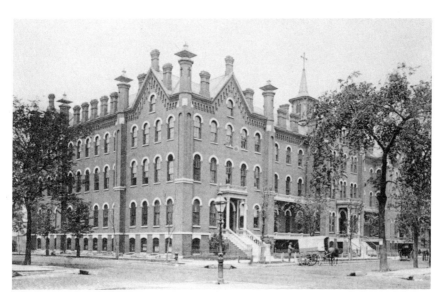

Mercy Hospital, 1892 (from *Select Chicago*, Courtesy of the Chicago Historical Society).

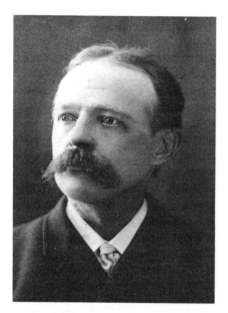

Christian Fenger (Courtesy of the Chicago Historical Society).

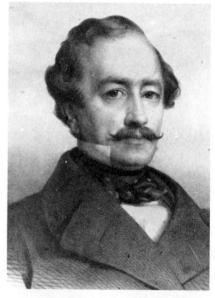

Daniel Brainard (by Leon Noel, after a painting by G. P. A. Healy, courtesy of the Chicago Historical Society).

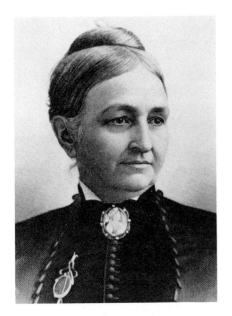

Mary Harris Thompson (Courtesy of the Chicago Historical Society).

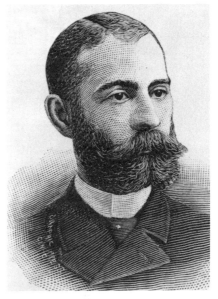

Daniel Hale Williams (Courtesy of the Chicago Historical Society, #ICHi-12921).

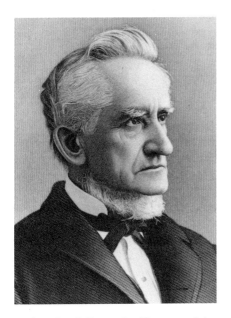

Nathan Smith Davis, Sr. (Courtesy of the Chicago Historical Society).

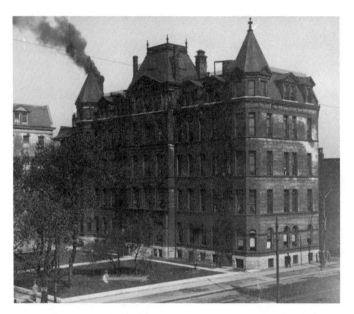

Mary Thompson Hospital, 1909 (Courtesy of the Chicago Historical Society).

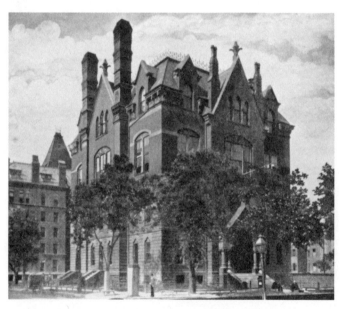

Rush Medical College, 1899 (Courtesy of the Chicago Historical Society).

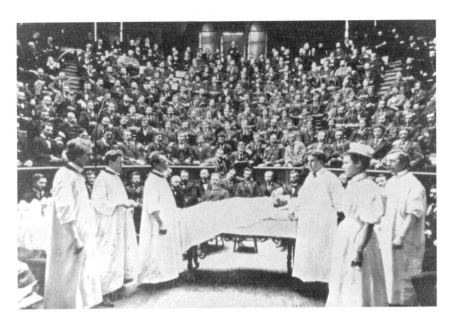

Senn's surgical clinic (Courtesy of the Chicago Historical Society).

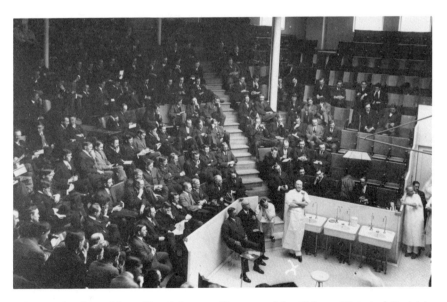

John B. Murphy at Mercy Hospital, 1910 (Courtesy of the Chicago Historical Society).

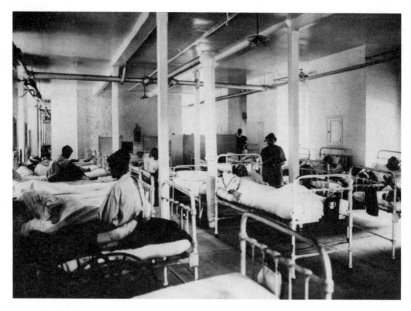

Old Cook County Hospital (Courtesy of the Chicago Historical Society, #ICHi-18718).

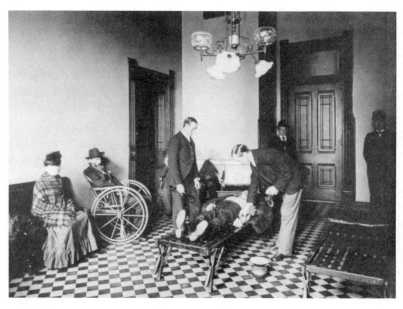

Cook County Hospital, examining room (Courtesy of the Chicago Historical Society).

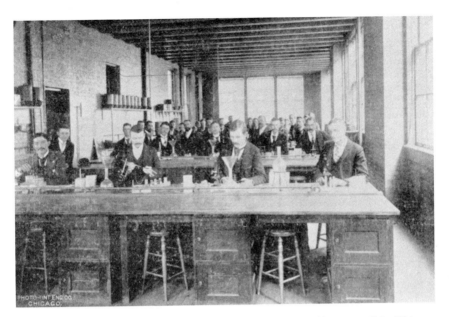

Chicago Medical College, ca. 1895, bacteriological laboratory (Courtesy of the Chicago Historical Society).

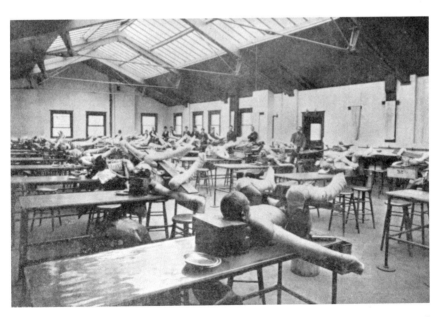

Rush Medical College, ca. 1895, dissecting room (Courtesy of the Chicago Historical Society).

| Chapter V | Professional Societies and Publications, 1850–1900 |

One of the striking features of modern medicine is the large number of societies, journals, and libraries devoted to informing the physician of recent developments affecting his art. The leisure time of the average doctor is occupied more fully with meetings, conferences, and reading than that of any other profession. In the United States, with its fast transportation, wholesale production of technical media, and remarkable zeal of its citizens for "joining," the physician is probably more alert to what is happening in his field of interest than any of his colleagues abroad.

This was not always true. The American physician of a century ago was likely to be not only poorly informed on the scientific work of Europe, but probably knew next to nothing about investigations being carried on in his own country, his own state, or even his own town. The doctor who came to the western prairies had to ready himself for constant calls for his service, calls that might take him along muddy, unmarked trails or across swollen, unbridged streams perhaps a day or two's travel from his own dwelling. Travel on horseback or by carriage was notoriously slow and painful, and if the patient was dangerously ill, the doctor might keep a week's vigil at the bedside rather than risk a retracing of his journey.

Under these conditions the doctor was understandably loath to spend his small and unpredictable leisure in riding to places of meeting convenient to his widely scattered colleagues. The professional organization of physicians in a given area depended not so much on the age of the community or the level of its culture, as on the achievement of a certain social and economic growth which made it feasible. The growth of cities, the coming of the railroad and the electric streetcar, and the development of cheap printing were more important in stimulating professional association than a particular location or the activity of certain individuals who only exploited opportunities made possible by these innovations. It was no accident, for example, that the American Medical Association was formed only five years after the British commenced their national organization, despite the differences in size and professional maturity between the two countries.

The dearth of medical and scientific associations of all types, coupled with the fluid nature of natural science during most of the nineteenth century, made it a common procedure for physicians to join with other scientists in organizational and publishing ventures. The first issue of Daniel Drake's medical journal in Louisville, for example, contained the announcement that "as there is not in this region, any Magazine devoted to the Physical Sciences, the Editors will be gratified to . . . make public, all kinds of original facts and observations on the Climate, Mineralogy, Botany and Zoology of the States, which lie between the Lakes and the Gulph of Mexico." [1] Similarly, when the need for an academy of sciences was felt in Chicago, Professor Blaney of Rush Medical College, a chemist and naturalist as well as a physician, was a logical choice for its first president. Other Chicago physicians played prominent roles; N. S. Davis served as vice-president, Hosmer Johnson was secretary, and the surgeon Edmund Andrews was given the strategic post of curator and librarian. [2]

With the coming of swifter and more dependable transportation in the 1840's and 1850's, a wave of organization for scientific purposes swept across the United States. While a number of states, notably in New England, had organized medically on a state level before this time, many new state societies appeared during these years. Among the older states, Pennsylvania, Ohio, South Carolina, Georgia, Alabama, and Kentucky all formed state medical associations in the period from 1846 to 1851, while in the West, Wisconsin, Indiana, Illinois, Iowa, Missouri, and Kansas organized societies before the outbreak of the Civil War. [3] The West of this period, once the barriers to easy communication began to fall, showed even keener enthusiasm for scientific organization than the eastern parts of the country.

The experience of Illinois in the development of medical societies was not greatly different from that of other western states. The lack of good transportation, busy practices, and low incomes

conspired to retard their growth. Those attending the first meeting
of the Illinois State Medical Society in 1850 found the trip to Springfield an arduous one. Most of the physicians drove their own vehicles,
but the Chicago delegation, in view of the distance, came by stagecoach. Under the most favorable conditions the trip from Chicago
to Peoria, where the second convention was held, could not be made
in less than two days.[4] Aside from transportation, the cost of attendance was the most serious obstacle to early medical organization.
The loss of income from practice on top of the expense of a trip to
Springfield or Peoria was more than most physicians could bear.
"Actual emoluments from practice," N. S. Davis complained, "will
scarcely equal those resulting from almost any of the mechanic arts."
Another pioneer doctor remembered that in Illinois "Money was the
hardest thing to get; even parties considered wealthy were compelled
to turn out produce in professional bills; wheat was tendered at 35,
oats at 10 and corn at 8 cents per bushel."[5] In consideration of all
these barriers, the promoters of early medical societies found it necessary to offer inducements to attend. The social and cultural, as well
as the scientific value of meeting in convention with one's fellows
was emphasized:[6]

Now, friends, why not break loose from your domestic and professional cares and anxieties for a few days, and attend the meeting;
visit Jacksonville, one of the most beautiful and pleasant spots in the
State; see its numerous State and other public institutions; enjoy its
intelligent and generous society; meet your professional brethren
from different parts of the State, and extend your acquaintance
among them; participate in the deliberations of the Society, and endeavor to improve the profession and yourselves?

The first call for a state medical convention in Illinois had
come in 1840. An announcement in the *Chicago American* stressed
the need for physicians to band together against irregular practitioners: "Hitherto we have been like a vessel cast upon a boisterous
ocean, without compass or helm; we have acted solitary and alone,
without harmony or concert; but when we see hundreds of our fellow citizens and worthy friends, annually sacrificed by the empirical
prescriptions of charletan [*sic*] professors, on the altars of ignorance,
erected within the very temple of Aesculapius, by rude and unskilful
hands, is it not time for us to act?"[7] The organizational meeting
was held in Springfield and a professional body known as the Medi-

cal Society of Illinois formed. After some discussion concerning the adoption of a fee table, the convention quickly adjourned; there is no record of any subsequent meeting or action. The present Illinois State Medical Society was formed ten years later, with seven Chicagoans among the twenty-nine founders. Professor Herrick of Rush was elected president of the Society, while Professors Brainard, Evans, Blaney, and Meek all won committee appointments.[8]

A number of regional and local societies were called into being during the 1840's in Illinois, but most of them were short-lived.[9] In Chicago there was no attempt at medical organization after 1836 when Dr. Levi D. Boone sought vainly to stir up interest.[10] Boone came to Chicago from the southern part of the state where he was doubtless aware of efforts to suppress quacks and imposters through professional action.[11] A relative of the explorer Daniel Boone, he had lived a pioneer's existence in western Kentucky, attended classes in medicine at Transylvania University, and served in the Black Hawk War before coming to Chicago. He was to have a noteworthy career in his new home. In 1848 he was elected city physician at the beginning of the great cholera epidemic; shortly thereafter he was chosen alderman from the second ward. He was elected mayor of Chicago in 1855 on the "Know-Nothing" ticket. As mayor, he introduced a new sewerage system, and established a high school, but was better known for the "lager beer riots" which he precipitated by his discriminatory policy toward German and Irish taverns.[12]

Though Boone failed to excite any action toward a medical society in 1836, his interest in bringing the medical fraternity of Chicago closer together continued. When later arrivals, such as N. S. Davis and W. B. Herrick, took up the campaign, Boone co-operated with them; he offered, for example, the use of the office he shared with Brockholst McVickar as meeting place for the city's doctors. In the fall of 1850, consequently, he played host to about fifteen physicians interested in forming a professional organization. Dr. David Rutter of Rush, a future founder of the Chicago Medical College, was chosen temporary chairman until a constitution and by-laws could be drawn. Though the scientific goals of the new body were stressed in the constitution, the society was also to enforce "proper ethical rules and a more courteous standard of professional intercourse." It was hoped that the society would put to an end the antagonism between physicians and bickering over patients which had been the bane of friendly relations between them. The new organization was denominated the Chicago Medical Society and Levi Boone was elected its first president.[13]

The choice of Boone as president set off a chain of events which brought to an end the society's existence before the first year was over. The influential President Brainard of Rush Medical College was dissatisfied with Boone's election and attended no further meetings. A number of others followed Brainard out of the society, including Philip Maxwell, the former Fort Dearborn surgeon. Brainard, almost alone among early Chicago medical leaders, never cherished any respect for medical societies; he probably attended the initial meetings of the Chicago association more from curiosity than any other reason. Most societies, Brainard felt, were simply "trade unions" in their concern for fee standards, or "punitive leagues" in their desire to enforce professional ethics.[14]

The membership of the Chicago Medical Society dropped sharply during the first year. The weaknesses of the new organization were readily apparent: it lacked sufficient support from the profession and it needed more power to enforce the professional standards resolved upon. A Dr. J. E. McGin, for example, was charged with using "very abusive and unprofessional language" to describe President Boone, but an investigating committee only met McGin's prompt invitation to Boone and the entire society to depart for the nether regions. After the second election of officers in 1851, it was impossible even to secure a quorum though informal meetings continued to be held.

A reorganization was effected in 1852 by N. S. Davis in an effort to revive the moribund association. Rules of procedure were simplified, the number constituting a quorum was reduced, and the society's name was changed to Cook County Medical Society to attract physicians from outside the city. From this point, membership began to level off and even to rise. In 1858, when the lone non-Chicagoan in the organization died, the name reverted to Chicago Medical Society; when it again became a county society in 1903, the Chicago title was retained.[15]

For many years the Society's only rival was the Chicago Academy of the Medical Sciences, founded in 1859 and composed largely of Rush faculty members.[16] Founders of the Academy intended to model it along the lines of New York's Academy of Medicine, organized in 1847 and in flourishing condition by 1859.[17] Significantly, Dr. Brainard of Rush lent his support to the early meetings of this body, while N. S. Davis, Edmund Andrews, and several others who seceded from Rush did not immediately join. Emphasis was placed on scientific papers and reports in the new organization, according to the announcements; a library and anatomical cabinets were also contemplated. About 1862, however, only three years after its founding, the Academy "died of inaction" according to its historian.[18]

For the first thirty years the scientific papers read before the Chicago Medical Society dealt chiefly with the epidemic diseases which swept periodically across the city. An essayist was appointed at each meeting to deliver an address on the diagnosis of diphtheria, the control of typhoid, the danger from smallpox, or some similar subject. Occasionally a meeting was brightened by the appearance of a distinguished guest, such as W. T. G. Morton, Marion Simms, or Sir William Osler.[19] But reports of individual cases normally occupied the major part of each meeting. These were usually long and earnest, warmly personal in their common-sense advice drawn from experience, and full of warnings to professional brethren against repeating their own unhappy errors. Sometimes a report added a touch of humor to the otherwise heavy proceedings, as the following must have if the secretary's account was accurate: "Dr. Davis related a case in which insensibility had been produced by chloroform on a patient laboring under Delirium Tremens—he so far recovered as to drink a tumbler ¼ full of brandy & water with gr I of morphine. Nothing unusual was noticed till just after taking the drink when he died." [20]

The first discussion of the germ theory of disease took place at a meeting held in June, 1877, though many members had doubtless considered the news from Europe privately before that date. The lack of knowledge on the subject among members of the Society caused one doctor to pronounce it a "disgrace that the profession of our country were not more alive to the importance of the advantages of the microscope." [21] In other respects, however, members of the Society were better informed on what was happening in Europe. Dr. Edward L. Holmes, for example, reported extensively on the use of the ophthalmoscope in 1858, showing a close study of the work of Helmholtz, Graefe, Jaeger, Arlt, and others. Once it was known that marvels were being accomplished in European surgery following the work of Pasteur and Lister, the Society heard detailed accounts of these developments.[22] Professor De Laskie Miller of Rush was present at Pasteur's address before the International

Medical Congress in 1881, and he also heard the classic plea for vivisection delivered by Rudolph Virchow. His subsequent report to the Chicago Medical Society stirred an enthusiastic interest.[23]

Members of the Society were stimulated to do more original work by the description of events across the Atlantic. The number of scientific essays, original contributions, and reports of unusual cases recorded in the Society's annals increased markedly during the 1880's and 1890's. Papers dealing with surgery, internal medicine, and nervous diseases jumped in number from next to none in 1880 to more than thirty in 1889; four years later, twenty-three papers in surgery alone were presented. During the year 1893, sixteen microscopical exhibits were presented to the Society, while ophthalmology and otology, always popular in earlier years, were the subjects of only four papers.[24]

The growing complexity of medicine and the difficulty in keeping informed of new developments gave professional organization in Chicago a tremendous boost. Doctors who had never attended a medical meeting flocked to a demonstration of the cholera bacillus or a report of a visit to Pasteur's laboratory. The membership of the Chicago Medical Society shot up to 560 by 1890, a threefold increase over the preceding decade. By the end of the century, nearly a thousand doctors were on the Society's membership rolls. Complaints from downstate members of the Illinois State Medical Society, fearing that the growth of the Chicago Society meant Chicago domination of the state group, were heard for the first time. The State Society, according to those who resented Chicago men occupying important committee jobs, was but another name for the Chicago Medical Society. By 1913 their fears were fully justified: Chicago physicians were in virtual control of the state group.[25]

With the rapid growth of the Society in the latter part of the nineteenth century, a place of meeting became a persistent problem. In the past, meetings had been held in physicians' homes or offices, the Washingtonian Home or Bill Sloan's Commercial College, the Court House or the Masonic Temple, and at least twenty-five other places. The Chicago Public Library provided a new refuge for the Society in the 1880's, but soon proved too small for the expanding membership. Beginning in 1875, plans for a permanent home were first discussed, but the fluctuating size of the Society, in addition to a lack of funds, prevented their fulfillment. Indeed, the Society has today no permanent building.

The Great Fire of 1871 destroyed the center of the city and therewith all places of meeting convenient to the whole membership. The Society split into two groups, one on the west side, the other on the south, until the damage could be repaired. The group on the west side, which retained the name of Chicago Medical Society, suffered heavily from the division and was barely able to muster a quorum at its infrequent gatherings. During the greater part of 1873 only seven or eight physicians appeared at each meeting. To stimulate attendance, dues were lowered from six dollars to two, but interest and support continued to lag.[26]

The restoration of the downtown section of Chicago permitted the reunion in 1878 of the Society with the southern section, which had called itself the Chicago Society of Physicians and Surgeons.[27] The recombination of forces did not satisfy all of the doctors of the growing city; many complained that the distances involved in attending meetings were becoming too great. Some of the west side members refused to make the trip downtown and instead formed a West Chicago Medical Society, which became eventually the Chicago Pathological Society.[28] One member, in resigning from the Chicago Medical Society, protested that "as I have only one life to live on earth, I cannot afford to pass the greater part of my time in journeying to and from the Grand Pacific Hotel." [29]

Regardless of location, members of the Chicago Medical Society showed early an awareness of the socio-medical problems which lay around them. Only four years after its founding, the organization had selected N. S. Davis as chairman of a committee to investigate sanitary conditions in the city.[30] In one early report, Davis charged that the "Sanitary condition . . . is about as bad as Nature and Art can Make it." [31] The Society interested itself also in the indigent. A Committee on the City Poor, established in 1864, recommended that Chicago support dispensaries and visiting physicians for the needy.[32] Other committees undertook investigation of Chicago's orphan home and insane asylum; patent medicine advertisement and condensed milk were also brought under the Society's scrutiny.[33] Sometimes the Society over-reached itself in its concern for the health and welfare of the community, as in 1891 when representatives were appointed to force "legislation to prevent the erection of high buildings at the expense of air & health." [34]

Leaders of the Society never hesitated to fight corruption in public medical institutions, though their efforts were usually futile.

Beginning in 1869, protests against the political nature of appointments to the Cook County Hospital were periodically made, but with no significant results. The county insane asylum was investigated by members of the Society on a number of occasions and its methods roundly criticized each time, but public authorities still saw fit to make only the thinnest differentiation between insanity and pauperism. The insane of Cook County had no building separate from paupers until 1871.

Contemporaneous with the growth of the Chicago Medical Society after the Great Fire came the beginnings of more specialized associations. It was observed earlier that the Chicago Pathological Society had its origins in the splitting of medical groups attendant upon the Fire. Not only in medicine, but in all scientific activity, the key tendency in organization after the Civil War was the growth of special societies reflecting the overall triumph of specialization.[35]

The pathologist, because he was away from general practice in the laboratory or morgue much of the time, was usually the first to join with his fellows in some sort of association. A "curator of the dead house" had been appointed at the Cook County Hospital as early as 1865, but the lack of such elementary equipment as microscope, alcohol, and specimen jars made it impossible for him to conduct more than gross autopsical examinations. Specialization became more pronounced with the election of the pioneer bacteriologist, Isaac Danforth, to the staff in 1873. Danforth's work prepared the way for the inspiring demonstrations of Christian Fenger, from whose appointment in 1878 modern pathology in Chicago may be dated.[36] The year that Fenger began his work at the County Hospital the forerunner of Chicago's first association of pathologists held its first meetings on the west side; three years later, in 1881, the name of Chicago Pathological Society was formally adopted. By 1900 the society boasted a membership of two hundred, second only to that of the Chicago Medical Society among medical associations in the city.[37]

During the 1890's the division of physicians into specialized societies proceeded rapidly. A Chicago Ophthalmological and Otological Society was begun in 1892; those interested in otology later transferred their allegiance to the laryngologists.[38] Pediatricians also held their first meetings in 1892. Those interested in internal medicine organized for the first time in 1898 as a protest against the lack of professional recognition given their specialty. This society failed in 1903 because it was simply "a replica of the Chicago Medical Society," according to one informed guess; not until 1915 did Chicago internists again reconstitute themselves as a distinct specialty group.[39] Still other specialty societies devoted to surgery, orthopedics, and dermatology were organized around the turn of the century.[40]

A number of neurologists met in the office of Dr. Sanger Brown in 1898 to draw up plans for an association. Since neurology was just separating from internal medicine at this time, a number of internists, notably Frank Billings, Henry Favill, and William Quine, became early members of the Chicago Neurological Society. This organization has had an interesting history. One might trace the evolution of neuropsychiatric thought and endeavor in the initial attention to individual case reports, the later emphasis on clinical analysis, psychoanalysis, and child psychiatry, and the still more recent interest in neurosurgery, anatomy, and pathology.[41]

Aside from specialty societies, social organizations of physicians, such as the Practitioners' Club and the Doctors' Club, came into existence; these two groups merged into the Physicians' Club of Chicago in 1895.[42] There were, too, organized groups of doctors of European extraction, notably the German, Scandinavian, and Bohemian medical societies. Sectarian practitioners had their own fraternities. A homeopathic association, for example, was inaugurated in 1857 and was succeeded by a more successful county organization in 1866.[43] By 1900 well over twenty-five Chicago physicians' groups of all types were competing for the doctor's leisure time.[44]

But professional societies were, of course, only one means of self-education and communication available to the doctor. The medical journal had developed by 1900 from a literary curiosity to an indispensable record of what was happening in the world of medicine. The physician who wanted to be well informed had not only to attend medical meetings, but also to read several of these technical publications each month.

American medical literature was not held in high esteem during much of the nineteenth century. In the famous first report of the American Medical Association's committee on medical literature in 1848, Oliver Wendell Holmes, the presumed author, analyzed brilliantly the weaknesses of American journals: lack of original articles, poor writing, and dependence for ideas upon Europe.[45] The fate of an article written by a professor at Rush Medical College in 1850 illustrated Holmes's charges and demonstrated the poor editing of American journals as well. It was copied from a Chicago journal by the *Ohio Medical and Surgical Journal,* where it looked so much like an original report in its new surroundings that the *New Jersey Medical Reporter* reproduced it, giving full credit to the Ohio periodical.[46] Other American Medical Association reports, one of them by the Chicagoan N. S. Davis, criticized the shortcomings of medical literature in the United States, citing the meager and fragmentary reports of cases, the neglect of hospital and clinical experience, and the use of edited European works as American texts.[47]

Chicago's first journal was typical of the average publication of the day. Established in 1844 by Professor James Blaney of Rush, it was called first the *Illinois,* then the *Illinois and Indiana Medical and Surgical Journal,* to promote circulation in as wide an area as possible. In the opening number Blaney explained that his journal was not in competition with existing publications but was designed for those parts of the West which were inaccessible to other media. His periodical would provide, he continued, a vehicle for disseminating valuable local news, such as statistics on epidemics or information on botanical remedies indigenous to the Northwest; it would also expose any "new-fangled impostures" preying on western communities.[48] Few original articles were published in Blaney's journal, save for those by the Rush faculty; most of the material came from eastern or European journals. But the value of this pioneer publication was nevertheless considerable. For several years it was the only medical periodical published in the states of Illinois, Michigan, and Indiana, as well as the large territories of Wisconsin and Iowa. The material published, whether reprinted or not, brought information to frontier practitioners who might otherwise never have been reached.

The editorship of this pioneer journal fell to John Evans in 1848, who changed its name to the *North-western Medical and Surgical Journal* during his campaign to publicize the activities of Rush Medical College. The editor wrote a number of papers himself, many of them dealing with cholera, and urged other faculty members to do likewise. President Brainard's surgical clinics during these early years were a fruitful source of firsthand reports on new techniques and operations; Brainard also joined Evans and Blaney in composing editorial comment covering a wide range of subjects.

When Evans gave up his duties in 1852, he was followed by a succession of Rush faculty members. In 1854, Dr. N. S. Davis fell heir to the post and conducted the journal's affairs until his split with Rush in 1859.[49] The title of the publication, meanwhile, was narrowed to *Chicago Medical Journal,* registering the rapid growth of other western periodicals. The editorial problems which Davis faced were not greatly different from those of his predecessors. Original medical writing was difficult to find in a community where practitioners lacked the time, even if they had the inclination, to make a serious investigation of any subject. "Write! write!" readers of the journal were exhorted, "if you do not begin early, you will never begin at all: just allow the first decade of your professional life to pass in unbroken silence, and you are dumb for all future time." [50]

When Davis left the Rush faculty in 1859, he turned the editorship of the journal over to Brainard, who promised to exclude "all discussions of a personal nature, speculations of a purely theoretical character, and dull, worthless matter generally." [51] Brainard did not succeed in all his objectives, however, for barely had Davis left Rush when the Rush president began the literary feud which was to last until Brainard's death in 1866. Davis started Chicago's second medical periodical the year following, and the two journals became the battleground where the tournament of clashing ideas between the two men was fought. Davis retained the editorship of the second publication, the *Chicago Medical Examiner,* until 1871; four years later it was united with the Rush organ as the *Chicago Medical Journal and Examiner.* The combined periodical was printed until 1889 when, fifty-five years after the *Journal's* first appearance, it ceased publication.

The passing of Chicago's first medical journal was scarcely noticed in the flurry of medical publication excited by events of the last quarter of the century. The specialization of medical knowledge demanded new media for the ever finer gradations of professional interest. The first specialized medical periodical to appear in Chicago, the *Journal of Nervous and Mental Diseases,* was not inaugurated until 1874. This journal was owned and edited by James S. Jewell, a pioneer neurologist of the Middle West; in 1883 it was removed to New York where another proprietor continued its publication.[52]

Numerous other journals began publication before the century was over. With the selection of N. S. Davis as first editor of the *Journal of the American Medical Association* in 1883, the importance of Chicago as a center of medical publication was enhanced. In 1887 the *Medical Standard,* a medium-size monthly devoted to general medicine, was established. The *Clinical Review*, specializing in clinical and postgraduate studies, commenced operations in 1892. The Post-Graduate Medical School started an outstanding journal known as the *North American Practitioner* during the 1890's. The homeopaths, too, were active in medical publication. Their first journal, the *Northwestern Journal of Homoeopathia*, was published in 1848, but lasted only four years. It was followed by the *United States Medical and Surgical Journal* and a number of others.[53]

The Chicago Medical Society undertook the publication of a periodical entitled the *Chicago Medical Record* in 1891. A monthly, it was filled largely with papers read before the Society, as well as reports of the proceedings of its meetings. After twenty-four volumes were issued, the *Medical Recorder*, as it was then known, was surrendered into private hands. Under the able editorship of Archibald Church, it became an outstanding Chicago journal and one of the more important in the United States. The Chicago Medical Society, in the meantime, commenced the publication of a weekly bulletin in 1902.

Despite the enormous expansion of medical publication, much criticism of American periodicals remained at the beginning of the present century. The very multiplicity of journals meant that many would be found wanting in comparison with European or eastern models. The number of poorly edited publications bereft of significant or original writing remained high in the West; many Chicago men chose to send their manuscripts to the *New York Medical Journal* or to the new *Journal of the American Medical Association*, rather than bury their work in an inferior periodical. Plagiarism continued to be a problem, even for respectable journals, though wider circulation and consequently speedier detection, made the practice more uncommon. Few victims of plagiarism, unfortunately, had the happy gift of satire of Chicago's Dr. Lydston, who was the victim of a literary steal by a Georgia physician:[54]

In the first paragraph of the parallel columns [Lydston produced the two articles side by side] it will be noted that Dr. Fitch [the plagiarist] has substituted the word "practice" for "field of labor" and "specialist in venereal diseases" for "venereal specialist." The implied adverse criticism of my verbiage is accepted in the same spirit in which it is given. The delicate compliment to the specialist in venereal diseases implied in the intimation that Dr. Fitch does not consider him "venereal" is worthy of a Chesterfield.

The insertion of the word *"demimonde"* in the second paragraph shows a literary finish to which Dumas, himself, the coiner of the word, could not take exception. The word lightens up the gloom of the otherwise turgid and heavy style for which I am noted, and illumines the pages with a brilliant forecast of future improvement in my composition for which I shall never cease to thank my confrère. I use the word confrère advisedly, not to be outdone in generosity, for I am sure my learned friend could ill spare the word *demimonde*, and I, therefore, reciprocate from my own scanty store of "furrin things."

Beside medical societies and medical journals, another means of informal education had become important by 1900: the public medical library. The problem of storing medical books, periodicals, and other materials had first become serious in Chicago in the 1880's. The rapid growth of professional journals made it next to impossible for the doctor to keep on hand more than the most useful of the older issues. The increased number, moreover, rendered it financially impossible for any one physician to subscribe to all the periodicals which might prove useful to him in practice or research. The problem was much the same with books. Cheaper printing and increased activity in medicine brought a plethora of new books for which the average physician lacked money and space on his library shelves.

There was no public medical library in Chicago until 1883, when the Chicago Public Library established a medical department. Prior to this time no large collection of books and periodicals was freely available to the doctor except in university medical schools. Not more than two or three sets of the great German year books, such as Schmidt's *Jahrbücher* or the Virchow-Hirsch *Jahresbericht*, could be found in the entire city and these were not available except by personal favor to the ordinary physician. Dr. Bayard Holmes recalled that many were forced to make a journey to Washington to complete a subject under investigation.[55] So struck was Dr. J. M. Toner, a national figure in medicine and public health, with the inadequacy of reference facilities in Chicago, that he offered in 1878 his large personal library to the profession of the city, provided a fireproof building was built to house the collection.[56] N. S. Davis canvassed the possibilities for such a project, apparently without success, since Toner wrote him shortly thereafter of his disappointment that "the profession of your state did not secure the library." [57]

An association for the purpose of establishing an adequate medical library was organized in 1889, with N. S. Davis as president and Bayard Holmes secretary. The initial plans called for a new library building financed from the contributions of physicians. The association, however, did not raise much money, though it did succeed in collecting a large number of books. An agreement was eventually reached with Newberry Library later in the year whereby the library would establish a medical department and the association was to turn over its collection of books.[58] The department at Newberry was subsequently swelled by the munificent gift of Dr. Nicholas Senn, celebrated Chicago and Milwaukee surgeon, of ten thousand volumes on surgery and medicine.[59] The Chicago Medical Society, in the meanwhile, arranged for the transfer to Newberry of the medical books at the public library.[60]

But the most important step in assuring a first-rate medical library to Chicago was taken by the trustees of the estate of John Crerar, a wealthy railway magnate, who in 1890 willed two million dollars toward the launching of a scientific library.[61] They authorized in 1906 the purchase of Newberry's medical collection of over sixty-five thousand volumes and pamphlets, and subscriptions to four hundred periodicals.[62] Thus did Chicago's economic and medical growth come together in philanthropy, a pattern which became familiar in the following years. The medical collection at John Crerar Library grew rapidly from this time, and today the library ranks among the world's largest storehouses of medical knowledge.

| Chapter VI | The Emergence of Chicago as a Force in Twentieth Century Medicine |

By 1900 Chicago was claiming the attention of the medical world. Its medical schools and journals, its societies and libraries, as well as its growing army of surgeons and specialists, brought the city a considerable measure of fame. Its unprecedented growth from frontier outpost to busy metropolis in a single lifetime effected a revolution in medical, as well as in cultural and scientific life generally. In Chicago, as elsewhere, the crowding of thousands of people into a great city stimulated intellectual and scientific development. The very size of a modern city meant that every person, no matter how obscure his vocation or special interest, could join with like-minded people in mutual discussion and action. It was in the great cities that the wealth of the nation was congregated; here were the places where civic-minded philanthropists might be persuaded to found institutions devoted to art, music, or the sciences. Here also were the powerful publishing houses whose support was often vital to the success of cultural and scientific enterprises.

The rapid development of Chicago was the key to understanding that burst of medical activity which brought it to the forefront among American cities in exploiting the opportunities opened by Pasteur, Koch, and their co-workers. The first recognition of Chicago's successful climb to national fame in medicine came about 1890; in that year it could boast four regular medical schools, two post-graduate institutions, a dozen medical societies, numerous hospitals and clinics, ten medical journals, and more than twelve hundred regular practitioners of medicine. A large and variegated population was of critical importance in supplying an endless stream of patients, with an infinite variety of afflictions, to the city's clinics and teaching institutions; with the passage of the anatomical law of 1885 there was also no shortage of material in dissecting rooms. At the Cook County Hospital in Chicago at the turn of the century a visiting physician might see more cases of diabetes, cancer, or meningitis in one day than in a lifetime of practice in his home town. The large number of physicians and surgeons in the city, moreover, permitted a specialization impossible in smaller communities. As early as 1885, Dr. Charles F. Sinclair told the Chicago Medical Society that specialization was the "distinguishing characteristic of recent medical study," while another paper a year later warned that "specialists are apt to become egotistic, and give rise to utterances which they will afterwards regret." [1] By 1900, certainly, specialization in Chicago was far advanced.

Surgery was the first specialty to reflect the city's new position in the world of medicine. During the 1880's a group of older surgeons, headed by Moses Gunn of Rush and Edmund Andrews at the Chicago Medical College, still held the center of the stage, but a decade later their influence was all but gone. Charles T. Parkes, who succeeded Gunn in 1887, became the first western surgeon to carry on experimental research in gunshot wounds of the small intestines. Other energetic young men—Christian Fenger, John B. Murphy, Roswell Park, Albert Ochsner, Lewis L. McArthur, and E. Wyllis Andrews—were attracted to Chicago's hospitals and had gone far by 1890 in making the city a recognized center of surgical progress and teaching.[2]

By far the most important of this group was the Danish surgeon and pathologist, Christian Fenger. Although Fenger spent only half of his life in Chicago, his influence on the development of surgery and general medical practice was such that the evolution of scientific medicine in Chicago has often been dated from his arrival. Fenger's medical education was begun at the University of Copenhagen, where he studied under the physiologist Panum, a former pupil of Claude Bernard, and the pathological anatomist Reisz, who had worked with Rudolph Virchow. He was doubtless influenced, too, by his uncle, Emil Fenger, a noted pathologist credited with the emancipation of Danish medical education from humoral pathology. After service in the Danish-Prussian War, where he performed important work on the endoscopy of bullet wounds, Fenger was authorized to continue his experiments in the Franco-Prussian War of 1870–71. He served, too, in Egypt, where he was a member of the national board of health. Finally, in 1877, he arrived in Chicago, so penniless that he was forced to sell for sustenance a mummy he had brought with great trouble from Egypt.[3]

Fenger's success in Chicago was almost immediate. He secured a place on the staff of the Cook County Hospital in the spring of 1878 and inaugurated lectures and demonstrations in pathological anatomy, a science then in a rudimentary stage of development in Chicago.[4] So impressed was Isaac Danforth, the hospital pathologist, with Fenger's postmortem demonstrations that he tendered his resignation to make his position available to the remarkable newcomer. From this time on, the autopsy room of the County Hospital became a mecca for medical students, interns, and practitioners who, for the first time, according to Frank Billings, "had an opportunity to witness scientifically conducted autopsies and to learn the fundamentals of morbid anatomy and pathology."[5] In the person of Fenger, Chicago medical men were coming into contact with the best of European study, practice, and investigation, and many were eager to benefit from the experience. As a rational diagnostician, Fenger had no peer in his ability to correlate the vast knowledge he gained from the deadhouse with clinical findings. His feats of diagnosis have become so legendary that it is difficult to separate fact from fancy. James B. Herrick, a well-known cardiologist, recalled a case where he and Ludvig Hektoen, both avid students of Fenger's techniques, were puzzled and consulted Fenger. The Danish surgeon announced, after a brief examination, that the patient was suffering from multiple myelomata. After he left, Herrick asked Hektoen: "What in the world is a myelomata?" "Damned if I know," Hektoen replied, "but I'm going to find out."[6]

Fenger was much sought after to read papers before the various medical groups in the city; it was at these meetings that he reached the general physicians and specialists who were unable to be present at his clinics. He was early invited to attend the sessions of the West Chicago Medical Society, where interest in pathology ran high. Before that group in 1879 he demonstrated the bacterial nature of endocarditis, the first such exhibition on this side of the Atlantic. He invited his listeners to examine "under the microscope some of the exudate from the heart valves in which were myriads of micrococci." The performance was all the more exciting because it was one of the first demonstrations of pathogenic bacteria of any kind in Chicago.[7] By 1881 he was reading papers frequently before the Chicago Medical Society; one of them, on extirpation of the uterus, was loudly praised as the best paper on the subject ever presented to the Society.[8]

As a surgeon, Fenger was remarkably, almost exasperatingly, thorough. So intense was his interest in pathological problems that he occasionally neglected the welfare of his patients; not a few of his operations resulted in fatality from surgical shock. The preparations which he underwent were unheard of in his day and age, and remarkable even today. For a major operation he reviewed thoroughly the literature on the subject in three or four languages, then drew up a résumé of his studies on the night preceding the event. The following day he outlined the whole procedure on a blackboard in the hospital, as, for example, the seventeen steps involved in removing a bronchial cyst. Four, five, or six-hour operations did not deter him; he sometimes paused to serve beer and pretzels to attendants and students. The aseptic precautions which he habitually observed were far more advanced than those of his colleagues. He pioneered in Chicago in the use of rubber gloves, and was one of the first to change street clothes and shoes for clean cotton clothing in the hospital.[9]

But much of Fenger's widespread influence must be attributed to his personality and character. Despite a speech impediment and a gruff, often tactless manner, he won by his kindness, honesty, and fairness the love and admiration of hundreds of medical practitioners in the Middle West. The friendliness and consideration which he showed for his interns gained him a group of disciples whose devotion and loyalty to their master has few parallels in modern medicine. His humility and lack of dogmatism endeared him to a generation schooled at the feet of didactic lecturers. His closing remarks in a discussion, one observer recalled, were likely to be: "But that is only what I think. That does not matter." [10] It was Fenger's severe integrity, however, which struck his contemporaries with greatest force; only a man deeply devoted to the search for truth could emulate Fenger's honesty in reporting his failures. He once reported eleven deaths in thirteen operations for general peritonitis following appendicitis, a proportion seriously damaging to the prestige of the operator, yet a fact that in fairness should be known to those who followed.[11]

Fenger's self-sacrifice and capacity for hard work stirred his assistants to amazement. One of them, John Clark, who had assisted Kelly and Halsted in the East, found Fenger's endurance incredible. To his students the Chicago surgeon repeated often his credo that "Every surgeon is a soldier; he must never complain while there is work to do." He once told a drooping assistant that he was too young to be tired, that he himself had for thirty years following his entrance into the *gymnasium* rarely removed his clothes. Fenger felt a moral obligation to keep posted on all American and foreign medical literature. He spoke eleven languages and subscribed to journals in many tongues, especially those dealing with bacteriology, pathology, genito-urinary disorders, nervous and mental diseases, internal medicine, and surgery. Most of the physicians and surgeons who knew him echoed Coleman Buford's tribute to the fallen leader: "Christian Fenger was the greatest man I have ever known. He possessed so many admirable qualities that I am sorry every medical man of his time did not come to know him well, for a slight acquaintance was likely to create an erroneous impression of him." [12]

In a sense, Fenger was the Osler of the Middle West. Like the great Canadian, he made some contribution to the furtherance of scientific truth, but it was the personality of both which raised them above their fellows. Just as the historian Sigerist was unable to understand Osler's fame except in terms of the impact of his personality upon his loyal and devoted adherents, so is it impossible to grasp Fenger's significance without realizing what his presence meant to a whole generation of Chicago medical men. Much of the professional change associated with Fenger's advent in Chicago preceded or was contemporaneous with similar development in New York, Boston, and Philadelphia; much was accomplished in Chicago before Osler, Welch, Kelly, and Halsted began to win acclaim for Baltimore. If Chicago's growth was the key to her new importance as a medical center, it was Fenger who actually opened the door to the vistas which lay ahead.

The remarkable influence of Christian Fenger on midwestern medicine was nowhere more clear than in the contributions of his students. A list of Fenger's disciples reads like a "Who's Who" in American medicine at the turn of the century, though it might be questioned whether, by 1900, Fenger attracted these students to Chicago or the attraction of Chicago led them to Fenger. At any rate, such celebrated surgeons as J. B. Murphy, William J. Mayo, and Lewis L. McArthur learned their surgical diagnosis and pathology from Fenger; three widely known pathologists, Ludvig Hektoen, E. R. Le Count, and H. G. Wells, received part of their training in Fenger's autopsy room; and many practitioners of internal medicine, notably James B. Herrick and Frank Billings, gave Fenger credit for their own success.[13]

Perhaps the most brilliant of Fenger's followers was the world-famous surgeon, John B. Murphy. In his lifetime Murphy achieved a renown unknown by his master; many surgeons considered him the greatest operator in the world of his day. William J. Mayo hailed him as "the surgical genius of our generation." [14] A man of boundless energy and aggressive self-reliance, Murphy sought to live the strenuous life advocated by his famed contemporary. His individualistic philosophy informed him that man could achieve any goal with push and determination, and Murphy went far to justify his own faith in a fiercely competitive civilization. Like most men of hypertensive energy, Murphy did not know how to relax; he could not even talk calmly, his voice was fiery and high pitched, and his tone was argumentative.[15] His egotism was so intense that many found it difficult to remain on friendly terms with him. A conflict over clinic hours with N. S. Davis, Jr., for example, brought the following communication from Murphy: "You occupy but one hour, while my clinic lasts from 4½ to 5 hours. Your class is composed practically of students of the college; the men who attend my clinic are from the world. It will, therefore, be easier for you to notify the smaller and more circumscribed circle than it would be for me to notify the class of people who attend my clinic." [16]

Like so many of the great medical leaders in Chicago during this period, Murphy was a Wisconsinite.[17] As the son of poor Irish settlers, he knew early the sting of poverty and made no secret of his desire for riches. The sacrifices of his parents enabled him to get an education, but he never forgot the scrimping and starving of his medical student days at Rush. After study in Germany, he returned to Chicago where he received his first opportunity for fame in the aftermath of the Haymarket Square explosion of 1886. Murphy was equal to the test; with herculean endurance the young surgeon operated on victim after victim of the massacre, outlasting assistants whose bodies demanded sleep during the long ordeal. His labors and subsequent trial testimony brought Murphy a flood of publicity, though many of his colleagues accused him of deliberate histrionics. In 1892 came his successful experiments in anastomosis of the gastro-intestinal tract by means of the "Murphy button," thus opening up a whole new field of surgery. Although this mechanical device lost much of its usefulness after Murphy's death, its pioneer value in making anastomosis simple was great.[18]

After 1892 Murphy was besieged with honors and invitations to speak, many of them from foreign countries. Some of these he accepted, but others he rejected in order to concentrate on his surgical studies of the abdomen, bones and joints, and circulatory system. It was Murphy, probably more than any of his contemporaries, who pioneered in early operation for appendicitis, a procedure invoked only in extreme emergency before this time. His interests were uncommonly broad and restricted to no special fields of surgery; George Crile could think of no operative field which was not influenced by Murphy, no problem which he had touched without leaving some significant contribution.[19] As the Chicago surgeon's fame spread throughout the world, however, his egotism and selfishness increased. Already a wealthy man, he declared to a prospective assistant that "some time previously he made up his mind to spare himself as much as possible the obligation of a charity service." [20]

As teacher and operator, Murphy was without peer in his generation. Though his voice was shrill and high pitched, his mastery of every phase of surgery more than compensated for this shortcoming. His Socratic questioning of students and interns at the operating table left them with indelible impressions of the fundamental anatomical and pathological features of any operative procedure. His personal technique inclined toward conservatism and thoroughness rather than brilliance and speed; one observer described him in action in the following manner: "He was infinitely careful in preparation, and compared with many was inclined to be slow, but every step in every operation which I ever saw him do was completed deliberately, accurately . . . without haste; that step completed, another followed. And so when the end came, a review of the operation showed no false move, nor part left incomplete, no chance of disaster; all was honest, sage and simple; it was modest rather than brilliant." [21]

Murphy's love of audiences and the limelight did not endear him to his Chicago colleagues. As he never shunned publicity of any kind, many felt that the free advertising he received placed them at an unfair advantage in professional competition with him. The feeling of the Chicago profession, according to Murphy's biographer, was that he was "a sensationalist, an opportunist, a publicity seeker, and what newspapermen called 'a trained seal'—a prominent person who is willing to be quoted on any subject at any time." For many years Murphy was refused membership in the Chicago Medical Society. Even after his admission he was haled before the judicial council of the American Medical Association in 1912 on the charge of inviting publicity by his officious handling of the wounded Theodore Roosevelt.[22]

Murphy's death in 1916 brought tributes from all over the world. No Chicago surgeon, before or since, has received such plaudits from his confrères. Even the Chicago Medical Society staged a special memorial meeting to pay homage to his memory.[23] His ability as a clinical teacher and his dexterity as an operator, almost all agreed, placed him among the greatest surgeons of all time. The most stirring tribute came from an Englishman, Sir Berkeley Moynihan, who ranked Murphy with Galen, Hippocrates, Harvey, and Lister in his contributions to the race: [24]

As we look backward upon the long history of the science and art of medicine we seem to see a great procession of famous and heroic figures, each one standing not only as a witness of his own authentic achievements, but also as a symbol of the traditions, ideals, and aims of the age which he adorns. . . . They have lost their nationality in death. They are men whose deeds will not be forgotten, and whose names will live to all generations. Among such men, few in number, supreme in achievement, John Benjamin Murphy is worthy to take his place.

While Murphy was bringing attention to Chicago in surgery, others of Fenger's students were building the city's reputation in other fields. Another young man from Wisconsin, who came to Chicago's College of Physicians and Surgeons in the mid-eighties, was to win a name for himself in pathology. Ludvig Hektoen, whose parents had migrated to Wisconsin some years earlier, found an early interest in pathology under Fenger's inspiration at County Hospital, where Hektoen had won an internship. In 1889 the youthful pathologist left the hospital for a position as curator of the museum at Rush Medical College. He subsequently taught in several of the city's medical schools during the 1890's and was also appointed pathologist at County Hospital in 1895. In 1903 there came an excellent offer from the University of Pennsylvania which Hektoen rejected in favor of Chicago, despite the urgings of Osler, Welch, and Simon Flexner, a choice hardly conceivable a score of years earlier.

In Chicago, Hektoen won a notable reputation by his contributions to immunology, especially blood grouping, and by his many important assignments in the battle against cancer. His associates and students now hold many of the key pathological and research positions in Chicago's medical institutions, thus assuring the continuity of Fenger's influence.[25]

Bayard Holmes and James B. Herrick were two other figures of importance who worked under Fenger during their formative years. Notice was taken earlier of Holmes's pioneer investigations in bacteriology and his collaboration with Fenger on studies in experimental asepsis. Herrick began his association with Fenger at County Hospital after graduating from Rush Medical College in 1888. He had come to Rush after a boyhood in Oak Park, Illinois, and a liberal education at the University of Michigan. At Michigan he had enjoyed the stimulating educational atmosphere created by James B. Angell and had acquired an abiding interest in Chaucer from the distinguished professor of English literature, Moses Coit Tyler. He finally decided on medicine over English as a career and elected Rush as his medical school. He won an internship at County Hospital, where he came under Fenger's influence, and was appointed in 1890 to the attending staff of the institution. The first ten years of his professional career were spent in general practice, but he subsequently focused his attention on internal medicine and later, still more narrowly, on cardiology. His contributions to the study of coronary thrombosis and other cardiac afflictions are widely known.[26]

Another of Fenger's associates in the 1880's was a young intern named Frank Billings, whose role in developing Chicago as a medical center was in some respects more important than that of any other man. The twin influences in Billings' life which did most to shape his unique character were his friendship for Fenger, from whom he learned thoroughness, accuracy, and intellectual honesty, and his association with William Rainey Harper, first president of the University of Chicago, whose superhuman energy and farsighted wisdom made a profound impression on him. Billings went from his internship under Fenger at County Hospital to a position on the faculty of Northwestern University Medical School. As secretary of the faculty from 1886 to 1897, the young doctor lent his support to the construction of Wesley Hospital, which provided needed clinical facilities for the school, and encouraged the drive for a new classroom building. He was personally responsible for the campaign which resulted in the erection of N. S. Davis Hall on the Northwestern campus.

When Rush Medical School affiliated with the University of Chicago in 1898, Billings was called by President Harper to a professorship in medicine. He was soon appointed dean of the school, where for the next twenty years he provided leadership in developing the clinical work at Rush and adjoining Presbyterian Hospital. His fondness for clinical and laboratory investigation, derived from his experience with Fenger, caused him to concentrate on providing facilities for these studies at Rush. It was largely through his influence that in 1902 the John McCormick Memorial Institute for Infectious Diseases was established and important experimental work begun. When Presbyterian Hospital, which was associated with Rush, began to suffer from a shortage of beds, Billings appealed to his wealthy patients, who were many, for money. More than a million and a half dollars was collected through him.[27]

Billings also found time to undertake a number of personal scientific investigations, the most significant of which culminated in his theory of focal infection. According to this theory, chronic infection in some part of the body sometimes produced such systemic manifestations as arthritis, neuritis, cardiovascular degeneration, and even nephritis. The physician, therefore, could check likely sources of such infection, notably teeth and tonsils, and if found diseased, extirpate them.[28] In practice, Billings' theory of focal infection produced some good results but was carried to such extremes that a few practitioners seemed to believe that all arthritis or nephritis might be cured by removing tonsils and teeth. The failure to distinguish clearly between certain types of recurrent arthritis and chronic osteoarthritis, for example, was responsible for a good many needless operations. Though discredited by some because of these attempts to overextend its applicability, the theory has nevertheless become a standard procedure in the practice of medicine.[29]

Perhaps Billings' greatest importance, however, was as a builder of medical institutions. At Rush he continued to expand facilities for education and research. He was instrumental, for example, in securing the affiliation with Rush in 1911 of the Home for Destitute Crippled Children and the County Home for Convalescent Children, both later joined to the University of Chicago. When plans were devised in 1916 for a clinical school on the University of Chicago's south side campus, Billings personally secured almost all the money necessary to meet the pledges required by Rockefeller's General Education Board. Over five million dollars were raised in the campaign, of which one million alone came from the Billings family for the erection of the Albert Merritt Billings Hospital. After his retirement in 1924, Dr. Billings was induced to head one more fund-raising drive, which was successful in raising more than two million dollars for the medical care and education of Negroes at Provident Hospital.[30]

As a medical practitioner, Billings' warm, vibrant personality enabled him to win the complete confidence and co-operation of his patients. He was a tall, genial, and sympathetic man, who radiated an impression of bigness and power. His large frame and strong face inspired confidence, and his ready sense of humor was infectious. He was a "doctor's doctor," the type of physician who could encourage even an ailing colleague, the most difficult patient a medical man can face. Billings' passing in 1932 was mourned by public and profession alike.[31] He was, according to James B. Herrick, the "biggest, best balanced, all-round doctor we have ever known." [32]

Not all important landmarks in Chicago medicine and surgery after 1890 can be traced to the influence of Christian Fenger and his students. There were significant independent lines of development; to consider only the Dane's disciples would be to omit one of the truly great Chicago surgeons of the late nineteenth and early twentieth centuries. A decade before Fenger came to County Hospital, Nicholas Senn graduated from medical school; he was studying in Munich when Fenger began his work in Chicago. Senn was a native of Switzerland whose parents had come to Wisconsin in the 1850's. After graduating from Chicago Medical College in 1868, and serving for several years as a resident physician at County Hospital, he returned to Milwaukee to practice.[33]

Independently of Fenger, Senn grasped early the importance of clinical microscopy, animal experimentation, and antisepsis.[34] He constructed his own laboratory in Milwaukee and carried on investigations there, usually alone, almost every evening for years. His most significant experimental work was accomplished in the treatment of gastro-intestinal lesions and bone tuberculosis. In 1878 Senn was called back to Chicago as professor of surgery at Rush; his teaching there was characterized by a combination of the practical American with the analytical German delivery. He excelled, according to a contemporary, as a diagnostician, but lacked the slow, broad analysis of a Fenger in leading students to the understanding of a case.[35]

Senn was notable for his courage, his zeal for work, his pride and sensitivity to criticism, and his cool impersonality.[36] His courage was of heroic proportions; at a time when the inoculability of cancer was at best an undecided question, Senn implanted several carcinomatous growths in his forearm to test current theories that the disease was transmissible in that fashion.[37] If the experiment had succeeded, his life might well have been lost. Senn was an indefatigable worker. Professor Quine, who knew him well, said that he never knew a man who drove himself harder. But his capacity for work had an unfortunate corollary; he wanted to see the results of all his labors published. So great was his passion for authorship, indeed, that much of his writing was short-lived, since he dashed it off in great quantity, while traveling or vacationing, without access to reference books or other materials. A friendly critic called him a "latter-day S. D. Gross" in his zeal for speech and publication, attributing this quality to Senn's "exalted preëminence in the West." [38] Another feature of Senn's personality which many found annoying was an inclination to make hasty judgments and then endow them with all the finality of a papal bull. A visit by Senn to the celebrated gynecologist, Lawson Tait, for example, was followed by a frank and harshly critical report of the experience in the pages of the *Journal of the American Medical Association*. Tait was so outraged by Senn's report that he called him "a typical specimen of the medical tramp, one of the most vulgar I have met with." [39]

Senn had a number of redeeming features, however. His operations and experimental work revealed a brilliant and original mind. He had an extraordinary memory and could cite chapter and verse in medical literature on a wide range of topics. His passion for publicity and stubbornness of judgment, moreover, might be attributed to his proud and sensitive nature; seeing himself as a man of heroic mold, he loved honors and adulation. His coldness, too, was probably overemphasized; he was at least friendly to acquaintances and at ease in all social situations. Professor Quine summed up his personal impressions of Senn as follows: "He was delightful if you were going his way and following; but you were in a very undesirable position if you were in his way. He was too preoccupied and self-centered to be habitually magnanimous to his competitors, but he was a prodigy of generosity to those who called him master. He was by nature autocratic, and to be on good terms with him you could not question his supremacy." [40]

By 1910 the work of Fenger, Senn, and their associates had made Chicago a center for medical research, study, and treatment. The growth of the city, improvements in the medical colleges, expansion of physical facilities through public interest and philanthropy, and the emergence of Chicago as a favored site for publishing and organizational ventures, were all important factors in the final result. In 1910 J. B. Murphy returned triumphantly from London to announce that Europeans were now admitting American superiority in surgery, and that it was to New York and Chicago that foreign students of surgery were now flocking. No longer did wealthy Americans find it necessary to go to Europe for major operations, for some of the world's outstanding specialists were now in Baltimore, New York, Philadelphia, and Chicago.[41]

In the first and second decades of the new century another Chicagoan was inaugurating projects in medicine which brought still further attention to the city. Like Senn, Murphy, and Billings, Franklin H. Martin came from Wisconsin to make an important contribution to the fame of his adopted city. He became a widely known gynecologist, but it was as journalist and organizer that he won greatest renown. He saw early in his career the need for a journal of practical surgery free of commercial control. His own experience convinced him that the best interests of surgery were not served through periodicals managed by professional publishers and littérateurs.[42] In 1905 with the enthusiastic support of John B. Murphy and other noted surgeons, Martin launched a new journal: *Surgery, Gynecology and Obstetrics.* The publication was almost immediately successful; Will Mayo pronounced it "the greatest surgical journal in the world." [43]

Martin's second project was the establishment of a Clinical Congress of North America in 1910. Practically, this meant the periodic meeting of leading surgeons for the purpose of pooling knowledge and effort in attacking disease. Martin again met with success and the Congress was launched with fanfare and praise for its founder. Two years later, Martin proposed carrying the institutionalization of surgery a step further through an American College of Surgeons. Consciously modeled after the Royal College of Surgeons in England, the American body was to enforce high standards of professional and ethical requirements for the practice of surgery, grant degrees to qualified surgeons, and make public the list of its members, so that everyone might know those best equipped to perform an operation. In an almost single-handed campaign, Martin carried his plan to the country's surgeons.[44]

He met this time with considerable opposition. Many feared that his program would produce a European-type aristocracy of surgeons, some thought the whole plan unnecessary, while still others deplored the professional distinction inherent in setting up a special college for surgeons. A branch of the Chicago Medical Society branded Martin's idea as "un-American" and "un-democratic," declaring its belief that founders of the college were simply appointing themselves judges of who was to practice surgery.[45] The *Illinois Medical Journal* warned that the new group would not only compete with the American Medical Association, but might eventually gain the power to determine who should practice surgery at all.[46] A letter to the *Journal* from an opponent of the plan epitomized the feeling against it: "The college represents the old temptation felt by men of ability, who see mediocrity held as highly as talent by the public, to proclaim by direct statement that they are the ones best fitted for the work—that is, to let self-praise, however disguised, rather than their achievements speak for them." [47]

The suspicion that the college was being organized for undemocratic purposes was reinforced by Martin's unfortunate infatuation with the traditions, academic regalia, and customs of the Royal College of Surgeons. He even went so far as to have Messrs. Ede and Ravenscraft, official gownmakers to His Majesty the King, design a gown suitable for the Fellows of the American College.[48] Even today one is struck, upon entering the college building, by the Great Mace in the foyer and other evidences of a traditionalism incongruent with the age of the college.

Despite this pretentiousness, Martin's goal was fundamentally sound. His main purpose was to raise the level of surgical practice and thus spare the lives of those who yearly became the unknowing victims of incompetent surgery. Martin had one real obstacle, however, to hurdle before the college became a reality: the charge that the whole plan was a "Chicago affair," because of the important roles played by Martin and his Chicago boosters, especially Murphy and Ochsner. This problem was skillfully handled by the nomination of a non-Chicagoan, John T. Finney of Baltimore, for the presidency of the new organization. The maneuver was successful; in

May, 1913, the American College of Surgeons came into being. The rigid standards enforced from the outset were largely responsible for the disqualification for fellowship in the college of all but 1,059 of the 4,200 surgeons who registered for the Clinical Congress in 1913.⁴⁹ Four years later the Clinical Congress was incorporated into the younger organization.

Surgeons were not the only specialists to mark off and cultivate a narrow field of endeavor in the years before 1913. By this time, virtually all of the specialties familiar today had come into being. Pathology, as observed earlier, was a subject of concentration in the 1860's, though not until the coming of Christian Fenger to County Hospital in 1877 did it take on distinctly modern characteristics. Fenger's influence on the evolution of pathology in Chicago was decisive until his death in 1902, when his splendid work was carried forward by Ludvig Hektoen, Edwin R. Le Count, H. Gideon Wells, Frederick Zeit, Richard H. Jaffe, and a host of others. In the twentieth century, pathology took on a new importance. It was the most stressed of basic courses in Chicago's medical schools; many men devoted full time to its advancement in research institutions; a number of hospitals installed pathology departments. The course of medical theory and investigation and the heritage of Fenger were probably jointly responsible for the new emphasis. At mid-century about one hundred Illinois specialists were certified by the American Board of Pathology, most of them serving in hospitals, cancer institutes, private laboratories, research institutions, coroners' laboratories, and medical schools.⁵⁰

The evolution of the other specialties was gradual and halting. Most of the famous teachers in Chicago in 1890 were not trained specialists but general practitioners who had become proficient in a certain line of medicine. The Chicago Medical Society, though it had committees on certain specialties as early as 1874, was still likely to hear from an all-around family doctor when the topic was obstetrics, laryngology, or pediatrics.⁵¹ Dr. N. S. Davis, whose knowledge of all phases of medicine was unusually broad, had only contempt for the complete specialist.⁵² It was not uncommon for an aspiring specialist of the 1890's to engage in general practice for some years before concentrating on his chosen department of medicine; James B. Herrick, for example, spent ten years in general medicine before turning to internal medicine and cardiology. The public, too, tended to be skeptical of the physician who restricted his practice. When a young intern intent on studying pediatrics consulted J. B. Murphy in 1895, the great surgeon advised against it, because "people knew nothing about pediatrics and would not take their children to a child specialist." [53]

Pediatrics as a separate subject was first taught in Chicago schools in the 1880's. In this respect Chicago was not far behind eastern schools, though Harvard had offered a course in pediatrics beginning in 1871. When Isaac Abt enrolled at Chicago Medical College in 1889, he found only one child specialist, Marcus P. Hatfield, on the staff, while at Rush, pediatrics was not separated from obstetrics until 1892. Alfred C. Cotton was first professor of pediatrics in the latter school.

No special hospital accommodations for children, except at Mary Thompson's Hospital for Women and Children, were available until 1884, when Children's Memorial Hospital was founded. A year later, a special ward for children was set aside at Cook County Hospital, but poor ventilation and lack of cleanliness made cross infection frequent. No special precautions in handling infants' milk were taken in any of these early children's wards. Mortality rates, particularly for children under five, were frightfully high. Dr. Abt recalled leaving County Hospital for a weekend during a severe hot spell and returning to find that all the infants had died during his absence. In the twentieth century a concerted compaign against infant mortality, involving infant welfare stations, parent education programs, improvements in general sanitation and hygiene, and a vigorous propaganda campaign by the Chicago Health Department resulted in a greatly decreased death rate. Too, pediatrics became more definitely established as a specialty. Undergraduate training in child care was greatly improved, better texts, notably Abt's remarkable *System of Pediatrics*, made better instruction possible, and scientific interest in child nutrition grew rapidly.[54]

The splitting off of pediatrics from obstetrics and gynecology enabled specialists in the latter branches to concentrate more fully on the problems of childbirth and diseases of the female organs. The development of these studies, as other branches of medicine, was a gradual process. John Evans, when he taught obstetrics at Rush in the 1840's, had found time for extensive investigations of cholera, mental disease, and other subjects, in addition to teaching all he knew of the process of parturition. His successor at Rush was De Laskie Miller, who founded the first gynecological clinic in Chicago in 1862. Other clinics were established in the medical schools and hospitals in the 1870's and a woman's hospital was founded by the surgeon A. Reeves Jackson in 1871. The first textbook on gynecology in the Chicago area came from the pen of William H. Byford in 1865; his text on obstetrics appeared five years later.[55] Despite this growing interest in the medical problems of women, however, a majority of the city's births were still unattended by physicians as late as 1883.[56]

The leading obstetrician in Chicago in the closing years of the century was W. W. Jaggard, whose pupil, Joseph B. De Lee, was to make a veritable crusade of saving women's lives in childbirth. Jaggard had enjoyed the benefit of European training and his clinics were frequented by physicians and students from all over the city. He unfortunately became addicted to narcotics and alcohol in his later years, ending his career in Chicago by entering a lecture room and shooting indiscriminately at his students.[57]

Ophthalmology developed somewhat earlier than the other specialties, both because of the delicacy of treating the eye, and because the basic anatomical and physical studies for eye specialization were worked out early by Helmholtz, Graefe, Bowman, and others. Courses in ophthalmology in the United States began at Harvard in 1850, five years before Elkanah Williams introduced the ophthalmoscope to America. In Chicago, the first departments of ophthalmology and otology were opened at Rush in 1869, and at Chicago Medical College in 1870, though E. L. Holmes had accomplished important work in the study of eye disease before this time. Holmes and J. S. Hildreth were the pioneers in ophthalmological work in the Chicago area; they were associated, respectively, with the founding of the Illinois Eye and Ear Infirmary and the Cook County Hospital. Hildreth was in charge of County Hospital during the Civil War, when it was controlled by the army as the Desmarres Eye Hospital. Another early ophthalmologist in Chicago was Henry Gradle, whose exploratory work in general bacteriology was discussed in another connection. The first professional society devoted to the advancement of eye study was inspired by the labors of Boerne Bettman, a former assistant to the famous Elkanah Williams of Cincinnati, who had come to Chicago in 1881.

In the twentieth century ophthalmology became a full-time specialty; rarely was it combined with laryngology, otology, or rhinology as in earlier days. A Chicago surgeon, William H. Wilder, took the lead nationally in attempting to raise standards in eye practice to defeat the growing army of optometrists who sought to infiltrate the domain of the physician. His proposals for an American Board of Ophthalmology won approval in 1908, when a distinguished panel was set up to pass on the qualifications of those practicing this specialty. By 1939 only 1,642 of the country's 7,200 eye physicians had passed the Board's stringent requirements.[58]

The development of neurology and psychiatry in Illinois followed a pattern familiar in the West. Neurology was not introduced into the medical curricula in Chicago until 1871, though interest in mental and psychiatric problems began with the first towns and cities. The reason for this discrepancy was clear; in the West, and to a lesser extent the East, the practical problem of what to do with the insane took precedence over more theoretical and less urgent problems. Thus it was that early western neurologists and psychiatrists were almost exclusively concerned with the care and management of mental patients. Many early Chicago physicians were well trained in neurological theory before coming west, but once settled in the new country they found their sense of humanitarianism forcing them into institutional upbuilding.[59]

Dr. James S. Jewell held the first chair of neurology in Chicago. He accepted this position at the Chicago Medical College after a long period of indecision between medicine and biblical history as his life's work. Having traveled extensively in Palestine and Egypt, he seemed on the point of deciding on the latter when his mind was suddenly changed in 1871.[60] Once decided on a career, Jewell plunged into his new work with energy. Two years later he founded the *Journal of Nervous and Mental Diseases* with the help of another early neurologist, Henry M. Bannister.[61] Meanwhile, a third specialist, Walter Hay, was engaged in 1872 to lecture on diseases of the brain and nervous system at Rush; this pioneer triumvirate of Jewell, Bannister, and Hay long dominated neurological development in Chicago.

At Rush, neurology was not made a separate department until 1910, when it was granted a quasi-independent position in the curriculum. One explanation of this delay was the great interest which Henry M. Lyman, head of the department of medicine, took in the subject; he was understandably loath to see a special department of neurology created. Lyman himself made important contributions to the study of the organization of the human nervous system; he-became in 1893 the first Chicagoan since Jewell to be elected to the presidency of the American Neurological Association. His successor at Rush, Frank Billings, continued to teach neurology as a part of internal medicine for a number of years. At the Chicago Medical College, however, the independent status of neurology made possible the selection of such outstanding specialists as Archibald Church and Hugh T. Patrick to occupy the chair of nervous and mental diseases.[62]

Other specialties emerged for the first time in the latter years of the nineteenth century. A successful text on *Diseases of the Skin*, for example, was published in 1883 by James Nevins Hyde, who assisted in other ways in the development of dermatology as a separate branch of medical study and practice in Chicago.[63] The arrival of Joseph Zeisler from Vienna, where Skoda, Rokitansky, Hebra, and Billroth were gaining international fame, and the experimental work of Emil Grubbé and William Allen Pusey in X-ray therapy in Chicago also stimulated greatly the growth of dermatology.[64] Roentgen's discovery of the X-ray was also adopted by other specialties; in a short while another study, that of radiology itself, evolved out of the growing maze of overlapping specialties.[65]

As a result of increasing specialization, the practice of general medicine in the twentieth century suffered, but not to the extent that the fame and publicity of the specialists might indicate. As late as 1928, indeed, 74 per cent of America's physicians reported themselves as still practicing general medicine, while 26 per cent were divided between those who classified themselves as full and part-time specialists. The trend toward particularism, however, has accelerated in recent years; a poll in 1942 revealed only 49 per cent of the country's physicians to be general practitioners.[66] In Chicago, only 45 per cent of doctors in private practice in 1950 devoted themselves solely to general medicine.[67]

Another reason for Chicago's advanced position in medicine was its changing attitude toward original research. It is from the laboratories and research institutions, after all, that progress in medicine normally comes, and no amount of technical brilliance or accumulation of physical facilities can supplant for long the necessity for original investigation. The tendency in a newly settled area was to concentrate on the immediately practical to the neglect of fundamental studies, and it was not strange, therefore, that America, and especially the West, lagged in its attention to medical research. The result of this neglect was a long dependence on Europe for fundamental discoveries and progress in medicine and surgery, a dependence which has come to an end only during the past generation. As late as 1933, when the noted medical historian Henry Sigerist compiled a work on the "Great Doctors" of history, no American's biography was included.[68]

There were a number of reasons why America lagged in medical research. During most of the nineteenth century, American physicians lacked the hospitals, laboratories, and clinics necessary for effective investigation, yet they were prone to look askance at government subsidization of research. Medicine suffered, too, from its inability to deal efficiently with the great epidemics which swept the country; philanthropists were understandably reluctant to give their money to medical institutions. The religious orientation of many of the wealthy, moreover, inclined them to dedicate their fortunes to the building of churches or to church-supported charities.[69] Nor were physicians themselves, busy as they were and dependent for their entire incomes on practice, likely to be interested in research. The practical problems met with at the bedside dictated the preference of American physicians in medical papers and essays. When Nicholas Senn, for example, together with a colleague from another city, read papers on fracture of the femur at a meeting of the American Surgical Association in 1883, the reporter praised Senn's patient experiments and prodigious scholarship, but concluded that his essay was "decidedly 'German' in its character" and inferior to "the paper of Dr. Moore, so full of practicability." [70]

By the last decade of the century, however, the value of medical research had been dramatically illustrated in the exciting achievements of European scientists. American interest mounted throughout the 1880's and 1890's, just at the time when America's new millionaires were beginning their unprecedented distribution of millions of dollars to philanthropies of all kinds. Sometimes the capricious interest of these benefactors turned to medicine: in the new century an increasing number of medical institutions and enterprises were endowed with the funds of a Rockefeller, Carnegie, Armour, or McCormick. This trend toward private subsidization of medical research was noticed by the *Chicago Tribune* in 1910, which commented on the gifts of Mrs. W. K. Vanderbilt, Nathan Strauss, John D. Rockefeller, and in Chicago the recent example of Thomas Murdoch and Mrs. Nelson Morris in giving to Presbyterian and Michael

Reese hospitals, respectively, large sums for medical investigation.[71]

An outstanding early research center in Chicago was the Mc-
Cormick Institute for Infectious Diseases erected from philanthropic
funds in 1902. Ludvig Hektoen, an early director of the institute,
gathered many able men and women around him. Under his supervision, the famous studies of George and Gladys Dick in scarlet fever
were done. Others of his associates made important discoveries. Howard Taylor Ricketts, despite his premature death in the fight against
disease, achieved brilliant results in his investigation of the method
of transmission of Rocky Mountain spotted fever. Hektoen himself
was the first scientist to make the direct suggestion that by properly
selecting blood donors, the danger of blood transfusion could be
largely averted. He was also the first in Chicago, and probably in the
United States, to make blood cultures from living patients, now a
procedure of great diagnostic value.[72]

It would be impossible to consider all of the significant research and discoveries which have come out of Chicago, but mention of some will indicate the wide scope of investigation in which
Chicagoans have been engaged. Notable was the work of Bertram W.
Sippy in gastro-intestinal diseases, of David J. Davis in hemolytic
streptococci, of Rollin T. Woodyatt in metabolism and water bal-
ance, of Allen B. Kanavel in surgery of the hand, of C. A. Jennings
in chlorination of water, of H. Gideon Wells in chemical pathology,
of G. Frank Lydston in gland transplantation, of Arnold C. Klebs
in a variety of infectious diseases, of Arno B. Luckhardt in anesthesia,
of Maud Slye in the heredity of cancer, of William F. Petersen in
meteorological medicine, and more recently, the experiments of S. S.
Rosenthal with BCG vaccine in tuberculosis, the work of Roger
Harvey and others with the betatron in cancer treatment, and the
widely heralded achievements of the research men at the Armour
laboratories and elsewhere with ACTH and cortisone.[73]

The dependence of American medicine on German research
and laboratory techniques was clearly at an end by the close of the
First World War. German laboratories and medical education, ideal-
ized and revered in America before this time, fell in popularity after
1918 as the realization struck home that there was much in German
medicine that was inferior or undesirable from the American point
of view. German professors of medicine, while economically secure
as employees of the state, were forced to publish to make their repu-
tations in research; this resulted, according to one report in a Chicago

journal, in the dehumanization of the profession and the conception of patients as simply data in a research report. Another objection which the report emphasized was the tendency in the German medical system to gear school and clinic to the pace of the outstanding student. This meant the encouragement of original minds but it resulted also in inferior training for the average practitioner who had to apply the lessons of the laboratory.[74] America, at any rate, declared her medical independence from Europe at this time and the cry went up for more original work from Americans. In the wake of the First World War, pleas were heard in Chicago for the development of a great research center. The need for more original research was constantly stressed at meetings of the Chicago Medical Society; one speaker noted particularly the need for investigation in diseases of the eye, nose, and throat, where Germany had been outstanding.[75] Scarcely a month passed in the years between the two world wars that someone did not ask for faster progress in building up Chicago's medical resources.

Much was accomplished: in vastly expanding the facilities of the medical schools, in increasing the opportunities for medical research and clinical study, and in consolidating existing resources. During the second quarter of the twentieth century, Northwestern University was provided with a whole new campus for medical, legal, and commercial studies; the University of Chicago built a new medical school on its south-side campus; and the University of Illinois greatly improved its overall facilities for the study of medicine. The University of Chicago Clinics, embracing a children's hospital, an outpatient department, a lying-in hospital, and a general hospital, provided means for study and research almost without parallel in the United States. The consolidation of Cook County Hospital with a number of other institutions added greatly to its value and usefulness; the last to affiliate was the bankrupt McCormick Institute for Infectious Disease, which became in 1943 the Hektoen Institute for Medical Research and began immediately to work on problems connected with leukemia, pernicious anemia, and several other diseases.[76]

The size and central location of Chicago attracted many national professional and lay organizations to the city. Aside from the American Medical Association, Chicago became the home of such groups as the American Dental Association, American Hospital Association, American College of Surgeons, American College of Radiology, American Society of Anesthesiologists, Association of American Physicians and Surgeons, American Association of Industrial Physicians and Surgeons, College of American Pathologists, and numerous other medical and allied organizations.

In recent years Chicago has become a leading center in the fight against cancer and heart disease. At the University of Chicago, Northwestern University's Rheumatic Fever Institute, Herrick House, La Rabida Sanitarium, and the Cardiovascular Research Institute of Michael Reese Hospital, important research in cardio-vascular afflictions has been inaugurated. Somewhat boastfully, but nevertheless with considerable accuracy, the chairman of the Chicago Heart Association campaign for 1950 declared that "Chicago today occupies the position in medicine held by Vienna a generation ago. Our community is one of the few great centers of cardio-vascular research. Medical authorities have predicted that when the problems of heart disease are solved, they will almost certainly have been solved in Chicago." [77]

The resources thrown into the battle against cancer in Chicago have multiplied rapidly since 1940. The city became in 1943 the third community in America to have a cancer prevention clinic; the Chicago Tumor Institute became an important center for research and treatment, notably in cancer of the larynx; and in June, 1950, the Nathan Goldblatt Memorial Hospital, providing fifty-two beds for cancer sufferers, was opened at the University of Chicago.[78] Almost half of the new Goldblatt Hospital was devoted to laboratory space; it was hoped that a "team attack" by scientists from thirteen departments of the university would make some inroad against the dread disease. A companion hospital to Goldblatt, the Cancer Research Hospital, financed by the Atomic Energy Commission, was scheduled for completion in December, 1951.

The educational programs sponsored by the Chicago Medical Society were also factors in bringing attention to the city in the 1940's. Beginning in 1943, Chicago became the site of annual clinical conferences which attracted thousands of physicians and members of allied professions. Significant papers, supplemented by panel discussions, were read by authorities from all over the country. Not the least important feature of these conferences was the consistently outstanding technical exhibits, which proved to have considerable educational value. In 1947 the Society undertook a second educational activity with the commencement of post-graduate courses for practicing physicians. Two courses in subjects of wide interest were given each year. By 1951 the Society was hoping to expand still further its program in this direction.

The city's new position in medicine was quickly acclaimed by the Chicago press. Almost all daily papers published series of articles dealing with Chicago's institutional and scientific advances in medicine. The *Chicago Tribune*, for example, in 1949 pointed proudly to the large number of foreign patients attracted to the city's clinics and hospitals. Physicians from all over the world, said the editorial writer, now sent their dear ones, as well as their patients, to Chicago; in some cases, rather than to New York, Baltimore, or even the Mayo Clinic.[79]

The climax of modern efforts to make Chicago a great medical center began in 1941 with authorization by the state legislature to create a special Medical Center District, which would have power to buy and clear land in congested slum areas on the city's west side. The nucleus of the Medical Center District was to be composed of existing institutions already located on the west side: Cook County Hospital with its affiliates; the University of Illinois hospitals, institutes, and schools of medicine, dentistry, and pharmacy; Presbyterian Hospital; Loyola and Chicago medical schools; and the State Bacteriological Laboratories. New projects contemplated in the district's plans were a Veterans Administration hospital, a new campus for Loyola Medical and Dental School, a state tuberculosis hospital and research institute, a Cook County graduate school of medicine, as well as extensive housing, wooded, and parking areas.[80]

| Chapter VII | The Expansion of Medical Education in the Twentieth Century |

Not the least important factor in turning the attention of the nation's doctors to Chicago was the rapid growth of facilities for undergraduate instruction in medicine. Beginning in the 1890's, existing facilities were consolidated, curricula were reorganized, and numerous new courses and departments were added. In the early decades of the twentieth century, Chicago began to concentrate on large-scale building programs for expansion of her medical schools. By 1936, more third- and fourth-year medical students were being educated in Chicago than in any city save Philadelphia.[1] At mid-century, the city boasted two of the largest schools in point of enrollment in the country, while her five accredited institutions made her an unrivaled center for undergraduate education in medicine.

A number of reforms were undertaken in the 1890's which prepared the way for later growth. At the Northwestern University Medical School, Dr. N. S. Davis, Jr., bore an increasing share of the administrative responsibility, as his venerable father became less and less active; finally, in 1901, the son became dean in his own right. The final union of the Chicago Medical College with Northwestern University which the elder Davis had consummated in 1891 forced several significant changes in the medical school. Admission requirements, for example, had to be gradually raised to conform to university standards. By 1897 the premedical education required of a matriculant in the medical school equaled the four years of high school demanded of an applicant for admission to the College of Liberal Arts.[2]

Teaching was still the province of practicing physicians and specialists in the 1890's. Northwestern University Medical School employed during these years only three full-time men on its staff:

the registrar, janitor, and professor of chemistry. All other professors were unpaid; reward came only in the form of prestige and research opportunities afforded by the college connection.[3] To find even one salaried professor on a medical faculty anywhere at this time was unusual; it was a credit to the wisdom of N. S. Davis, Sr., that he had hired as professor of chemistry a layman trained only in pure chemistry, John H. Long. Professor Long began his career at Northwestern in 1881 when he commenced the first systematic laboratory course in chemistry in a Chicago medical school. The stress he laid on training in pure chemistry as an antecedent to practical work, in addition to his own notable contributions to biochemistry, was an important influence on other departments of the college.[4]

The affiliation of Rush Medical College with the University of Chicago in 1898 had an enduring effect on the fortunes of the former school. One of the first adjustments that Rush was forced to make was the adaptation of its curriculum to the quarter system in use at the university, in order to ensure the full use of costly equipment and to promote the "systematizing and grading of courses." A more radical innovation was the transfer of the freshman and sophomore medical classes at Rush to the University of Chicago campus, ten miles away, where they were to receive regular instruction in the basic medical sciences from full-time professors in these studies.[5] President Harper was thus one of the first to separate the scientific or preclinical subjects from the practical or applied aspects of medicine. Only clinical subjects were now taught at Rush during the junior and senior years, the medical course having also been lengthened from three to four years, a step taken in 1890 by Northwestern. The Rush faculty was greatly strengthened before the affiliation by the appointment of Nicholas Senn and Arthur Dean Bevan to the department of surgery, Daniel R. Brower to the chair of mental diseases and therapeutics, and E. Fletcher Ingals to a professorship in laryngology.[6]

Many aspects of medical education at the two schools, however, remained unchanged. The system of class recitation, for example, wherein a student committed to memory Schaefer's *Histology* or Delafield and Prudden's *Pathology*, was still a fixture in educational technique. Arthur Hertzler remembered memorizing Gray's *Anatomy* "so that we could recite it like a devout man saying his prayers."[7] There was still very little obligatory practical or laboratory work, though both Rush and Northwestern instituted a number of practical courses during the 1890's. By the mid-nineties manual training in auscultation and percussion, obstetrical manipulations, surgical operating, bandaging, and other maneuvers was the subject of special courses at Rush.[8]

Some of the most significant reforms in medical education before the turn of the century were undertaken at the reorganized College of Physicians and Surgeons. This school was established in 1881 as a typical proprietary college; the condition of employment of each professor was the purchase of two thousand dollars' worth of stock. An instructor, however, was asked to contribute only five hundred dollars. Despite this requirement, the desire for the prestige and legitimate publicity attendant upon a college connection attracted sufficient applicants to enable organizers of the school to select a creditable faculty. Though avowing improvement of medical education as their aim, the founders sought in reality, according to William Quine, an early faculty member, "to provide teaching positions for ambitious members of the profession who could not find accommodations in the colleges then existing." [9]

Dr. Quine was himself elected to the board of directors of the college in the late 1880's to succeed Charles W. Earle, who was expelled for his opposition to the tight control of the dominant officers. Earle, along with Quine and A. Reeves Jackson, had pledged his private savings against the growing debt of the school; the debt amounted to thirty thousand dollars by the end of the first decade of operations. In 1892 the desperate financial situation caused a breakup in the solidarity of the controlling clique and two of the board members, Jackson and D. A. K. Steele, appealed to Quine to lead a reorganization movement. Quine undertook the assignment solely on the condition that the corporation and the college, that is, the business and educational aspects of the enterprise, be separated so far as possible. One of his first acts was to secure the services of Bayard Holmes as college secretary; under Holmes's wise direction, the faculty, curriculum, and physical plant of the College of Physicians and Surgeons were thoroughly renovated.[10]

Holmes was largely responsible for the laboratory building added in 1892, the first such structure erected by a private medical school in the United States. The emphasis on laboratory work contemplated by Holmes was so new to American schools that the curriculum he devised surprised even Quine, who remarked, upon seeing the new catalogue: "*This is not a catalogue, it is a treatise on medical education. It will alarm students and drive them to other schools.*" [11] Holmes sought colleagues who were believers in the "new medicine," who would give students the opportunities for witnessing and performing laboratory exercises which they themselves had missed in medical school. Although the laboratory approach to medicine was perhaps premature, the zeal of the men involved in this venture was infectious; the school gained considerable attention at the American Medical Association meeting in 1892 in Detroit, where the drawings and exercises of its students were exhibited.

Holmes also displayed unusual wisdom in his choice of faculty members. He hired Albert P. Ohlmacher, a pioneer bacteriologist, to teach embryology and pathology; Ludvig Hektoen was persuaded to teach pathology; and Weller Van Hook taught surgical pathology. Holmes himself taught courses in bacteriology, while John B. Murphy, Henry T. Byford, and William A. Pusey were added in 1893 to teach surgery, gynecology, and dermatology, respectively. The college adopted an obligatory four-year course in 1895, each year consisting of a required winter term of twenty-eight weeks and an optional spring session of eleven weeks. A loose affiliation with the University of Illinois was negotiated in 1897, just as the prosperity and popularity of the reorganized institution was reaching a new peak. The enrollment jumped from 235 in 1895 to 710 in 1900. Although Holmes later thought the whole experiment a failure, there was little doubt that in his insistence upon adapting the curriculum of his school to the most recent changes in medicine, he had taken an important step toward a functional medical education.[12]

Despite the reforms in the older schools and the bold experimentation at the College of Physicians and Surgeons, there was much to be criticized in the existing state of medical education. Perhaps the greatest problem facing medical educators at the turn of the century was the growing number of third-rate, poorly equipped, inadequately staffed institutions which were empowered by law to confer the medical degree. Ten medical schools of various description were in operation in Chicago by 1889; one journal jeered that the "medical man who has escaped a 'professorship' deserves congratulation." [13] A score of years later, Chicago was suffering from an even more bewildering assortment of schools, night and correspondence, missionary and sectarian, homeopathic and regular, osteopathic and chiropractic, ophthalmic and chiropodic, each of which sent dozens or even hundreds of graduates into the practice of medicine each year. Many were nothing more than "diploma mills" which made no pretense of giving the student more than a superficial indoctrination in the fundamentals of medical science.

During John Rauch's tenure as secretary of the State Board of Health, an honest attempt had been made to expose the incompetent and fraudulent institutions, but after his removal in 1891— for political reasons, according to his friend Victor C. Vaughan—the number of low-grade schools multiplied rapidly.[14] Occasionally, even the regular schools received requests for diplomas in the mistaken belief that they were diploma mills. The applicants were commonly men already in practice who wanted their offices dignified by an elaborate diploma. The following letter, displaying less erudition than most, was received by Rush in 1910:[15]

Please accept of My hand writting though I hav'nt been in touch with you as to write you before.

But at this time I write you for a Diploma of being a family Doctor. I have purchase a family Medical Book from Sears Roebuck and I have Studied it for two (2) years and I have been Examined by Doctor—and I Desires to Give Rush Medical College Honor for what I know, and that is why I asked for a Diploma from that College. I have been Teaching for twelve (12) years and I believe I am Prepaired to do the work. I will give you One Dollar and a half ($1.50) for the Diploma if you will Except of My request Please let Me hear from you by return Mail.

Most of the poor schools were honest in their intention of giving students the preparation necessary to practice medicine; they simply lacked the necessary facilities and staff. These schools felt they were performing a useful function in providing opportunities for young men who could not otherwise afford a medical education. The one single factor which best explained the mushrooming of these low-grade schools at the turn of the century was the high tuition fees and expenses of the better schools. Northwestern, for example, was charging an annual tuition fee of $175 for its four-year medical program in 1908, in addition to separate laboratory, hospital, examination, and diploma charges.[16] These rates made it impossible for the families of many boys desiring to study medicine to support a son in college. Those from poor families who did attend spent long hours in caring for doctors' offices, delivering newspapers, lighting street lamps, reading gas meters, waiting on tables, or performing the offices of a janitor.[17] The *Medical Standard* declared in 1915 that an "aristocracy of education" already existed, that only the rich could afford a medical education, and that able young men were being driven into business, where they were accepted on the basis of ability alone.[18]

One solution to this dilemma which appealed to a generation schooled by William Rainey Harper in the value of adult education, was the evening medical school. A number of such schools—Dearborn, Harvey, and Jenner medical schools—inaugurated evening classes in Chicago, so that students might combine productive employment with their education. Some graduated large numbers of students in the early years of the twentieth century; there were men practicing in Chicago in 1950 who received their degrees at one or another of these schools. Contemporary feeling regarding evening education was reflected in a panel discussion held in 1904 at the Physicians Club of Chicago. At that meeting Dean Billings of Rush declared himself opposed to all such schools on the ground that medical work was too exacting for the tired student who must perforce slight his studies. Some of those present agreed with Billings, but many favored the schools for the democratic reason that they gave opportunity to those denied it by the regular colleges. Those who had the courage and ambition to undertake such a program, these doctors agreed, would be successful physicians.[19] The argument, of course, was but one phase of the quality versus quantity controversy in medical education, a problem now largely resolved in favor of quality because of the great complexity of medical knowledge and skills. But the economic discrimination involved in training only those able to bear the costs of a decade or more of higher education remains today a vexing social question.

The campaign for better medical schools in the twentieth century had its beginnings in 1904 when the American Medical Association appointed a Council on Medical Education and Hospitals, destined to become one of the most powerful private regulatory bodies in the country. When the council was formed, only five schools in the United States, one of which was Rush, required two or more years of preliminary college training as a condition of admission. Rush had taken this step only a few months earlier. There were, in 1904, 158 medical schools in the United States, which granted annually 5,600 degrees. Illinois was particularly notorious for low-grade medical colleges; at least fifteen schools were in operation in the state in 1904 and their graduates scored close to the highest percentage of failures in state board examinations of any group in the country.[20]

In 1906 the council undertook the investigation of medical schools with the intention of grading them. In their inspection, the doctors took special notice of the medical school plant, curriculum, laboratory, dispensary, and hospital facilities. On the basis of their ratings in these particulars, the council graded eighty-two schools as satisfactory, forty-six as satisfactory but needing improvements, and thirty-two as unsatisfactory. The council sought approval and publication of its survey by the Carnegie Foundation in 1908; it was felt that the report would be accorded greater respect if it bore the stamp of a disinterested foundation. The Carnegie Foundation was convinced of the necessity for a published investigation of conditions in American medical schools, but decided on a research project of its own under the direction of Abraham Flexner. The resulting "Flexner Report," published in 1910, became an invaluable aid in the fight to raise the education level in America's medical colleges.[21]

With regard to medical education, Chicago was termed by Flexner "the plague spot of the country." He found adequate the state law requiring four years of secondary education and certain course requirements in the medical school, but he castigated the flagrant violations of the law which, he suspected, were carried out with the "connivance of the state board." He found that ten of the fourteen Chicago schools he visited were contraverting the law, yet only one had been deprived of its "good standing" status by the State Board of Health. If the law were efficiently administered, he concluded, only Rush, Northwestern, and the College of Physicians and Surgeons would survive.

In teaching facilities and scientific work, Flexner found Northwestern and the College of Physicians and Surgeons "distinctly inferior" to Rush, though there was little difference on the clinical side. All three of these schools made use of the Cook County Hospital, but the frequent turnover in the staff there, according to Flexner, made this institution unreliable for clinical instruction. The author reserved his sharpest barbs for the ten substandard and evening schools which he found in operation.[22] Most of these schools, he reported, accepted any amount of education as the "equivalent" of four years of high school, and not one offered anything resembling proper clinical training. The facilities of the evening schools were characterized as farcical. He noted, for example, that several taught anatomy without dissection.[23]

Many of Flexner's claims were exaggerated. Most of his conclusions were based on observations made on hurried inspection tours and were not borne out by more thorough investigations conducted locally. Furthermore, many of Flexner's conclusions were *a priori* in nature, the whole purpose of his survey being to expose certain shortcomings in medical education in America. For his purpose, the sensational charge, the ringing phrase, and the sweeping generalization were far more useful than a strictly dispassionate analysis of the accumulated data. Finally, Flexner's conclusions for the country as a whole belied his striking characterization of Chicago as "the plague spot of the country." Only a small fraction of the nation's schools were providing proper medical training in 1910. Less than one third, he found, were integral parts of universities. Privately owned schools, with third-rate faculties and inadequate hospital and laboratory facilities, constituted the great bulk of American medical colleges.

The results of Flexner's remarkable book were nevertheless striking and immediate. The initial reaction was one of resentment at his severe strictures on Chicago schools and what seemed to his critics to be a warm adulation of German educational techniques. Those men who disliked the strong trend toward the standardization and regimentation of American medicine tended to oppose the report, while the *Illinois Medical Journal* and organized medicine in general supported it. Dr. James Egan and other members of the State Board of Health protested what they felt was a gratuitous attack on the board, particularly in view of the lack of co-operation they had received from the profession in trying to raise educational standards.[24] But the general reaction to Flexner's work was favorable; the Chicago Medical Society undertook an independent investigation in attempting to correct the conditions scored in the report.[25] In the following years, as the education necessary for the competent practice of medicine grew in quantity and complexity, most of Flexner's critics saw the futility of continuing the fight.

In the fifteen years following publication of the Flexner Report, enormous progress was made in bringing Chicago's medical schools into line with the best of contemporary educational philosophy and technique. Northwestern acted swiftly to bring her admission requirements up to those of Rush and other leading schools by demanding in 1911 that every successful applicant show two years of college preparation.[26] This requirement was gradually extended to three years in all Chicago medical schools; an increasingly high level of scholastic achievement was, in addition, insisted upon.[27] The question of compulsory internship at an approved hospital was dealt with at Rush in 1918, when senior students were given the alternative of an internship or a fifth year of advanced work in a clinical department.[28] In 1920 the Illinois State Medical Society announced that by 1922 every graduating medical student would be required to intern for one year in a hospital of at least twenty-five beds, with normal equipment and staff.[29]

Another step in the educational advance inspired by the Flexner Report was the consolidation of the medical schools and their incorporation into universities. Homeopathic schools were particularly hard hit by the rising premedical and curricular standards. The two homeopathic colleges in Chicago had reunited in 1905 in the face of these pressures.[30] Homeopathic education was subsequently doomed by the adoption of the one-year and then the two-year premedical requirement in physics, chemistry, and biology; a student trained in these basic sciences turned naturally to scientific medicine when he came to choose a medical school.[31] Other sects felt the sting of rising standards. Bennett Medical College, home of Chicago's eclectics, joined in 1910 with two other failing institutions to form the medical department of Loyola University, later renamed the Loyola University School of Medicine.

More importantly, the regular medical colleges began to merge with universities. The Chicago Medical College had been the first, having become an integral part of Northwestern University in 1891.[32] The Woman's Medical College of Chicago followed in 1892, also affiliating with Northwestern. In 1913, the College of Physicians and Surgeons was joined permanently to the University of Illinois, the physician-stockholders surrendering voluntarily their ownership after the state legislature equivocated and finally rejected their offer to sell.[33] The last medical school to be incorporated into a university was Rush, which turned over all its holdings to the University of Chicago in 1924.

Despite the closer connection with the universities, few fundamental changes were made in the organization of the medical curricula during the first quarter of the twentieth century. The Rush program for 1924, for example, was almost exactly that of

1898: freshmen were still taught anatomy, physiology, chemistry, pharmacology, and bacteriology; sophomores took further courses in these subjects and studied pathology, *materia medica*, medicine, and surgery in addition; emphasis in the clinical years was shifted to surgery, obstetrics, gynecology, pathologic anatomy, and clinical medicine. When the first two years of study were transferred to the University of Chicago, neurology and embryology were added to the subjects taught in the preclinical years. A system of electives was also introduced; all junior and senior courses were left to the choice of the student, subject only to a modern system of majors and minors. Students were invited after 1908 to take courses in psychology at the university, where James R. Angell and J. B. Watson were giving outstanding instruction in that subject. A department of ophthalmology was also created in 1908 at the university, while otology was joined with laryngology to form a second department.[34] At Northwestern, the course arrangements were nearly the same. Unlike those at Rush, however, the student was not required to take bacteriology or pharmacy the first year but was given more intensive training in anatomy, chemistry, and physiology. Students were permitted some choice of courses at Northwestern, but the number of required studies was greater.[35]

After 1925, the emphasis on the clinical side of undergraduate study was increased even more. At both Northwestern and Rush, virtually all academic and laboratory courses were crowded into the first two years, thus leaving the remaining two free for intensive practical training. The emphasis on the clinical aspects of training was carried even further at Northwestern by the introduction in the sophomore year of physical diagnosis and other clinical studies. The third year at Northwestern was largely devoted to mastering the principles of medicine, surgery, gynecology, and obstetrics, while the senior year was almost entirely practical; most of the fourth-year student's time was occupied with clinical clerkships, outpatient service, and ward walks.

Just before the Second World War, all Northwestern courses were organized into twelve major divisions: anatomy, bacteriology, chemistry, pathology, physiology and pharmacology, medicine, obstetrics and gynecology, pediatrics, surgery, bacteriological research, the institute of neurology, and eye, ear, nose, and throat. Since then, a separate division of pharmacology has been set up, reflecting the new importance attached to drug therapy in the last decade. Ophthalmology was also given divisional status recently, as were also physical medicine, nervous and mental diseases, radiology, urology, and bone and joint surgery.[36]

Probably the main efforts of medical educators in the last quarter-century have been concentrated on the expansion of physical plant and the provision of greater opportunity for special research and graduate work. The growing public interest in medical education has assured the schools a large measure of co-operation in raising funds for these purposes. Philanthropists, too, have become increasingly generous in their attentions to medical projects. In the case of the University of Illinois, the state itself has recognized the need for providing outstanding facilities for medical study, care, and investigation. The state-supported hospitals, institutes, and schools of medicine, dentistry, and pharmacy which form the University of Illinois group in the Medical Center District provide opportunities which are not surpassed by those existing at any other state university in the country.

Under the leadership of a series of very able deans, Northwestern has greatly expanded its medical facilities in the past twenty-five years. Irving Cutter was primarily responsible for the development of the new McKinlock campus (now called Chicago Campus) on the north side after 1927. Finding no hospital in the immediate area, Cutter negotiated successfully with hospital officials for the erection of Passavant and Wesley Memorial hospitals adjoining the medical school. Cutter's literary interest caused him to play an important role in developing the resources of the school's library; from nine thousand volumes the library's holdings rose steadily to 119,000 in 1951.[37] Under Cutter's successor, J. Roscoe Miller, Northwestern developed plans for expansion which dwarfed even these remarkable achievements. At mid-century the university was planning a twenty-story institute for medical research and, more important, hoped to attract eminent medical scientists to carry on special research there. In time the medical school was to add a cancer clinic, a neuropsychiatric clinic, a urological institute, an eye hospital, a women's hospital, a school of nursing, a children's hospital, a university clinic, and another general hospital. When completed, this ambitious long-term program would make Northwestern one of the leading research institutions in the United States.[38]

The final union of Rush with the University of Chicago in 1924 produced a concentration of medical facilities surpassing even

Northwestern. Rush boasted at the time of union two buildings, one devoted to classrooms, the other to laboratories, as well as the privilege of using the clinical resources of Presbyterian Hospital and the Central Free Dispensary; the latter had for years offered free outpatient care to the indigent as well as affording medical students an opportunity to acquire practical experience. The university, on the other hand, was far advanced by 1924 toward its ultimate goal of an undergraduate medical school on the south side campus. Abraham Flexner, representing Rockefeller's General Education Board, had worked out a plan with university officials in 1916 for the development of medical education in the university as a whole. According to this Flexner plan, which was substantially the one agreed to by Rush in 1924, the university was to develop its own four-year medical curriculum on the south side, while Rush and Presbyterian Hospital were to form the nucleus for a postgraduate department on the west side of the city.[39] In 1927, therefore, clinical departments, in medicine and surgery only, were established on the university campus, while Rush continued to give undergraduate instruction until such time as the university was able to complete a medical school of its own.

The first clinical instruction on the University of Chicago campus was begun with the opening of Billings Hospital and the Max Epstein Clinic in 1927.[40] From the outset, emphasis was laid on teaching and research; for this reason, the University of Chicago Clinics, as the combined hospital and clinical facilities were called, were operated on a noncharity basis. In order to obtain the clinical material necessary for proper training and investigation, university officials felt that patients from all economic classes should be received, in accordance only with the medical interest of their afflictions.[41]

During the 1930's, several new buildings were added to the University of Chicago Clinics. A children's hospital, adjoining Billings Hospital, was dedicated in 1930, and a year later, the Chicago Lying-in Hospital was provided with a new building on the south side campus. The Lying-in Hospital was largely the work of Joseph B. De Lee, who hoped by the university affiliation to insure the hospital's continuation after his death. The orthopedic unit of the University Clinics was formed by the merger of three institutions concerned with the welfare of crippled and convalescent children.[42]

While these hospitals and clinics were being added to the

university, corresponding departments of pediatrics, obstetrics and gynecology, and orthopedics were organized to conduct teaching and research. These departments were staffed with full-time, salaried men to permit more time for research.[43] By 1936 the university felt ready to undertake the clinical instruction of all its students; Rush was asked to submit a plan for post-graduate education in the west side buildings. The plan drawn up underscored the deep differences in educational philosophy between Rush and the university. Rush was clearly interested in training good practitioners of medicine, while the university's concern, as one trustee phrased it, was in the "advancement of science in medicine."[44] Research and graduate training were stressed at the university; practical instruction in diagnosis and therapeusis were the aims of the Rush professors. The university then made the suggestion that Rush and Presbyterian Hospital move to the south side; an earlier offer to turn over Billings Hospital with all its equipment to the Board of Managers of Presbyterian Hospital was repeated. While the Rush faculty tended to favor the move, the Presbyterian trustees felt they could not leave the community which the hospital had served so long. The plan was dropped. Finally, in 1937, the university indicated to Rush that undergraduate teaching there would be terminated in about five years; Rush was to be restored to its status as an independent medical school.[45]

The Rush alumni and faculty attacked the university's decision to abandon the west side school. Many claimed that the university had given the impression that Rush was to be the only medical school of the University of Chicago. Some evidence existed to show that President Harper had intended the affiliation to be a permanent one. He wrote the dean of Rush in 1900, for example, that fears that the university might ever desert the school were without foundation. "If there is anything certain in the future," he assured Dean Dodson, "it is that nothing of this kind will ever happen. I think I can speak with authority on this question."[46] But it was equally certain that Harper intended that the university should have its own medical school sometime in the future, and that it was E. Fletcher Ingals of the Rush faculty who persuaded Harper of the advantages of an affiliation with Rush. Harper had not sought it out. He wrote of the merger in 1902: "It is unquestionable that the results came at last in the largest possible measure because of Dr. Ingals diplomatic labors."[47] The provisions of the actual articles of affiliation, however, gave the final answer to Harper's intentions:[48]

It is mutually agreed and understood:

1. That nothing in affiliation as described by these articles shall be understood to give encouragement that Rush Medical College is ever to become the Medical School of the University.

2. That it is the distinct purpose of the University to establish such a Medical School when funds shall have been provided.

With the refusal of Rush to move to the south side campus and amalgamate with the medical school there, the University of Chicago had no choice but to discontinue its connection with Rush. This step was taken in 1941; the university returned all of the Rush properties together with improvements and funds accumulated since the merger.[49] The Rush faculty was promptly invited to join forces with the University of Illinois; since 1941 some of them have constituted a group known as the "Rush faculty" on the clinical staff of the medical school there. As of 1951 Rush continued to exist as a corporation but did not engage in any classroom instruction. The meager endowment funds were used to finance research at Presbyterian Hospital, which also enjoyed use of the college buildings. Such was the status at mid-century of the oldest medical school in Illinois.[50]

Meanwhile, at the University of Chicago, an expanded program of medical research and training was inaugurated. Forty-five days after Hiroshima, Chancellor Robert M. Hutchins announced plans for an Institute of Radiobiology and Biophysics to study the use of radioactive substances against human disease. The medical school became the only such institution in the United States where the entire staff of approximately two hundred was engaged in full-time teaching and research. An announcement by the dean of the Division of Biological Sciences in 1946 revealed that the principles upon which the school was founded remained unchanged: "THE MEDICAL school is concerned with the advancement of medical science, and though it trains practitioners, it stresses the training of medical scientists who will engage in teaching and research." [51]

In 1950 there were five recognized medical schools in Chicago: University of Chicago School of Medicine, Northwestern University Medical School, University of Illinois College of Medicine, Stritch School of Medicine of Loyola University, and the Chicago Medical School. This last school rose from a merger of the Chicago Hospital College of Medicine and Jenner Medical School in 1912.

It was frowned upon for many years by the American Medical Association, first because of its evening medical classes, and later for its lack of hospital and university connections. Graduates of the school were barred from practice in all but two states. Later, however, an unusual arrangement with Mount Sinai Hospital was reached, whereby every patient might be used for didactic or clinical purposes. In 1948, largely through the courage of Dean John J. Sheinen, the college won full approval from the American Medical Association.

Chapter VIII | The Chicago Medical Society

in the Twentieth Century

The death of Nathan Smith Davis in 1904 registered the end of an important era in Chicago medicine. By the turn of the new century, many of the institutions and projects with which Davis had long been identified were developing along lines new and strange to him. The hospital which he had founded in a suite of rented rooms in 1850 might have made him feel uncomfortable with its cotton-uniformed nurses and spotless cleanliness in 1900; the college which had developed under his leadership now boasted a curriculum broader and more complex than anything he had envisioned; the medical journal which he had established in 1860 finally ceased publication in 1889. The Chicago Medical Society, another of his institutional progeny, had grown wide of the mark which Davis had set for it; by the time of the Society's special memorial services for him in 1904, the organization had split into component branches, with each branch similar in size and function to the whole Society as Davis had organized it.

In the years just preceding Davis' death the Society underwent a number of changes. It was finally incorporated in 1898 with a twelve-man board of trustees composed of the president, vice-president, and secretary, together with nine members elected by the affiliated specialty societies and the membership at large.[1] Much of the business of the Society was not turned over to the trustees, though short business sessions were still held in conjunction with the scientific meetings. There were eight specialty organizations, such as the Chicago Gynecological Society and the Chicago Surgical Society, affiliated with the Society by 1900. According to the new constitution, all members of these affiliated groups had also to be members of the Chicago Medical Society.

123

A more fundamental reorganization of the Society took place in 1903. The reforms of this period marked the end of the old Chicago Medical Society, where all members could meet together and vote personally on matters affecting the profession. By the Constitution of 1903 the Society was divided into component branches, where scientific and social meetings were to be held, while the business of the Society as a whole was transferred to a council of delegates from the new branches and the specialty societies. The number of trustees was reduced from twelve to five; they were given sole custody of all Society property and funds. The trustees' approval was now necessary for the expenditure of all monies. By 1904 eleven branch societies were in operation; the number increased gradually to fifteen at mid-century. Each of the branches, according to the new scheme, had its own officers and programs.[2]

A successful campaign for new members was launched in 1904 and the branch societies grew rapidly. A cardinal factor in the success of this drive was the medical defense plan inaugurated just before the Society's reorganization.[3] Each member, according to this plan, was entitled to legal and financial support from the Society's Medico-Legal Committee in malpractice suits. By 1906 the idea of a defense fund to aid doctors in malpractice cases and other legal difficulties was so popular that it was adopted by the State Society; the fund was an important feature in attracting physicians into medical organization in Illinois until 1937, when the program was reluctantly discontinued at the behest of the American Bar Association.[4]

The scientific meetings of the whole Society, where business was no longer discussed, attracted much larger attendance after 1903; larger and larger halls were necessary to accommodate the crowds. Eventually it became necessary to abandon these meetings completely in favor of the local scientific gatherings in the branch organizations. The federal nature of the Society, however, enabled it to enroll a membership far beyond most civic medical organizations. In 1905 President John B. Murphy announced with pride that the Chicago Medical Society was the largest local medical organization in the world, a position which it still holds.[5]

The financial stability of the Society increased with the membership. The treasury, which held assets of $0.25 in 1862 when there were forty-five members, contained $15,000 by 1905 when the membership reached two thousand. Both membership and wealth climbed after the reorganization; by 1950 the Society counted more than six thousand physicians and surgeons on its active rolls. The control of the Society's growing assets gave the trustees a position of considerable power and influence, and voices were occasionally raised in protest at the parsimony or conservatism of a particular group of trustees. A proposal was approved in 1946 enabling the council by a three-fourths vote to override the trustees when appropriations were refused. A few months later, however, the council voted down a formal move to amend the constitution in accordance with the proposal.[6]

For a number of years after the reorganization of 1903, the new council was the scene of endless wrangling over constitutional issues and electoral procedures. These debates registered what was already apparent: politics had become an important part of the operation of the Chicago Medical Society.[7] Disputes over minor points, such as places of meeting or the admission of particular applicants, occupied much of the time of the council. Occasionally a long-suffering member arose to protest that no business was being accomplished, but in general the meetings were dominated by a few—Drs. Corwin, Hess, Stubbs, Lydston—who subjected their colleagues to lengthy disquisitions on points of order and procedure. The real issue at stake, made almost indistinguishable by the smokescreen of language, was a struggle for power between two factions. One group was made up of members who had offices in the center (or Loop district) of Chicago, were fairly prosperous, and were likely to be specialists; the other group considered themselves "liberals," practiced in the suburbs and outlying sections, and were often suspicious of the specialists and leaders of the profession. The former favored strengthening the central organization of the Society at the expense of the branch societies; the latter sought decentralization of the Society and strengthening of the branches. The reorganization of 1903 was in itself a victory for the insurgent liberals, who deplored the tight control of both the Chicago Medical and the specialty societies by a small clique of close friends. It was the feeling of this dominant group, according to William A. Evans, leader of the insurgents, that the mass of physicians in Chicago were inferior intellectually and poorly equipped by education to handle modern technical problems in medicine; the better informed, therefore, should lead the way. Dr. Evans' branch plan was strongly opposed by Malcolm L. Harris and Hugh T. Patrick, most vociferous of the group of specialists dominating the Society; they could not be expected, of course, to vote themselves

out of control by supporting the branch scheme. Evans' only recourse was to compromise; the agreement of 1903 provided for specialty representation on the council in return for approval of his
branch society plan.[8]

But the compromise meant that the undemocratic practice
of mulitiple voting still prevailed. Since most specialists belonged to
a branch society as well as to a specialty organization, they voted for
council representatives in both groups. The election campaigns after
1903 were fought on this issue; they became so intense and fierce
that a retiring president warned of the dangers of factionalism and
pointed to what the Society might accomplish if its strength were
united.[9] The climax came in the election of 1910. The opposing
parties accused each other of being aristocratic or trying to "Russian-
ize" the Society.[10] The conservatives in control sought to stay the insurgents by ruling that only those whose dues were paid could vote,
but the liberals retaliated by paying the back dues of members in
return for votes. Victory went to the insurgents on their "One Man,
One Vote" platform, and multiple voting in the Society came to an
end.[11] Although the issue was at last settled, there were still reper-
cussions. The Gynecological Society withdrew from affiliation with
the Chicago Medical Society when its delegates to the council were
excluded, claiming "No affiliation without representation." [12]

The problems and responsibilities of the Chicago Medical
Society multiplied as the twentieth century wore on; the growth of
special and standing committees reflected the Society's efforts to
meet those problems. The four permanent committees of 1900—
membership, publication, judiciary, and auditing—multiplied steadily. A Public Relations Committee was established early in the
century, concentrating its attention at first on pure-food legislation
and the abolition of patent medicine advertising.[13] The medical
profession was opposed to patent medicines on the ground that many
of them were pure frauds, composed of cheap ingredients and sold
at exorbitant prices. The popularity of some such medicines, such as
Peruna, was due to their high alcoholic content; as "medicines" they
might be sold in prohibition areas where ordinary whiskey was not
readily available. Though successful in securing the stoppage of
abortifacient   advertisements in Chicago newspapers, the committee's campaign against patent medicines had few results.[14] The weakness of this particular drive lay within the ranks of the profession
itself, where doctors frequently approved the use of patent medicines

out of laziness or ignorance, or because they felt that self-medication was better than no treatment at all. In 1908 a special Committee on Patent Nostrums charged that physicians were "misled into using ordinary mixtures of unknown composition and actually fraudulent nostrums, and by doing so had aided in extending the use of patent medicines among the laity." [15] The influence of the great drug manufacturers was still another factor which rendered impotent the efforts of reformers. Even the medical journals of this period displayed extensive advertisements of patent remedies. The whole question was partially resolved when the American Medical Association's council on pharmacy and chemistry condemned journals carrying advertisements of patent or proprietary articles not approved by the council.[16]

Another function of the Public Relations Committee was to champion the Society's causes in the state legislature. The committee fought all legislation which it felt was inimical to the welfare of the profession and public, especially bills for licensing optometrists, osteopaths, and chiropractors. These lobbying activities in Springfield proved so effective that President George W. Webster was able to report in 1907 "that practically every bill in the legislature that was actively supported by this committee became a law, and . . . every one opposed by the committee was killed." [17] The boldness of the committee mounted with its successes until by 1910 it was soliciting pledges on medical issues from candidates for office, establishing temporary lobbies in Springfield when important medical legislation was on the docket, and exhorting individual members of the Society to take a greater part in politics through letters and telegrams. In 1910, 143 of 227 candidates for state office solicited by the committee signed pledges agreeing to support a uniform method of admission to medical practice in Illinois, meaning that all legislation setting up special standards for osteopaths and other irregular practitioners would be barred.[18]

The political influence of the Chicago Medical Society reached such proportions by 1914 that Harold Ickes, state chairman of the Progressive party, sharply attacked the campaign of the Public Relations Committee to force candidates for the County Board to agree in advance to accept the Society's recommendations in all medical matters. Ickes compared the pre-election pledges to outright bribery.[19] After the First World War, much of the Society's political activity was gradually transferred to the state organization. Under the guidance of John R. Neal, an effective state plan for influencing legislators through their family doctors was worked out. This so-called "Neal system" received the plaudits of representatives of other state societies in 1939; the Indiana delegate announced that his state had adopted the plan "on the theory that, all things being equal, no one has as much influence on a legislator as that legislator's own family doctor, and hence we bend our efforts in giving our story to the doctor, who in turn gives the story to the legislator." [20]

The Society was also active in other programs having a direct bearing on the health and welfare of Chicago's citizens. In 1907 a milk commission was established to assure a pure and reliable source of milk for infant feeding. This commission undertook the inspection of milk, dairies, and cows belonging to producers who wanted their product certified.[21] During World War I another direct health service was provided in organizing free medical care for the needy families of servicemen.[22] The Society sometimes co-operated, too, in giving free health examinations to school children. Since the end of the Second World War, the organization has taken the lead in fighting for such vital ancillary medical services in Chicago as adequate nursing and ambulance transportation. The war highlighted the need for emergency ambulance service, and under steady pressure the city increased the number of its emergency ambulances in operation to five in 1948.[23] Representatives from the Society had recommended twenty, but this was reduced to five by the City Council. The five ambulances compared very unfavorably with New York's 124 units. With regard to nursing, a special committee drew up a number of recommendations, all designed to make the profession of nursing more attractive and accessible, which were brought to the attention of interested public groups.[24]

In the twentieth century, the Society has expended considerable effort in trying to improve its relations with the public. As early as 1904, a series of public lectures, designed to enlighten laymen on a number of medical subjects, was arranged. Continued for a number of years, these lectures became eventually the responsibility of the branch societies. The attendance at these meetings was unusually good, considering the technical character of much of the material presented; an average lecture attracted about 150 persons.[25] In 1917 a further step toward good public relations was taken with the inauguration of a grievance committee which was instructed to "hear complaints and adjust differences between members of the Chicago

Medical Society and the public." [26] The committee served a useful purpose as a kind of "escape valve" for frustrated patients who felt that their physicians had mistreated them in some way. Another disturbing problem in the relations between profession and public was attacked, beginning in the 1930's, by a new committee on medical economics, which dealt with the whole vexing question of the cost and availability of medical care.[27]

From the standpoint of the physician, one of the most important committees of the Society was that dealing with the ethical relations of the profession. This committee was early given jurisdiction over the behavior of doctors in their professional relations with the public and with each other. It was given the power to recommend the expulsion of members guilty of advertising, fee splitting, malpractice, derogation of a fellow physician, or other unprofessional conduct.

No other aspect of medical organization has aroused so much controversy as the doctor's ethical code; yet nothing so distinguishes medicine from other professions and occupations. Many observers have felt that these regulations were reservations on the traditional right of free enterprise in America. Occasionally a Chicago physician has challenged the philosophy behind medical ethics and declared medical societies to be nothing more than glorified trade unions. Medical meetings, declared the sensitive Bayard Holmes, were invariably more interested in fee tables than any other item of business.[28] But most medical men have accepted regulation of professional behavior as proper and necessary. Without the prohibition of advertising, they argue, the public would be forced to bear the enormous cost of publicity which would be transferred as in other businesses to the consumer. Difficult as it may be for the uninitiated to select a satisfactory physician today, the problem would be infinitely more difficult if each doctor advertised, so far as his modesty and pocketbook would permit, his own virtues.

The questions which came before the Ethical Relations Committee were varied, and frequently challenging. A typical case might involve a doctor who advertised his own superiority, endorsed some commercial product, or was connected with some institution guilty of blatant advertising. In 1906, for example, two brothers were censured by the committee for their association with the Finsen Light Institute, which advertised extensively its purported successes in treating skin diseases.[29] A few years later a number of members were reprimanded for their recommendation of "Pau Cola" as a healthful and beneficial beverage.[30] The question of advertising by commercial laboratories was earnestly debated in the 1920's, the Society condemning particularly their tendency to circularize the lay public with misleading literature.[31] Complaints against the diagnosis of illness without adequate examination of the patient by private laboratories have also been frequent.

Sometimes the committee was forced to make decisions respecting the conduct of a leading member of the profession. John B. Murphy was frequently the subject of complaint because of the extensive publicity he received. One member was so incensed at the free advertising which always followed Murphy and others that he advocated the repeal of that section of the code of ethics which prohibited advertising. Medical regulations, he charged, "are for the little man to obey and . . . the great men will not or cannot obey them." [32] In 1932, Arthur Dean Bevan, a noted surgeon, was sharply censured by the Society for his widely heralded charge that more than 90 per cent of alcoholic prescriptions by doctors during the prohibition period were "bootlegging prescriptions." [33] Morris Fishbein, editor of the *Journal of the American Medical Association,* was reprimanded a year later for the publication in a lay periodical of an article on the high costs of obstetrical care.[34] The resolutions charged that Fishbein had followed "the irresponsible de Kruif in attacking the Medical Profession for personal profit." The Society's reaction to the sensational writings of Paul de Kruif has been consistently antagonistic.[35]

The interests of the Society expanded greatly in the aftermath of the First World War. Gradually the organization's activities were broadened to include the publication of a weekly roundup of medical information concerning Chicago medicine, the operation of an information service for persons seeking physicians or specialists, and the recruiting of doctors for war service. The Committee on Medical Preparedness played an important role in selecting physicians for military duty during World War II, as well as trying to retain men essential to their communities.[36]

The educational program of the Society was accelerated considerably after the Second World War in line with the attempt to bring Chicago to the forefront as a great medical center. Annual clinical conferences were inaugurated at the urging of Dr. Charles H. Phifer in 1943; registration for these events increased progressively until 1950 when over six thousand persons, including almost a thousand non-Chicago medical men, attended the conference of that year. At the conventions, papers were read, panel and round-table discussions held, and exhibits of a high order of scientific and technical excellence displayed. A second educational program was added in 1946 as the result of a suggestion by Willard O. Thompson that "short, intensive Post-Graduate courses of from one to two weeks duration in various fields of medicine and surgery" be conducted by the Society.[37] Thus there have developed special annual courses in cardiology, neurology, gastro-enterology, obstetrics and gynecology, allergy, and other subjects which have attracted physicians from other states and from Canada. Enrollment has been limited to somewhat over one hundred in each course, but the interest and enthusiasm of the participants promised an expansion of the program in the future.

A number of new specialty societies, reflecting the growth of medicine since 1900, affiliated with the Chicago Medical Society after its reorganization. A new Society of Internal Medicine was formed in 1915 by James B. Herrick along with such notable internists as Frank Billings, N. S. Davis, Jr., Arthur R. Edwards, Bertram W. Sippy, Robert B. Preble, and Ernest E. Irons.[38] The increase in the number of medical problems peculiar to industry resulted in 1920 in the organization of a Society of Industrial Medicine and Surgery. In their constitution, the industrial physicans announced their intention "To strive toward the conservation and enhancement of industrial health . . . [and] . . . to maintain the highest standards of fitness of the worker." [39]

In 1930 the allergy specialists elected to form a society which soon affiliated with the Chicago Medical Society. The concept of allergy during the previous decade had been, for the most part, unfamiliar to physicians, though Chicago was an early center for specialized work in this field. Allergy clinics were established at Rush in 1920 and at Northwestern in 1924. Only eight specialists appeared at the first meeting of the Chicago Society of Allergy in 1930; the group numbered over one hundred two decades later. In 1937 the society undertook a unique collaborative study on oral pollen therapy at a time when interest in the subject was restricted. Important work in public relations has also been accomplished by the society in promoting understanding by asthma and hay fever sufferers of their afflictions.[40]

The overlapping interest of medical and other scientific investigators in certain research problems led a group of men to form in 1915 an organization devoted to the closer co-operation of all research workers in the field of medicine. The Institute of Medicine of Chicago, as it was called, was unique in opening its doors to non-physicians who were doing research along lines of interest to doctors. The Institute has done yeoman service in dealing with the numerous socio-medical problems that beset Chicago. The Administrative Committee of the Central Service for the Chronically Ill, which the Institute has sponsored, has done pioneer work in the United States on the problems of the chronically ill. The percentage of the necropsies in Chicago hospitals has increased fivefold under the stimulus of another Institute committee. The Institute has also been concerned with such other community problems as ambulance service, medical care for the Negro, medico-legal legislation, and the teaching and medical services at municipal and county institutions in the Chicago area. Membership in the organization was composed of physicians in various specialties, in addition to a hundred scientists, chiefly from universities, who did not practice medicine.[41]

The Chicago Institute for Psychoanalysis was founded in 1932 to teach and carry on research. A number of physicians and psychiatrists have received training at the Institute. Its research program has thrown new light on such problems as homosexuality, gastric neuroses, glaucoma, neurodermatitis, and colitis; studies have also been undertaken in the field of social psychology and child study. Under the direction of Franz Alexander, the Institute has brought added attention from medical scientists to Chicago.[42]

Chapter IX	Some Socio-Medical Problems,
	1900–1950

As in other large cities, life in industrial Chicago was menaced by health problems which, if not unique, were at least magnified to new proportions. An infant might perish from infected milk in a rural area without causing a stir among local medical men, but a diseased milk supply in the great city meant that the lives of thousands of children were in mortal danger. The likelihood of infection increased, moreover, in proportion to the score of middlemen who now handled the milk in its trip from farm to consumer. Detection of a typhoid carrier, a relatively simple task in a rural area, might require the sleuthing of hundreds of investigators in a city of Chicago's size.

Some of the medical problems connected with life in a modern, industrial civilization were more subtle in making their appearance. Medical and technological advances enabled many more people to survive disease and reach old age. This, in turn, presented new problems. Aside from the economic burden of supporting increased numbers of the aged in a society itself grown older, medicine faced an additional challenge in the ominous rise in degenerative disease occasioned by the prolongation of life. The death rates for heart disease, cancer, and nephritis rose steadily, while the rates for the epidemic afflictions were falling to new lows; invalidism and chronic illness among the aged became the subjects of mounting public concern.

The health problems resulting most directly from urban industrial growth were probably those associated with poverty and low incomes. Slums, periodic unemployment, poor wages, long hours, and unsanitary workshops: all took their toll on the lives of the poorer inhabitants of the large cities. The statistical relation between sickness and economic status has been often shown. In Hagerstown,

Maryland, a survey conducted in the early 1920's proved the illness rate to be considerably higher for the poor than for those economically better situated. An investigation of ten communities during the Great Depression showed "a definite causal relation between lowered standard of living and high illness rate." Another study, based on 1930 census data, concluded that the mortality rate among male industrial workers was "greatly in excess" of that for business and professional men. A recent author of an important medico-historical work has commented that "There can be little doubt that the disparities in medical care . . . have contributed to the higher mortality rates among the lower income classes. That the death rate in the United States as elsewhere is correlated with income has long been known." [1] There are, of course, other factors involved in this correlation between income and illness besides economic status, *per se.* Such related social considerations as size of family, education, customs, familiarity with language, and dietary habits may play a role in the incidence of disease. It has frequently been noted that racial differences seem to play a significant part in predisposing persons to disease, the association between Negroes and tuberculosis, for example, having been observed early. But even here race itself is probably not responsible for the higher tuberculosis rates; it is more likely to be the economic, social, and cultural factors associated with racial differences.[2]

In Chicago, Nathan Smith Davis early recognized the role of economic and social factors in the origin of disease. As early as 1870, he attributed the causes of relapsing fever "to the wants of poverty and destitution in crowded and badly ventilated uncleanly habitations." [3] An American Medical Association report the same year cited the sharp difference in mortality rates in Chicago between the wealthy inhabitants of the high and dry areas along the lake shore and the artisans and laborers who lived in crowded, wooden huts along the river. The terribly high mortality of the second ward was attributed "to close confinement in small and badly ventilated rooms and workshops, to the depressing effects of venereal excesses and alcoholic stimulation, to the contaminating effects of syphilitic poison and their [*sic*] general devitalizing influences that manifest themselves among its paupers and lowest class of debauched inhabitants." [4]

But with the overcrowding that characterized the city after industry began to attract its hundreds of thousands of immigrant workers, the correlation between disease and social status became even sharper. With such living conditions as those described in the report of the Department of Health for 1893, it is not at all difficult to understand why this was so:[5]

August 11th, 11:45 p.m.—Called at No. 399 Canal street; found 15 beds in cellar, no plaster on ceiling or walls; dim, dirty lamp emitting sickening odors was the only light in cellar. Floor all rotted, sink used for urinal purposes; floor and wood work impregnated with urine. Room measured 6 feet 9 inches from floor to the bare joists. This is one of the filthiest of the whole lot. This cellar is run by a man who keeps a saloon upstairs.

August 12th, 11:00 p.m.—525 State street. Thirty-one bunks in cellar, all in small wooden partitioned, 4 x 7 rooms; damp, wet floor; bad odors; defective pan closet; low ceiling.

August 12th, 11:30 p.m.—515 State Street. Fifty double-deckers in cellar, 7 x 3 [sic]. Bare ceiling; damp, wet floor; no ventilation except from front door. Defective water closet; bare stone walls on side.

In the twentieth century a number of studies have been made in Chicago which show clearly the effect of sharp economic change on health. A survey made during the 1930's disclosed the mortality pattern in Chicago to be one of concentric circles with the highest rates at or near the center of the city, gradually falling off toward the outlying suburban sections. The Negro district fell almost entirely within the section of highest mortality, but a comparison with a chart showing median rentals revealed this to be an area of low rentals and therefore, presumably, economic status. The morbidity rates for adult communicable diseases provided the clearest correlation with general economic position, enabling the investigators to conclude that "as the economic level decreases, morbidity rates increase."[6] Exceptions to the concentric pattern were found in the high mortality areas along the lake shore; since these were districts where the median age was high, the steeper mortality rate might be attributed to the diseases of old age. Even the incidence of mental disorders in Chicago seemed to show a decline from the center to the periphery of the city, thus indicating a sociological approach to some of the problems of insanity.[7]

Despite the statistical evidence, very little has been done to correct these conditions. Regardless of the implications of such mortality statistics for social philosophy, it might at least be assumed that the most shocking and remediable of the factors promoting high mortality and morbidity rates would be immediately dealt with by public officials. But the politician has ignored the findings of the economist and the sociologist. He has found that in Chicago, at least, the articulate public is more interested in tax rates than mortality rates, in the demands of life than in the prevention of death. The pitiful results of attempts at housing reform were summed up by Edith Abbott in 1935: [8]

In every section of Chicago . . . are crowded tenement districts, with the same offensive and outlawed toilet accommodations, damp basements, dark and gloomy rooms, and, everywhere, wretched conditions of overcrowding. Many of the buildings in the districts investigated were old houses built before, sometimes long before, the tenement law of 1902, often overcrowded but not covered by the provisions relating to the construction of tenements. The same conditions, however, were also found in the buildings erected at a later date whose construction should have been regulated by the provisions of the code; but the results of one study after another showed how futile these provisions were and how frequently the law has been disregarded.

By 1951, housing conditions were worse than those described by Miss Abbott. The old tenements were fifteen years older, no new construction was attempted during World War II, and attempts to secure federal aid after the war were effectively blocked in the city council.

The disease which has proved most responsive to social conditions is tuberculosis. Though this "white plague" has passed from first in the list of causes of death in the United States to sixth or seventh, it still ranks high among the poorer classes, and is the second cause of death among Negroes. Social and economic influences play a tremendous part in the genesis of tuberculosis; bad housing, overcrowding, malnutrition, exposure, and failure to isolate open cases: all are important in determining who will fall victim to this largely preventable disease.[9]

The contagiousness of tuberculosis was long in dispute. During most of the nineteenth century, the disease was thought of as a debilitating hereditary affliction; it was "consumption, a wasting; euphemistically a decline." [10] The conception of tubercular communicability was not firmly established until 1882 when Koch reported his identification of the transmitting agent. But even after this date, many physicians were reluctant to accept the idea of contagion because their own observations taught them that certain types of people, living under certain circumstances, were more likely to acquire tuberculosis, germ or no germ, than others.

Gradually, tuberculosis was recognized as the product of a bacillus and a social condition; the germ was free to attack all persons indiscriminately, but the ill-housed and ill-fed were far more likely to succumb to the attack. In Chicago, researchers such as Theodore B. Sachs early recognized tuberculosis as a "social disease" since it "prevails most widely where social conditions are unfavorable . . . is especially a disease of poor people . . . living in crowded, insanitary quarters with insufficient food and unhealthful occupations." [11]

Sachs was active in the campaign for a municipal tuberculosis sanitarium and became its first director in 1909. His indefatigable labors in the cause of the tuberculous won him the praise and admiration of other workers in the field. But the political atmosphere which pervaded all municipal projects under the administration of William Hale Thompson proved too much for Sachs, who finally resigned from the city sanitarium. He advised the mayor in his note of resignation that "I do not believe in political management of hospitals, sanitaria, or similar institutions." A month later this pioneer in Chicago's anti-tuberculosis crusade was a victim of suicide, a discouraged and frustrated man who had given his all to a great cause without recognition or public support.[12] His death stirred a small tempest of indignation and revulsion in Chicago; the press and numerous civic groups belatedly castigated the mayor and his commissioner of health for their responsibility in forcing political appointees into the sanitarium. The guilty officials, however, had a ready explanation of Sach's suicide; a shortage, they said, had been discovered in his accounts.[13]

There were other pioneers in the anti-tuberculosis movement in Chicago. Harriet Fulmer, of the Visiting Nurses Association, for example, had an important part in the establishment of the Chicago Tuberculosis Institute, as well as the opening of an early camp for tuberculosis sufferers in Glencoe, Illinois. Dr. Frederick Tice, long Chicago's foremost authority on the disease, was another early worker in the field.[14]

Tice was born in Wisconsin in 1871. After years of farm labor, and a boyhood reminiscent of that described by Hamlin Garland in his *Son of the Middle Border*, he apprenticed himself to the village

physician until he was able to attend Rush Medical College. While
Tice was at Rush, his mother and sister both died of tuberculosis;
these sorrowful events caused him to dedicate himself to the study of
the "white plague." In 1899 the young physician himself developed
the disease and was informed he had only a year to live. The prog-
nosis, fortunately, proved mistaken; he returned to Chicago from a
self-imposed exile in Vienna. In the years following his return, he
became medical superintendent of Cook County Hospital, was appointed to a professorship at the College of Physicians and Surgeons, and later Rush, and opened one of the first tuberculosis clinics
in Chicago. In 1915 he conceived an outstanding reference work for
the general practitioner: a ten-volume, loose-leaf compendium of
medical practice which could be revised without necessitating a new
edition every few years. As president of the Municipal Tuberculosis
Sanitarium after 1931, Tice was largely responsible for the inauguration of a pneumothorax clinic for ambulatory patients, thus ignoring
older opinion that this procedure should be restricted to sanitarium
patients. A program of tuberculin testing of school children was
begun in 1936, with follow-up mobile X-ray testing. Tice was responsible for the first use of BCG vaccine in Chicago. A laboratory
was named for him at Cook County Hospital in 1932 and experiments in preventive vaccination of the newborn with the vaccine
were carried on there.[15] More and more, accent has been laid on prevention of the disease through the use of BCG, first discovered in
France in 1908. Under the direction of Dr. Sol R. Rosenthal, extensive experimentation has been carried on at the University of Illinois; in 1950 the vaccine was given federal approval for use in mass
immunization against tuberculosis.[16]

Despite the advances made in its management, much remained to be done with regard to tuberculosis in Chicago. In 1940
the city ranked sixty-ninth among ninety-two cities of over one hundred thousand population in mortality from tuberculosis.[17] During
the next decade, the number of deaths from the disease declined
faster in every state bordering Illinois, save Kentucky, than in Illinois itself. The mortality rate for the state in 1947 was 45 per 100,-
000, while Iowa recorded a rate of only 15. Chicago's mortality that
year was 58, a decline of 10 per cent over the preceding decade,
compared with a national decline of 35 per cent. For control measures, Illinois was spending at this time only $0.42 per tuberculosis
death, while the country as a whole was spending $3.09 per death.

Illinois, moreover, continued to be one of two states which lacked state-owned and operated sanitaria.[18] In Cook County, authorities were providing in 1946 less than one hospital bed for each death from tuberculosis; the minimum recommendation of the United States Public Health Service was two and a half beds. Another shortcoming of the anti-tuberculosis campaign in Illinois was the inadequacy of facilities for discovering new cases. This was evident in the fact that in the year 1942 nearly 30 per cent of all tuberculosis cases were unreported before death.[19]

The scourge of tuberculosis has fallen particularly hard upon the Negro in Chicago. While Negroes accounted for only 2 per cent of the city's population in 1910, their proportion rose to 7 per cent in 1940, and was considerably higher in 1950. The 1940 census showed the areas with the highest ratio of Negro inhabitants to be also the sections with the highest mortality rates. Tuberculosis was responsible for most of the Negro deaths. According to the United States Public Health Service, the conditions conducive to tubercular infection were "fulfilled notoriously in the Negro residential districts of Chicago." [20] Racial susceptibility has been claimed by some investigators as the cause for the great differential between White and Negro tuberculosis rates, but a total explanation would ascribe an important role to the standard of living among the Negro people. This was sharply demonstrated by evidence that death rates for Negroes, as well as Whites, go down as the economic level rises.[21]

Tuberculous Negroes have received less than their share of medical and institutional treatment in Chicago. Hospital and clinical facilities for Negroes at mid-century were limited out of all proportion to their needs. In 1939 a report to the Chicago Medical Society emphasized the "urgent" need of the Negro community for additional medical care, yet in 1946 the United States Public Health Service reported that the need had not been met. Since 33 per cent of tuberculosis deaths occurred among Negroes, Public Health Service investigators reasoned that a similar proportion of Negro patients would be found at the Municipal Tuberculosis Sanitarium; but they discovered that Negroes accounted for only 15 per cent of those treated with pneumothorax and only 24 per cent of all those under clinic supervision. Most observers were convinced by 1950 that any significant progress in handling the Chicago tuberculosis problem would have to begin with the Negro and his unique problem.[22]

Another problem which has been of concern to both medical

and public authorities since 1900 is that of infant and maternal mortality. "The care of the child-bearing woman," one writer has remarked, "is an index of the civilization of the community as a whole." [23] As in tuberculosis, a definite correlation has been discovered between low economic status and a high infant mortality rate. The squalor and filth of the tenements, coupled with the ignorance of the parents and a lack of adequate obstetrical care go far to explain the high death rate among the indigent. Large families have been the rule in the tenements, though parents have never expected all their children to reach maturity. If a mother of ten in 1900 steered six or seven children successfully through the perils of infancy, she might reasonably congratulate herself.[24]

The early campaigns against infant mortality in Chicago laid heavy stress on the importance of educating the mother. Under the supervision of physicians, summer clinics were held in the poorer neighborhoods and the Department of Health dispatched nurses to the homes of new mothers. The mothers were given instruction in the proper feeding and clothing of their babies, the sterilization of bottles and equipment, and the necessity for calling a physician at the onset of illness. The Chicago Medical Society established in 1909 a milk commission to inspect milk from certain dairies and farms to assure a reliable source of pure milk for infant feeding. Lay interest in the problem of infant care resulted in the formation of the Infant Welfare Society in 1911. This body directed the establishment of infant welfare stations around the city, where needy mothers could receive medical aid and advice concerning their children. By 1915, a survey showed, the Society was responsible for most of the charity work being performed in the field of infant health; the report concluded that Chicago was "distinctly backward" in supporting this important work. Under the direction of Herman Bundesen and his successor, Arnold H. Kegel, the Department of Health undertook an effective educational campaign on baby care in the early 1920's which brought marked results; the number of deaths per thousand live births dropped from 89.3 in 1921 to 76.9 in 1924 and to 53.4 in 1930.[25]

Chicago and Illinois doctors fought hard against outside intervention, particularly by the federal government, into their efforts to reduce the infant death rate. Congress had passed in 1921 the Sheppard-Towner Act, providing for grants-in-aid to the states for child and maternal health, but the state and city societies, as well as the American Medical Association, lobbied strongly against state compliance with the terms of the law.[26] The provision of medical care by the government, it was felt, was but a prelude to state medicine and the subjugation of the medical profession by an incompetent and irresponsible bureaucracy. The editor of the *Illinois Medical Journal* professed to see the advent of bolshevism in the Sheppard-Towner Act and expressed the feelings of many physicians when he wrote: "Born in the spinster confines of the Childrens Department of the Bureau of Labor, it was put into effect in a great many noncomprehending states simply because its proponents, mostly political workers in need of a job, sold the measure to the voters with the idea that when the Sheppard-Towner act was working no child would be born without its mother being in comfortable surroundings and with competent care during her ordeal." [27]

The death of women in childbirth had become virtually a national scandal by the 1930's. It was the subject of debate in the medical journals and the general public was aroused by articles in the popular magazines. Much of the controversy centered upon a Chicagoan, Dr. Joseph B. De Lee, whose whole life was devoted to a crusade against unnecessary death in parturition. As a young man, he had become obsessed with the irrationality of death resulting from a natural life-giving process. While interning at County Hospital in 1891, he was appalled at the low esteem in which obstetrics was held. Most births were still attended by midwives at this time, and none of the abler medical students thought of undertaking specialization in such a subject. De Lee realized that before the practice of obstetrics could achieve proper dignity, students of the art would have to be given practical training in confinement and receive careful instruction in pathological cases. For these purposes he opened a lying-in dispensary on Maxwell Street in 1895, and established a small hospital a few years later.[28]

The procedures which De Lee emphasized in dispensary, home, and hospital were patient care and scrupulous attention to cleanliness. The precautions which he took for a home delivery were extraordinary. He covered the floors and furniture with newspapers, scrubbed the area surrounding the delivery table, and permitted no one save assistants to enter the room during the entire labor. According to Isaac Abt, who sometimes assisted him, "He had not altered his technique to fit conditions; he had made conditions suitable for the practice of technique worthy of a hospital." De Lee was particularly anxious to get Caesarian cases, which he was studying; he became a pioneer in developing the modern technique for this operation. His early experience became even more important when he became director of the University of Chicago Lying-in Hospital; from 1931 to 1948 only eleven deaths among 2,729 deliveries by Caesarian section occurred at this institution.[29]

De Lee's experience and study convinced him that the maternity hospital should be separate from the general hospital. Much of his later life was spent in crusading for this idea. Why was it, he asked, that it was safer to have a baby outside of Chicago than in the great city, with its large hospitals, famed obstetricians, and trained nurses? Why did the deaths from puerperal causes in 1924 average one to every 150 births in Chicago, while the rate for the rest of Illinois was one to every 224 births? [30] De Lee made his first open attack on the general hospital maternity ward in 1933. Writing in the *Journal of the American Medical Association*, he stressed the danger to new mothers from infection in a hospital where all types of diseases were treated, and doctors and attendants rushed from one ward to another. "Home delivery," he concluded, "even under the poorest conditions, is safer than hospital delivery, if the hospital is a general one without adequate isolation precautions." [31]

This statement set off a hornet's nest of criticism and controversy. Two years later, De Lee incurred the further wrath of the Chicago profession and hospital authorities by collaborating with Paul de Kruif on a series of articles in a popular weekly which assured mothers of the safety of having babies at home under the care of a competent lying-in dispensary. Health Commissioner Bundesen also joined the attack on general hospitals, poor obstetrics, and unnecessary deaths during the 1930's.

As a result of the growing criticism, the Maternal Welfare Commission, composed of representatives from medicine, the general public, and welfare organizations, was established in 1937. Under the guidance of the new commission regulations for conduct of maternity wards in Chicago hospitals were drawn up. Improvements in hospital standards, personnel, and equipment followed; better isolation facilities for babies and mothers were found necessary in many cases. The new regulations were approved by the Chicago Medical Society, more apparently because members wished to avoid further public controversy, than because they agreed on the desirability of further supervision of medical and hospital work. Many thought the new regulations inconvenient and costly to hospitals, as, for example, the one requiring the obstetrical room to be a certain minimum distance away from laboratories and necropsy rooms.[32] Later critics of the De Lee-Bundesen campaign pointed out that mortality statistics in maternity cases at home and in hospitals were not comparable, since many fatal cases charged to the hospital were there simply because they were difficult cases and subject to complications.[33]

Maternal and infant mortality rates, nevertheless, dropped steadily in the decade following De Lee's campaign. Much of the improvement was due to the use of antibiotic drugs, which greatly lessened the dangers of infection; these drugs, many doctors declared, rendered the controversy over general hospitals largely academic.[34] But De Lee's supporters pointed to the fact that the Lying-in Hospital continued to boast one of the lowest maternal mortality rates in the world. Of 3,989 births occurring there in 1948, only two resulted fatally for the mother.[35] When De Lee died in 1942, he was widely considered the world's leading obstetrician; the Lying-in Hospital on the University of Chicago campus remains an enduring monument to a man who left an indelible mark on the evolution of his art.

Still another medical problem associated with the changing character of modern life has been the care of the aged. Medical discovery and advances in sanitation and public health work have combined to prolong the life of the average individual. This does not mean that the life span of the race has been lengthened—a man of sixty in ancient Greece could reasonably have expected fifteen more years of life, just as he could in 1950—but it did mean that more and more people survived the perils of childhood and middle age to reach senescence. This saving of lives, coupled with the stabilizing birth rate in the United States, resulted in the steady aging of the whole population. In 1840, for example, only 2.5 per cent of the American population was over sixty-five, while in 1900, 4.1 per cent had reached that age. In 1950 about 7.7 per cent of Americans were sixty-five or over, and estimates based on medium fertility and mortality indicated that about 11 per cent would be over sixty-five in 1975.[36]

This aging of the American population had increasingly important economic, social, and medical ramifications. It meant, for example, that a greater number of people reached a nonproductive age and were consequently dependent on family or public resources for their livelihood. By contrast, a smaller percentage of persons were to be found in the most productive period of life, from twenty to forty-five years. Socially, many older people now felt themselves useless or a burden on their relatives, despite the fact that many would be capable of productive work if given the opportunity. An anonymous letter to a Chicago newspaper in 1950 reflected the growing sense of futility and uselessness engendered by the callous policies of short-sighted employers:[37]

Are not the noble labors of medical science futile and pointless if not downright cruel when you consider that at 40 you are already thought too old for a job? Look at the prospects in store for you when you are 60.

When compassionate nature gives many of the aged a painless exit from this vale of tears via pneumonia, the doctors have to butt in and devise means of blocking nature and prolonging the heartaches and loneliness of the intolerable existence of old age.

From the standpoint of medicine, the rise in the number of older persons meant a higher incidence of those diseases which attacked the aged. In 1900, tuberculosis, pneumonia, infantile diarrhea, and enteritis—largely the afflictions of youth—were the leading causes of death; but a half century later heart disease and cancer—chiefly diseases of old age—were responsible for the greatest number of deaths. One statistician estimated that the incidence of cancer in 1960 would be double that for 1935.[38] In Chicago, the ratio of deaths from infantile diseases to all deaths dropped from 22.7 per cent for the four-year span 1897–1901 to 4.9 per cent in the period 1940–1944; while deaths from heart diseases leaped during the same period from 5.3 to 36.9 per cent. Pneumonia and tuberculosis accounted for 21.2 per cent of all deaths from 1897 to 1901, but for only 8.1 per cent in the four years after 1940; cancer and nephritis, by contrast, took the lives of three times as many people in the years 1940–1944 as in the earlier period.[39]

With the growth in number of the aged, the care of the chronically ill has become an acute problem. The social significance of a considerable segment of the population suffering from crippling and disabling diseases has not been generally realized. The permanent loss of income entailed by chronic illness, in addition to the heavy expenses for medicines, physicians, special diets, and appliances, has cast an intolerable load on many families. This "insidious modern plague," as one student of the problem has termed it, "not alone endangers the health, the working capacity and the lives of untold individuals; it jeopardizes the physical and mental health of the families of those stricken with a chronic illness; it places on society the great burden of caring for ever more families driven to economic dependency by the ravages of chronic diseases." [40]

The magnitude of the chronic-illness problem in Chicago can be seen from a glance at the following table: [41]

	Population 65 Years & Older	Number with Chronic Disease or Impairment	Number Chronically Ill
1940	197,079	94,998	11,741
1950	278,860	134,411	16,592
1960	338,250	163,037	20,126
1965	363,660	175,284	21,638

These statistics point up a problem for medicine and for all society which is as yet only faintly understood. An able report by the Institute of Medicine of Chicago on the subject of facilities for the care of convalescents, a closely allied problem, pointed out that Paris in 1859 had more beds for convalescents than did Chicago in 1938, that England was fifty years ahead of the United States in establishing homes for the convalescent, and that the Soviet Union had convalescent centers more adequately planned than existing facilities in Chicago.[42]

By 1950, however, there were a number of encouraging signs that the problem was not being completely neglected. A Central Service for the Chronically Ill, recently established, was playing an important part in educating the Chicago public and medical profession to the necessity for an over-all program for meeting the needs of the convalescent and the chronically ill. According to a survey which the Central Service made in Cook County, more than 750,000 persons were suffering from chronic diseases sufficiently serious to constitute some degree of handicap. Of this number, 50,000 were thought to be complete invalids. To meet this problem, the Central Service developed a comprehensive, well-integrated plan for satisfying the needs of these sufferers. The plan looked to the co-ordination of prevention and control, rehabilitation and long-term care, in a well-rounded attack on the problems of the chronically ill.[43]

The increase in degenerative diseases also aroused physicians to greater efforts to control them. Important research on cancer, for example, has been conducted in Chicago's hospitals and medical schools, as well as in the Chicago Tumor Institute. The opening of the new cancer hospital on the University of Chicago campus expanded considerably the research facilities available. To discover incipient cases of cancer, a number of prevention clinics have been opened in Chicago with the co-operation of the Chicago and Illinois medical societies. The state society has done excellent work in rousing physicians to the necessity of detecting cancer in its early stages. A plan for cancer detection in the doctor's office was inaugurated in 1946 by the society's committee on cancer, and has been copied by state societies in Virginia, Indiana, and elsewhere.[44]

Also in 1946, a survey of Chicago's total health resources was undertaken by the United States Public Health Service. Twelve thousand additional beds, it was concluded, were necessary to give adequate care to victims of chronic illness. Of these, 5,500 beds were needed for chronic invalids, 3,000 for tuberculosis patients, and 3,500 for those mentally unfit not institutionalized because of the serious bed shortage. With regard to cancer, a number of the recommendations made at that time have already been carried out. The United States Public Health Service suggested a special cancer hospital of 250 beds associated with a medical center, more cancer prevention clinics in general hospitals, a registry of cancer cases and of tumor tissues, a division of cancer control in the Chicago Health Department, and a general intensification of the cancer education program. The report cited, too, the urgent need for more facilities for the care of terminal cases of cancer.[45] Similar recommendations were made for the care of sufferers from the other degenerative diseases.

It is clear that a number of health problems have arisen in modern urban life which deserve careful study from the medical profession and general public alike. The interrelationship between medicine and society is nowhere more clearly seen than in the overlapping responsibility in meeting these problems. Medicine, more than one observer has commented, is basically a social science. In its broadest aspect, medicine is concerned not only with effecting cures but with readjusting the sick individual to his environment, whether this involves occupational therapy or psychotherapy, decent housing or adequate diet, recreational opportunity or prolonged rest.

Chapter X	The Origin and Development of
	Hospitals in Chicago, 1850–1950

The modern hospital has become an indispensable medium for the practice of medicine. When a patient requires treatment involving confinement, only a hospital is equipped to offer the efficient nursing and dietary service, the centralization of medical equipment, and the ready aid in emergency which all physicians now deem necessary. The general confidence of the public in hospitals today is such that few persons would entertain the idea of a major operation in any other surroundings. A century ago the public attitude toward hospitals was quite different. In 1850 hospitals were usually thought of as institutions for the accommodation of strangers or the sick poor. They were places for the care, rather than the cure, of patients. No self-respecting woman ever thought of having her baby in a public hospital. Most of the older hospitals in Europe had their origin in ecclesiastical enterprise, and all hospitals were looked upon as charitable establishments.

Conditions in some of these institutions, notably in the surgical wards, defied description, and improvement was to await scientific discovery, particularly regarding bacteria and their role in infections. Cleanliness was rarely invoked; a late eighteenth-century student thought his teacher excessively fussy if he prohibited spitting in the wards. Infection and cross infection were frequent; several diseases became so common in hospitals that they were identified as "hospital diseases," namely, erysipelas, pyaemia, septicaemia, and gangrene. Surgeons, before the discovery of antisepsis, frequently prided themselves on their blood-encrusted aprons, the degree of filth registering to some extent the experience of the operator. The nurses in these pioneer hospitals were normally drawn from a tough, charwoman class which regarded nursing as a distasteful drudgery rather than a humanitarian calling. The work of Florence Nightingale was yet a few years in the offing.[1]

The hospital development of the last century in Chicago is bound up with the growth of three types of institutions: the voluntary hospital, the public hospital, and the hospital for the mentally ill. The first was relatively unimportant in Chicago, except for the experience it afforded local medical schools, until well after the Civil War; the boost given public confidence in hospitals by the discovery of antisepsis and, later, modern asepsis, however, made the voluntary hospital the most numerous and significant type after 1875. The public hospital had its origins in the desire of citizens to provide medical care for the destitute of Chicago, as well as for travelers and homeless immigrants; the area of public responsibility for the health of the more unfortunate members of the community was steadily broadened in the course of the century. The hospital for the mentally ill, finally, was a product of humanitarian and scientific revolt against the practice of isolating the insane as special cases of pauperism.

The history of voluntary hospital development in Chicago begins in 1850 with the efforts of Dr. Nathan Smith Davis to obtain clinical material for his course in the practice of medicine at Rush Medical College. When he concluded that only a hospital could adequately serve the college, Davis undertook a series of popular lectures on medicine and sanitation to finance the project. There was great need for an institution which would care for the sick in the young city. A short-lived hospital had been opened in 1847, but after its closing there was no place where the homeless and friendless could be cared for in time of sickness. The city's poor, too, had to be treated individually in their widely scattered and usually filthy homes. Both the humanitarian and economic motives for establishing a hospital were cited by the *Chicago Daily Journal* in approving Davis' project. The county tax for the sick poor would be cut in half, the editor exulted, if these unfortunates could be brought together in one place.[2]

The opening of the Illinois General Hospital of the Lakes in the fall of 1850 was largely the result of Dr. Davis' initiative. Other members of the Rush faculty joined Davis on the staff of the new hospital; Daniel Brainard was placed in charge of the surgical ward, John Evans agreed to handle the obstetrics cases, while Levi D. Boone and Davis himself were responsible for the medical department. The hospital began operations in a suite of rented rooms in the Lake House Hotel on the corner of North Water and Rush streets. Medical students were at first assigned the responsibility for nursing patients at the institution, but this arrangement did not prove satisfactory. In February, 1851, an agreement was reached with the Sisters of Mercy, the first female religious order in the city, who consented to take over the management and nursing of the hospital. The Rush faculty reserved the right to use the clinical facilities offered by the institution, promising free medical care to all poor patients in return.[3]

Only a few years after they took over the administration, the Sisters of Mercy were faced with the panic and horror of a cholera epidemic. The disease had been introduced into Chicago by a train-load of Norwegian immigrants arriving in the spring of 1854. By midsummer, an epidemic was raging, hysteria was mounting, and a wave of emigrants was leaving the city. The Sisters performed heroic service during the days of panic. They stayed at their posts and ministered to the suffering victims of the plague. At the end of the attack, seven of them lay dead of the cholera.[4]

When Dr. Davis and several of his colleagues left Rush to found a new medical school in 1859, the agreement with Mercy Hospital was transferred to the new college. Later, when Davis' college affiliated with Northwestern University, Mercy was also brought into the university's orbit. During the closing decades of the century, the facilities of the hospital were greatly expanded. A school of nursing was added in 1889, the second such institution in the state. In 1901 a surgical pavilion and clinical amphitheater were completed; of the amphitheater, John B. Murphy, Mercy's most famous surgeon, said, "It is one of the most beautiful and perfect amphitheaters in the west."[5] In 1920 the long affiliation with Northwestern was ended, and an affiliation with Loyola was established.

After 1859, when Davis left the Rush faculty, President Brain-ard and his staff were dependent for clinical instruction upon the Rush College dispensary and the United States Marine Hospital. The Marine Hospital had been opened in 1852 on the site of the old Fort Dearborn reservation; a new site, midway between Chicago and Evanston, was chosen in 1867 for the erection of a new hospital.[6] During the 1870's, Rush was able to expand its clinical work by agreements with St. Joseph's Hospital, a young Catholic institution, and the Central Free Dispensary, organized at Rush in 1873 through a merging of two older dispensaries.[7]

In 1879 Rush purchased a site for a hospital of its own. The original intention of the faculty-trustees was to finance and maintain the building themselves, but it was soon apparent that Rush could not support the project alone. Dr. Moses Gunn, Brainard's successor in surgery, dickered at length with several Catholic sisterhoods which were willing, if not eager, to manage the proposed hospital on a basis similar to the previous arrangement with Mercy Hospital. Dr. J. P. Ross, however, convinced his colleagues that the Presbyterian churches of Chicago would finance the enterprise if given the opportunity. Ross was proved correct; Presbyterian Hospital was dedicated in 1884 with the Rush faculty maintaining control over all clinical instruction in the hospital. Fourteen years later Presbyterian Hospital joined Rush in its affiliation with the University of Chicago.

For a quarter of a century thereafter, Presbyterian was the only institution offering hospital training in the University of Chicago's medical program. With the completion of the Albert Merritt Billings Hospital in 1927, the university was equipped to begin clinical instruction on its south side campus. Several other hospitals— the Bobs Roberts Memorial Hospital for Children, the Chicago Lying-in Hospital, the Gertrude Dunn Hicks Memorial Hospital with its related orthopedic units, and the most recent addition, Nathan Goldblatt Memorial Hospital—have since made the university a center for clinical and hospital work. In 1941, with the separation of Rush from the University of Chicago and the discontinuance of medical education at the west side school, Presbyterian established a teaching affiliation with the University of Illinois College of Medicine.[8]

Northwestern, too, gradually increased its facilities for practical education in hospital work. Wesley Memorial Hospital followed Mercy in attaching itself to Northwestern in 1891. Wesley had its first home in the Chicago Training School in 1888, but after its affiliation with Northwestern it expanded steadily; the benefactions of William Deering made it possible for Wesley to support two hundred and fifty beds by 1910. In 1926, Northwestern moved its medical school to the new university campus on the north side of the city, where Passavant Memorial Hospital was already under construction. A number of Wesley's doctors left to join the staff of

Passavant. The trustees of Wesley thereupon decided to follow Northwestern to its new location and bought land across the street from the school in 1929. The great financial crash of 1929, followed by the years of depression, delayed construction. The new building was finally opened during the Second World War with a capacity of five hundred and fifty adult beds.[9]

When Passavant Memorial Hospital joined forces with Northwestern in 1925, it was already sixty years old. Founded in the summer of 1865 for the care of "sick and suffering strangers and immigrants," it had grown slowly during its early years. A laboratory and a training school for nurses were added around the turn of the century. After World War I it suspended operations for several years. When it affiliated with Northwestern in 1925, reactivation and construction of a new building began. Four years later the new building was dedicated on the university campus. According to the agreement with Northwestern, all members of the hospital's medical staff had also to be members of the medical school faculty.[10]

Not all hospitals founded before 1900, of course, were affiliated with the city's medical schools. Passavant led an independent existence for sixty years, as observed above, while Wesley was founded three years before it opened negotiations with Northwestern University Medical School. More important, there began to appear in the years following the Civil War a number of hospitals which had no expectation or desire to lose their identities through combination with one of Chicago's medical colleges.

A number of factors were responsible for this remarkable growth. The rapid increase in Chicago's population taxed existing facilities, while the expansion of the city over a wider and wider area meant that many communities had no hospital at all. Religious groups, moreover, vied with one another in establishing hospitals to meet the needs of their particular communicants. Catholics were especially active in this regard because of the importance they attached to receiving the final rites of the Church before death. Nationality groups, too, often built their own hospitals, where nurses and attendants familiar with the patient's language and background might make his sojourn more tolerable. Special hospitals for women, for children, and for Negroes also appeared in the years following the Civil War. But perhaps the most important reason for the increased attention given hospital development was the incorporation of the antiseptic technique into hospital routine during the 1870's and 1880's. The ability to control, or at least limit, the infections common to hospitals was a necessary preliminary to public confidence. Only gradually did hospitals lose their reputation as "vestibules to death." And before many years had passed, most persons began to realize that their lives were safer within the hospital than without, that the likelihood of contamination and complications was much greater at home than in the hospital ward.[11]

Among Catholic hospitals, Mercy Hospital was by far the oldest. Other hospitals administered by Catholic orders followed. In 1866, the Alexian Brothers, a religious order tracing its origins to service in the Black Plague of the thirteenth century, laid their plans for a hospital in Chicago. The building they erected was unhappily lost to the flames during the Great Fire, but the hospital was rebuilt on a larger scale. The present hospital at Belden and Racine avenues, erected in 1896, renders service only to sick and needy males. The institution is at present informally affiliated with De Paul University.[12]

In 1889 a Sister was struck by the appalling need of Chicago's Polish community (which was predominantly Catholic) for a hospital where Poles could converse in their own language and receive the final sacrament. Five years later, with the enthusiastic support of Polish-American groups, St. Mary of Nazareth Hospital was successfully launched.[13] Catholic hospitals were gradually established in other sections of the city; in 1901 St. Francis Hospital was opened in Evanston. By 1950 there were twenty-two hospitals under Catholic auspices in metropolitan Chicago. Catholics even had their own maternity hospital after 1931, where "Mothers of Catholic families of white race, living in legitimate wedlock, and whose husband's income is less than $2600.00 a year" were eligible for care. Catholics also had their own medical school in the Stritch School of Medicine of Loyola University. Affiliated with the Stritch School after 1938 was Loretto Hospital, first established in 1923 and subsequently known as the Frances E. Willard Hospital. One of the last Catholic hospitals to be built in Chicago was the Little Company of Mary Hospital, completed in 1930; its bed capacity in 1950 was approaching three hundred and fifty.[14]

Of non-Catholic sectarian healing institutions, St. Luke's Hospital (Episcopalian) was the first. St. Luke's was founded in 1865 by the Reverend Clinton Locke and his parish, who sought to create a "clean, free Christian place" for the housing of the sick poor. A cottage with seven beds was all that Reverend Locke's parish could support for the first few years. St. Luke's was one of the few hospitals fortunate enough to survive the Great Fire of 1871; its good fortune continued through the following years.[15] By 1950 the hospital contained 553 beds and bassinets, and occupied five buildings on Indiana and Michigan avenues.

In 1866, the Jewish citizens of Chicago raised funds for a hospital of their own. The building, like that of the Alexian Brothers, was lost in the fire of 1871. Several years later, a benefactor was found in Michael Reese, and the Michael Reese Memorial Hospital was opened in 1882 at the corner of Ellis Avenue and 29th Street. The present modern hospital was completed in 1907; a hospital for children and a Medical Research Institute were added in 1910, and a free dispensary in 1928. In 1950 the hospital represented an investment of ten million dollars; it was the largest voluntary hospital in the Chicago area with its 718 beds. In the field of medical education, Michael Reese undertook after World War II the conduct of a postgraduate school, which in 1947 gave courses to over five hundred practicing physicians from various parts of the country.[16]

The large influx of foreign-born in Chicago during the late nineteenth and early twentieth centuries accounted for much of the hospital construction of this period. The German Hospital of Chicago, for example, was incorporated in 1883, housing its first patients in a small private dwelling. During the First World War, the unpopularity of the German cause forced the renaming of the hospital. As Grant Hospital, this institution has continued to grow, maintaining in 1950 almost three hundred beds and bassinets.[17] The Norwegians were responsible for the building of several hospitals in the 1890's. The Norwegian-American Hospital and the Lutheran Deaconess Home and Hospital are both offsprings of enterprises begun by Norwegian immigrants.[18] Other nationalities built their own hospitals, some of them still vigorous and thriving today.

Beginning in the 1890's, some hospitals appeared which had no connection either with medical schools or with the city's immigrant or religious groups. Their founding marked the dramatic change which had occurred in the whole field of medical and surgical practice. With the advent of asepsis, hospital confinement was no longer a matter for the homeless, the friendless, or the poor, but was coming to be considered a vital necessity by enlightened members of the community. Charity became less important as a motive in the establishment of hospitals. When Evanston Hospital was opened in an eight-room cottage in 1892, the largest and most comfortable room was set aside for paying patients. Three years later, the Evanston Hospital Association was formed to support the institution as a necessary community enterprise.[19] Also in 1895 a group of physicians and citizens incorporated the South Chicago Community Hospital to meet the needs of the expanding population in the southern sector of the city.[20] Both the Evanston and South Chicago hospitals were nonprofit and nondenominational in their policies, thus inaugurating the trend which has since become dominant.

The educational motive in the founding of hospitals declined in importance, but remained a significant one. Hospitals were organized in connection with the two postgraduate medical schools started in the 1880's. The Chicago Policlinic Hospital was erected to facilitate teaching at the famous Policlinic school. With the death of Fernand Henrotin, noted surgeon and member of the Policlinic staff, the hospital was renamed after him. Though the postgraduate school was abandoned in 1920, as graduate work in medicine gravitated more and more toward the universities, Henrotin Hospital continued to offer service to the north-central section of the city.[21]

With the growth of the Negro population of Chicago in the last two decades of the century, a serious problem in hospitalization arose. The refusal of most hospitals to admit Negroes added another obstacle to the Negro's slow progress toward better health and prosperity. Many physicians and hospital administrators recognized their need but were stymied by the widespread prejudice and misunderstanding characterizing relations between the Negro and White races. Chicago in 1891 had a Negro population of 15,000, the majority of them living on the south side, from Wabash Avenue to Armour Avenue, and from Polk Street scattered down to 35th Street. A few of the city's hospitals accepted Negro patients, but only if they were brought by staff members. Negro physicians, of course, had no hospital facilities at all for their patients. In 1891, largely through the initiative of Daniel Hale Williams, regarded as the greatest Negro doctor of his day, Provident Hospital for Negroes was opened at the corner of 29th and Dearborn streets.[22]

Williams was a remarkable figure in Chicago's medical history. His accomplishments, marvelous by any standards, were magnificent when measured against the deprivation, discrimination, and lack of opportunity experienced by every Negro doctor. Williams was born in Pennsylvania in 1858, but was brought by his mother to Janesville, Wisconsin, at the age of five. She abandoned him there, and he was cared for by a humanitarian Negro family. The family helped him to get a preliminary education; by 1880 he was ready for medical school. He left for Chicago in the fall of that year to enroll at the Chicago Medical College. After graduation three years later he interned at Mercy Hospital, where he attracted the interest of J. B. Murphy and Christian Fenger. He soon won some little fame as a surgeon. It was through his drive, energy, and persistence that Provident Hospital was opened in small quarters in 1891. Two years later he brought the new hospital national attention when he performed an unprecedented operation in emptying and suturing the pericardial sac in a stab wound of the chest. Late in 1893 Williams was called to the Freedmen's Hospital in Washington as Surgeon-in-Chief. Under his supervision, the hospital completely reorganized its surgical services and established a nursing school. But discouraged by racial discrimination and disheartened by political machination, he returned to Chicago after a few years in Washington. The money he might have made in private practice never concerned him greatly; he toured the country after his return to Chicago, teaching surgery to interested Negro doctors. In his later years he grew increasingly bitter and taciturn. When a young Negro doctor asked his advice about accepting an internship at Freedmen's Hospital, Williams replied that he would rather see a boy of his selling newspapers. He died in 1931 in Chicago.[23]

Provident Hospital developed rapidly under the leadership of Williams and his successor, George Cleveland Hall. A new building erected in 1898 served the Negro community until 1934, when Frank Billings and Julius Rosenwald managed a successful campaign for a Greater Provident Hospital. A quasi-affiliation with the Northwestern University Medical School existed until 1930; a number of Northwestern's outstanding men—Fenger, Billings, Jaggard, Favill, De Lee —served at various times on the Provident staff.

The changed racial situation in Chicago beginning in the First World War was reflected in the greater proportion of Negroes using the hospital after 1915. The influx of 50,000 Negroes into the city to meet the needs of war industries placed a heavy burden on the institution. In 1903, 1,500 patients had been admitted to Provident, 1,169 of whom were white; but twelve years later whites accounted for only 7 per cent of those entering the hospital. During the race riots of 1919, Provident was one of the few hospitals to open its doors to all victims, regardless of race.

The affiliation of Provident with the University of Chicago in 1930 was a great boost for Negro medical education. The university provided a consulting staff, sent lecturers, and held clinical conferences at the hospital. Several of Provident's Negro staff members were sent to Europe for a year or more of graduate study. In 1936 a five-year resident training program in general surgery was inaugurated. Graduates of Provident have spread gradually into the white hospitals of the city. In 1944, there were six colored physicians working at the Billings Hospital, two at the Illinois Research Hospital, three at Children's Memorial, two at Loyola, one at St. Luke's, and one at Presbyterian. Twenty of Provident's staff were diplomates of specialty boards that same year. According to one estimate, Provident "has contributed more than any other so-called Negro hospital to the inspiration and accomplishment of colored physicians." [24]

The provision of special hospital facilities for women and children began even before gynecology and pediatrics assumed the status of independent specialties. Dr. Mary H. Thompson founded the Chicago Hospital for Women and Children in 1865 as a "home for women and children among the respectable poor in need of medical and surgical treatment." It was her intention to provide a haven for pregnant women and sick children who would otherwise be exposed to the coarseness and impersonality of a public ward at County Hospital. Many of the hospital's early patients were war widows, unwed mothers, and refugees from the South, but they were succeeded by employed women and the wives and children of laborers. Another feature of the hospital which attracted many women was the opportunity of consulting physicians of their own sex. A women's medical college was organized in connection with the hospital in 1870; both were burned completely in the Fire the following year. [25]

Since the Great Fire created a serious need for hospitals, the Relief and Aid Society, which controlled the money and supplies heaped upon the stricken city, financed the reorganization of the women's hospital. Rooms were rented on West Adams Street, and the sick, burned, and wounded were crowded into the structure. A semipermanent home was built in 1873 and twelve years later a new and improved hospital building was erected. [26]

During the 1880's the lack of hospital space for children was widely criticized and discussed. The pioneer pediatrician, Frank E.

Waxham, told the Chicago Medical Society that the city compared unfavorably with New York in this respect. Special hospitals, he advised, would do much to prevent the spread of contagious diseases and spare young lives.[27] A year later, another doctor exploded that "in this christian century there should be more hospitals built for children and a less number of large stone wall churches erected. These hospitals will do more to save them and their lives from the slums and alleys . . . than churches." [28]

The need was partially met by the provision of a children's ward in County Hospital, and by the founding of the Maurice Porter Memorial Hospital for Children. The Porter Hospital was opened to the public in 1882, declaring its intention "to care for children without discrimination against any race, color or creed or inability to pay." Infants under three years of age were not admitted until 1904, by which time enough was known of infants' afflictions to enable the hospital to help them. All hospitalization was free until 1926 when provision for paying patients was made. In 1948 the hospital, renamed the Children's Memorial Hospital early in the century, gave 65 per cent of all its services without charge. Mounting costs have caused the hospital considerable difficulty, but the Community Fund, welfare agencies, and wealthy individuals have combined to supplement the income from endowments and patients.[29]

Other special facilities for children have been provided by the city's hospitals in the twentieth century. The La Rabida Sanitarium, for example, is a nonsectarian, charitable hospital dedicated to aiding children in the fight against rheumatic fever. For more than a score of years this sanitarium has cared for rheumatic children without charge. It was one of the first hospitals to concentrate on this treacherous disease, long dismissed as "growing pains" and not recognized as associated with the serious heart damage which it fosters.[30]

In the twentieth century hospital building of all types, public, private, denominational, and special, has been greatly accelerated. By 1910 the attitude of the public toward hospitals, even among the superstitious and uneducated, had undergone a complete and wholesome transformation. During the two decades from 1910 to 1930, 131 hospitals were constructed in Illinois, representing about 40 per cent of the state's healing institutions still in operation in 1949. The provision of facilities for the care of the sick, long regarded as exclusively a local responsibility, became more and more a matter of state and national concern. Of 102,649 beds (and bassinets) in Illinois hospitals in 1949, 69,092 were in government- (including city) owned institutions; 16,471 were in church-related hospitals; 14,666 were controlled by nonprofit associations; and 2,420 were in proprietary institutions.[31] Governmental intervention in the field of hospitalization has been confined, on the state level, to long-drawn-out diseases, especially tuberculosis, while the federal government has been concerned only with special classes of patients, such as war veterans.[32] An example of federal provision of hospital care in the Chicago area is the Veterans Administration Hospital at Hines, Illinois. Begun as an army hospital during World War I, it was taken over by the United States Public Health Service in the postwar years, and later by the Veterans Administration. The Hines reservation in 1949 contained 138 buildings and 3,253 beds.[33]

Most of the hospitals built since 1910 have been nonprofit community institutions. The American Hospital of Chicago, for example, has since 1917 served the Irving Park—Broadway section of the north side; the MacNeal Memorial Hospital was organized about the same time as the first hospital in the community of Berwyn; the Mount Sinai Hospital opened its doors in 1918 to the Lawndale district of Chicago.[34] Mount Sinai has recently affiliated with the Chicago Medical School, giving that college some much-needed clinical facilities, and assuring the Lawndale community of competent medical and surgical care. A typical community enterprise was the Belmont Hospital, opened in 1927 as a neighborhood project on the northwest side. Comprising six stories, one hundred beds, and thirty bassinets, this hospital is well equipped to meet the emergency medical needs of the Belmont district. Belmont Hospital was financed by a stock and bond issue, beginning its existence as a profit-making corporation. The corporation was converted a few years later into a nonprofit institution with stockholders exchanging their holdings for second mortgage bonds. The change, of course, freed the hospital from the taxes to which profit-making corporations were subject.[35] The great majority of Chicago's hospitals in 1950 were organized on a nonprofit basis; only 47 of the state's 330 hospitals were still classified as proprietary enterprises in 1949.

The growth of public facilities in Chicago for the care of poor and certain other classes of patients has been quite different from that of the voluntary hospital. Public hospitals had their origin in the need of local officials for an institution where the sick poor could be brought together economically for treatment; they met, too, a need for a place where persons suffering from mental illness or from a contagious disease might be isolated from the rest of the community. Their expansion depended not so much on community interest, modern hospital development, or growth in medical specialization, as upon the incidence of epidemics, increases in population, and an enlarging area of public responsibility for the health of the city.

Public responsibility for the medical care of the poor, as well as sufferers from epidemic afflictions, was recognized early in the history of the city. A city physician, charged with the care of the sick poor, was appointed in the early 1830's, though a hospital was not erected for a number of years. Many of the workers on the Illinois and Michigan Canal during this period came to the young city to have their injuries or diseases treated at the expense of the local taxpayers. The *Daily American* complained in 1839 that it was unjust to expect the county on which the burden fell to bear it alone. The state, according to the writer, should erect hospitals along the route of the canal for these people.[36]

The first city hospital was authorized and constructed in 1843 to give shelter to epidemic victims in need of care. Two years later this simple structure burned; it was soon rebuilt in the face of a rise in the number of scarlet fever and smallpox cases in the city. The first general hospital in the Chicago area was established in 1847 in a large warehouse known as Tippecanoe Hall. Drs. Brainard, Blaney, and Herrick of Rush Medical College, the persons most responsible for the enterprise, served on the first medical staff of the institution.[37] Since the county authorities furnished most of the supplies, this project has been considered the first Cook County Hospital. It was short-lived, and after the establishment of Mercy Hospital in 1850, county patients were cared for there by special agreement. This arrangement was continued until 1863 when a new county hospital was established in the town of Jefferson, where buildings for the housing of the poor and the insane were already located.[38]

An early division of responsibility between city and county in health matters was made. A number of statutes and legislative acts pointed to city responsibility for epidemic control and for sanitary and prophylactic action in preventing disease, while other laws assigned the care of the individual sick to the Board of County Commissioners. The city hospital, which continued to function during epidemics after its reconstruction in 1845, was responsible only for the care and isolation of victims of epidemic disease. No provision was made there for cases of general illness, which were considered the obligation of the county.

The cholera epidemic of 1854 sorely taxed the facilities of both the city and Mercy hospitals; it was found necessary to erect another temporary structure for cholera victims. Dr. Levi D. Boone, elected mayor of Chicago in November, and Brockholst McVickar, the city physician, joined in urging the Board of Health to construct a large permanent city hospital. Plans were quickly approved and the cornerstone was laid in 1855.[39]

When, two years later, the structure was completed at a cost of $75,000, the Board of Health proceeded to select a medical and surgical staff. A number of Chicago's prominent citizens had petitioned the board to allow homeopathic physicians a separate staff at the hospital, so that patients might choose homeopathic treatment if they desired, and the board decided in favor of the petitioners, appointing both a homeopathic and an "allopathic" staff to the new institution.[40] The decision was fought savagely by the regular physicians. Dr. N. S. Davis immediately declined his appointment to the staff. But the homeopaths were strong—a large percentage of the world's homeopaths were congregated in Chicago at this time—and the battle was stalemated. No patient was admitted to the hospital in the next two years; the City Council left it unoccupied and uncared for. The absence of epidemic disease and the consequent reluctance of the council to maintain the hospital help to explain the abandonment of the project. In 1859, when Dr. Davis left Rush, taking the clinical privileges of Mercy Hospital with him, the Rush professors leased the vacant structure from the city.[41] With the Rush faculty as staff members, the hospital was operated for three years as a private hospital, caring for some charity patients under contract with the Board of County Commissioners. In October, 1862, the building was commandeered by military authorities and administered for the duration of the Civil War as an army hospital.[42]

Soon after the war, Drs. Joseph P. Ross and George K. Amerman, who had served on the staff of the hospital during the war, conspired to have the institution taken over by Cook County authorities as the county hospital. After 1863, the county hospital was located with the buildings for the poor and insane at Jefferson, being neither convenient nor adequate. Amerman succeeded in getting himself elected in 1865 to the County Board of Supervisors and he promptly persuaded his colleagues to lease the premises of the city hospital as a county hospital. Thus did the ephemeral city hospital become officially Cook County Hospital in 1865.[43]

The county's charges were removed from Jefferson to the new hospital the following year. The medical board of the hospital was composed of an equal number of representatives from Rush and the Chicago Medical College, in addition to a majority of doctors having no connection with either college. Trouble arose in 1867 when Dr. Edwin Powell upset the equilibrium between the two medical schools by resigning from Rush, securing an appointment to the staff of the hospital as an independent, and then being re-elected to the Rush faculty. The ensuing discord and wrangling caused the county authorities to dismiss the entire board in 1871. The subsequent political degeneration of the hospital began with this single act of the Rush professor, since it ended hopes for a self-governing and self-perpetuating medical staff. The hospital has never realized its full potentialities as a great teaching institution because of the political controls over appointments, tenure, and procedures resulting from the failure of the doctors themselves to exercise self-discipline.[44]

The early equipment of County Hospital was meager, the number of beds was inadequate, and frequent complaints were made of the large number of infections acquired by patients. There was no microscopic or clinical laboratory; antisepsis was not introduced until 1878; and the obstetrical ward had to be closed several times for disinfection because of deadly attacks of puerperal fever.[45] The coming of Christian Fenger to the staff in 1878, however, did much to develop the hospital as a center for medical study, despite the conditions. The number of nurses employed by the county was five, three men and two women, but these were assisted by convalescent patients. The capacity of the hospital was 130 patients in 1870; there was scarcely a day when there was a bed to spare. The exterior of the institution that same year was vividly described by a *Chicago Tribune* reporter: [46]

It is a large brick building, of a dirty red color, planted in a low and badly-kept lot, at the corner of Eighteenth and Arnold streets. The outside appearance and surroundings of the building are not calculated to cheer the spirits of a sick man. . . . A low, rickety fence, inclined at an angle of 45°, runs around the lot. Outside the fence the landscape consists of the rear of some shanties which bound the horizon; of mud puddles in vacant lots; of a badly kept road; a sewer, a sidewalk and the tottering fence. . . . To the north, stretching out to the fence, is a vacant space full of rubbish, garbage and all manner of unsightly things.

By the early 1870's County Hospital was vastly overcrowded. Admission became extremely difficult; a large number of qualifications were introduced to keep the number of eligible patients down to the capacity of the institution. To make matters worse, thousands of immigrants were streaming into the city every month, all of them homeless and without resources, and many of them in need of medical attention. The city's newspapers and medical publications pointed to the great need for a new and larger structure to house the numbers demanding entrance. "Let us have no more strangers, or even vagrants," urged the Chicago Medical Journal, "dying in the Armory, Bridewell or station houses, because there is no room for the sick or wounded poor in the hospitals of this great city of Chicago." [47]

In 1876 the two central pavilions of the present structure were completed on the west side of the city. But more than twenty years were to elapse before completion of even the initial plans. Two thousand beds were provided in the completed hospital. Still more pavilions were started in 1912, and the Cook County Psychopathic Hospital was established two years later.[48] A number of buildings have been added to the Cook County group since 1914, the latest being the Hektoen Institute for Medical Research, formerly the McCormick Institute of Infectious Diseases, bought from the University of Chicago in 1943.[49]

An agreement regarding the attending staff was reached in 1877: one third to be appointed by Rush, an equal number by the Chicago Medical College, and the remaining third by the County Board.[50] This arrangement lasted only five years. In 1882, when the board attempted to interfere in some skin-grafting experiments being carried out at the hospital, the whole staff resigned in protest. After this time there was no further college representation on the medical board of the hospital. County authorities appointed the entire staff until 1905 when civil service regulations were adopted for both attending and resident physicians. The homeopaths and eclectics, who were given jurisdiction over portions of the hospital in 1881 and 1889, respectively, were no longer recognized after 1905. Medical students never enjoyed after 1882 the benefit of County Hospital facilities. For many years they were not even allowed inside the institution since it was believed that their presence would be inimical to the welfare of patients. They have been admitted in recent years under conditions of close supervision.[51]

The history of Cook County Hospital illustrates some of the shortcomings of a politically controlled medical institution. For many years the management and policies of the hospital were governed by political considerations alone. Favoritism in the appointment of the attending staff, interference with research and the teaching of students, and outright graft were some of the problems which the medical profession and public alike faced in their relations with the hospital. Corruption was particularly widespread during the years from 1876 to 1887. Positions on the staff in these years were obtained only through political influence or outright bribery. Christian Fenger borrowed enough money to buy his appointment in 1878; David W. Graham later confessed that his appointment was obtained "through the political influence of a friend"; James B. Herrick recalled that his position on the attending staff was secured through a friend sitting on the County Board.[52] The only price that the fortunate Herrick had to pay for his appointment "was an annual note of thanks, with a box of cigars to my sponsor."

The hospital's expenses mounted curiously during the 1870's. The expenditure for liquor in 1876 was almost twice that for clothing and bedding, three times the amount spent for surgical supplies, and more than half the expense for drugs and medicines. Over 10 per cent of the budget went for unspecified miscellaneous charges.[53] The nonmedical employees, chosen from among the political friends of the regime in power, were paid much larger salaries than their meager experience and performance on the job warranted. The hospital was branded by one medical journal an "almshouse for the scum of the party who get beaten in the local elections." In 1888 several members of the medical staff were criticized by the Chicago Medical Society for their collaboration with the politicians. The *Medical Standard* characterized these doctors as a "collection of servile tools of the vilest political ringsters. In place of upholding the dignity of the profession, the County Hospital staff has made the name of hospital physician a byword and reproach." Even the State Board of Charities, which was powerless to act against the political mobsters, described the hospital as the "best built and the poorest managed . . . in the country." Eventually Warden McGarigle and a number of his colleagues in corruption at the hospital were brought to trial and found guilty. Conditions began to improve toward the end of the century; the adoption of civil service in 1905 did much to erase the remaining abuses.[54]

The years of political control saddled the hospital with a bad reputation. The public was understandably suspicious of an institution where political hacks were given administrative positions, and where money for necessary foods and medicines was declared lacking, despite an overflowing liquor cabinet. The maternity ward, in particular, suffered severely from the lack of competent personnel, adequate supplies, and a serviceable sewerage system. The incidence of puerperal fever was higher than at any other of the city's hospitals; the Chicago Medical Society heard repeated criticisms and uncomplimentary reports on the maternity care afforded by the institution.[55] Ludvig Hektoen, who served as an intern in the obstetrics ward in 1888, left this revealing notation on the obstetrical records: [56]

The necessary supplies have sometimes been obtained with difficulty, at other times not at all. There have [sic] been no intra-uterine irrigating-point in the ward during the present service, it being impossible to obtain a supply in spite of vigorous and constant demands.—The fumigator at one time officiated as night morgue-keeper, but it is thought not for some time past.—The sanitary condition of the ward is imperfect; the sewerage is bad and during rain water leaks through the ceiling in torrents into the large north-east lying-in ward especially, and then into W'd 12 below. Attention of the authorities has been directed to these defects over a month ago, and until they are remedied a perfectly normal course of the lying-in period cannot be hoped for.

The Cook County Hospital has come to enjoy a fuller measure of public confidence in the twentieth century. Political influences have been markedly reduced, while the medical and surgical services provided have been of consistently high caliber. Complaints heard in 1950 were more likely to center on the shortage of nurses and other trained personnel, or on the rapid turnover of staff members, which discourages extensive teaching and research projects. The hospital today is the scene of prodigious activity measured by any known standard. About eighteen thousand operations are performed there each year; blood for an average of thirty transfusions daily is taken from its blood bank; one of every ten babies born in Chicago is brought into the world there. The number of beds in the hospital now totals more than 3,400. The physical plant embraces a psychopathic hospital, a men's medical building, a children's hospital, a contagious disease hospital, a tuberculosis hospital, a medical research institute, a power plant, and a laundry.[57]

A special type of public hospital, differing considerably in its purposes and development, was that provided for the mentally ill. The isolation and treatment of the insane has become in the course of the past century almost completely a function of the state, rather than a supplementary service for those unable to attend private hospitals. The necessity of special quarters for those suffering from mental illnesses was not recognized for many years by public authorities in Illinois. But with growing public recognition of mental illness as only a special type of general illness, one that would respond to hospitalization and medical treatment, there came the realization that only the state could support the hospitals, medical staff, equipment, and personnel for the sustained period of treatment which mental disease required.

The early treatment of the insane in Illinois did not differ greatly from that in other states. Insane persons incapable of caring for themselves were considered only a special category of the poor. Until the 1840's, the insane poor in Illinois were cared for chiefly by private citizens, usually under contract. They might be locked up or chained in solitary cabins, or given some degree of freedom, depending on the extent of the mental affliction and the enlightenment of the keeper. William Blair of Cass County, for example, was allowed eighty-five dollars in 1840 for the erection of a small frame house "for keeping a deranged woman." Larger communities cared for their demented paupers at the county poor farms, where the more violent inmates were given separate rooms.

When a differentiation began to be made between insanity and pauperism, the insane were usually given the worst quarters available. The basement or attic of an almshouse often served as their habitat. Where a building was constructed especially for the mentally diseased, it was likely to incorporate the worst features of a prison. According to one description, departments for the insane "had solitary cells seven or eight feet square, improperly heated or without any heat, not ventilated, often dark and destitute of furniture, sometimes in an outrageously dirty state, filled with foul odors arising from cesspools underneath, built commonly in the cheapest possible manner, sometimes of weatherboarding, not lined and opened to the weather, and infested in time with vermin." There was little medical care provided in the almshouses, and the mentally ill could expect no specialized attention at all. Although a state insane asylum was erected in 1847, the transfer of the mentally diseased from the poor houses was a slow and gradual process. As late as 1900 over three thousand of these unfortunates were still cared for in almshouses. In 1909, however, care of the mentally ill was made exclusively a matter of state concern.[58]

Some persons recognized the inhumanity of early methods of treating the insane in Illinois and began to work for reform in the 1840's. When Dorothea Dix, the famed benefactor of the mentally ill, addressed the Illinois legislature in 1847, she found that her words fell on ears made receptive by local reformers and physicians. For this was the great age of Jacksonian democracy; the leaven of democratic preaching and a common experience in building a new country had alerted the masses to their rights as human beings and taught them the democratic basis for helping the underprivileged and unfortunate among them; this was to be an era of reforms and reformers.

Dr. Edward Mead provided perhaps the best example of the humanitarian striving toward better care of the insane in Illinois. Although born in England, Mead had come to America at an early age and was essentially American in his outlook and attitudes. After graduating from the Medical College of Ohio in 1841, he came to the faculty of the short-lived Franklin Medical College in St. Charles, Illinois. In 1846 he accepted an invitation to join the faculty of the Illinois Medical College at Jacksonville. Mead began his labors on behalf of the insane almost immediately after his arrival in the state. As early as 1842 he began advocating a state hospital for their care. Only five years later the Illinois State Hospital was inaugurated, significantly, in Jacksonville. But Mead's work had only begun. He left Jacksonville in 1847 for Chicago, which lagged far behind in the matter of agitation and interest concerning the mentally ill. There he established the Chicago Retreat for the Insane, an institution which would, he announced, "rely on moral agencies for their restoration to reason,—a library of 300 volumes, music, lectures, exercises, and amusements to divert the mind from subjects of hallucinations." In the absence of any public institution, Mead's Retreat was used by county authorities as an asylum for the insane poor. In 1852, five years after its founding, this pioneer hospital for the insane burned to the ground, and Mead moved on to Cleveland to continue his work.[59] With Mead's departure, Chicago reverted to its previous indifference to the problems of the insane. Jacksonville's lead in the establishment of charitable institutions—the city also had a shelter for the deaf and dumb—can only be attributed to the humanitarian spirit and enlightened sense of responsibility which that progressive community manifested. They were local leaders, after all, who had brought Mead to teach at Illinois College and who had invited Dorothea Dix to come to Illinois.[60]

Only John Evans among the early medical men of Chicago displayed any real interest in the problems of the mentally ill. This resourceful pioneer had played a key role in the establishment of the Indiana Hospital for the Insane before coming to teach at Rush Medical College. He commenced petitioning for a state hospital soon after his arrival in Indiana, addressing the legislature in 1843.[61] His interest in the insane was probably more humanitarian than medical, though he composed several scientific articles on mental disease. "The laws of humanity and of kindness," he asserted, "are the only ones that should be applied for their [the insane's] government. However much the reason may be dethroned, there are few, very few, who cannot be made to feel those heaven-born influences that flow from the benevolent heart." [62] When the state hospital was built in Indiana, Evans designed the building and supervised its construction. Dorothea Dix found conditions much better in this state than elsewhere and gave full credit to Dr. Evans.[63]

During the 1860's, Illinois became the center of a national controversy regarding the commitment of the insane to hospitals. A Mrs. E. P. W. Packard wrote several widely distributed "exposés" charging that she had been confined while perfectly normal at the Jacksonville institution at the instigation of her minister-husband who deplored her unorthodox religious views.[64] The allegations inspired a national sensation and a demand for legislative safeguards to protect from incarceration persons not actually insane. The Illinois legislature in 1867 made a jury trial mandatory in all cases of alleged insanity. But this law was universally condemned by psychiatrists and physicians since it placed in the hands of laymen the decision as to the insanity of an accused person. The law, moreover, deterred many families from presenting mentally ill persons for institutionalization because of the publicity attendant upon a jury trial.[65] Nevertheless, this system remained in effect for twenty-five years before its repeal in 1892. Dr. Richard Dewey, a superintendent of the Kankakee State Hospital, said later of this so-called "personal liberty" law: "The entire annals of the insane in the state of Illinois furnish no greater evidence of cruelty to the insane and their friends than this so-called 'reform' so zealously promoted by Mrs. Packard. As a matter of fact, more sane persons were found insane by jury trials, as shown by the reports of institutions from year to year, than were ever wrongfully committed under the earlier system." [66]

In the early 1870's a campaign for the introduction of the "cottage system" in caring for the insane was begun in Illinois. According to this plan, inmates at a mental institution were separated into small buildings where, it was felt, they would feel more at home than in the huge, prisonlike structures where all lived together. A compromise with proponents of the conventional, one-building arrangement was agreed upon in the construction of Illinois' second insane hospital at Kankakee in 1877; a group of small cottages was scattered around one large central building. This represented the first large-scale application of the cottage scheme to a mental institution in the United States. [67]

Not until 1870 did Cook County authorities erect a separate building for the insane on the grounds of the county poor house at Jefferson. Previously, the more violent of the mentally ill were housed in a small brick building adjacent to the poor house. This structure was described as one "with small barred windows, iron doors, and heavy wooden doors outside, with apertures and hinged shutters for passing food. The cells were about seven by eight feet; they were not heated, except by a stove in the corridor, which did not raise the temperature in some of them above the freezing point." At the time of the construction of the new building, there were 301 inmates in the poor house, of whom 136 were declared to be insane. After 1870 the population of the new insane asylum began to increase at a faster rate than that of the poor house, reflecting the repressed need for such an institution. Within three years the capacity of the new building—three hundred persons—had been filled, and the asylum was overcrowded. Nevertheless, with only minor additions, the same structure was accommodating 592 persons in 1883 and 1,071 in 1890. [68]

Almost from the outset the good intentions of the promoters of the new asylum were frustrated and corrupted by political knavery. As at County Hospital, the staff of the asylum enjoyed a bounteous liquor supply; maintenance funds were grossly mismanaged; needed drugs and foods were denied the medical attendants; the responsible position of ward attendant was filled by political appointees whose coarse brutalities went unnoticed in an insane asylum. Three reputable neurologists—James S. Jewell, Daniel Brower, and Henry M. Lyman—clashed with the political ring controlling the hospital and quickly left its service. The medical superintendent complained heartily in 1877 of interference by the warden of the institution in dietary matters. He reported that he was not allowed to make recommendations with regard to the preparation of food; he was told that "the physician's duties did not extend into the culinary department." He complained also of overcrowding and the resultant fire hazard.[69] The warden, meanwhile, was complacently reporting on the general well-being of the asylum.[70] Gradually the public became aware of conditions and protests were heard from medical and civic groups. The *Chicago Times* in March, 1876, attacked the political corruption which was riddling the institution's effectiveness: [71]

Who enters there must leave hope behind, for the object of its management is not to bring the inmate . . . back to the light of reason, but to make as much out of him as possible during the tenure of the term of the manager, who may be supplanted at any moment. If the wardens and physicians of the insane asylum were something more than mere creatures of a political board, if they had really at heart the mental improvement of the unfortunate people committed to their charge . . . they might make a decided change in the asylum, rendering it immensely more beneficial to the unhappy insane and materially less costly to the general taxpayer.

In 1883 a young man was appointed to the medical staff of the asylum who did not give up the fight against corruption as easily as his predecessors. Shobal V. Clevenger had been recommended by Drs. N. S. Davis and R. L. Rhea for the appointment, but the superintendent of the asylum, J. C. Spray, was forced to take him to Chicago's political boss, Michael McDonald, for confirmation. The following dramatic description of his meeting with "King Mike" is borne out by Clevenger's own account.[72]

To CLEVENGER's astonishment he brought him into a drinking-saloon on Clark street; the proprietor, an ordinary-looking fellow, was leaning on the customer's side of the long counter. SPRAY went over to him and CLEVENGER heard him whisper, "This is the doctor I was telling you about." At these words the saloon-keeper raised himself, looked at CLEVENGER for a moment, nodded quietly, and put out one finger for him to shake. "I congratulate you," smiled SPRAY to CLEVENGER.

Clevenger found the asylum worse than he expected. It was a veritable cesspool of corruption and horror. He was repelled by the bestial treatment of the inmates, the drunken bacchanalian revelries at the taxpayers' expense, the insulting of physicians with impunity by employees sure of their political jobs. Everywhere he found that King Mike's was the ultimate authority. Theft he learned was a common occurrence. The institution was surrounded by "fence houses" and all-night saloons where blankets, food, and the clothing of patients might be exchanged for drink or rendered in payment of gambling losses. He discovered that thousands of curious sight-seers were allowed to tramp around the grounds on Sunday, greatly disturbing the inmates. But his attempts to halt this practice failed because of the effect such a ban would have on certain saloons in the area in which one of the trustees was interested.

The division of authority between laymen and physicians was intolerable to Clevenger. The lay superintendents he characterized as "purely business agents of politicians in the worst sense of the term." On one occasion, when the warden refused to buy some needed medicines because of their high cost, he noted that the next drug account concealed forty-eight cases of beer, ten barrels of whisky, twenty thousand cigars, and other liquor and wines under the appellation "sundry drugs." Complaints about the preparation of food brought no more attention than they did earlier. When Mike Wasserman, later convicted as one of the "boodle commissioners," was shown an iron ring from a pig's snout found in the soup of a patient, he retorted: "Well, what would you have; gold watches?" The mistreatment of inmates Clevenger found the most galling feature of political control of the asylum. Brutal natures, he commented in one paper, were common enough, and it was not strange that their possessors were sometimes given appointment in mental hospitals, but the deliberate appointment of uneducated hoodlums to guard the insane was close to murder: "These weakest and most helpless of humanity are not only liable to be neglected through their filthiness, repulsiveness and burdensomeness, but their irresponsible aggressiveness has often aroused the brutal retaliation of the none too patient or considerate savage, who, all too often, happened to be in charge." [73]

Clevenger sought a hearing from the county commissioners, and then from the State Board of Charities, but these pitiful attempts to combat entrenched corruption were drowned in the furor surrounding the election of 1884. The crusading psychiatrist published during the campaign of that year a request that citizens not vote for the gamblers and thieves who controlled the insane asylum. Following the election he was shot at through the window of his study at the hospital.[74] Clevenger sought the help of the Chicago Medical Society in his drive, but that body, while sympathizing with his objectives, shrank from bold action; only a few doctors, such as Gerhard C. Paoli, strongly supported his crusade. Late in 1885, almost two years after Clevenger began his campaign, the Society appointed a committee to formulate a plan for turning the asylum from its "present authorities to the State Board of Charities." Several months passed before the State Board of Charities came to Chicago for an investigation. Their report, despite its restrained language, confirmed most of Clevenger's charges: [75]

We found that the institution was in effect a part of the Cook County political machine; that the power of appointment . . . was virtually in the hands of the county commissioners; that the inevitable result was laxity of discipline, insubordination on the part of the employees, conflict of authority between the officers, and general bad management. A good deal of intemperance in the use of ardent spirits . . . was clearly shown. The food furnished to patients was . . . inferior. . . . The clothing and bedding were insufficient, especially in view of the fact that the building was insufficiently heated. There appeared to be an unnecessary amount of mechanical restraint of patients, and some cases of absolute cruelty on the part of attendants was brought to our notice under oath. The cost of the institution was found . . . to have been very largely in excess of what it should have been. . . . We were embarrassed in this investigation by the impossibility of obtaining all the evidence we desired. . . . Enough, however, was proven, to confirm our minds in the conviction that the care of the insane should not be entrusted to county authorities. . . .

This report marked the beginning of the end for the political grafters who controlled Chicago. Several of them fled to Canada, including King Mike himself, while the remainder were jailed under the "omnibus boodler" bill. Conditions at the insane asylum improved, but were still far from ideal. Julia Lathrop of Hull House sharply criticized the failure of county authorities to correct all the evils created by their predecessors.[76] The institution of civil service and the appointment of an able staff with complete jurisdiction over the medical care of the inmates did much to improve the morale of employees and patients alike after 1895. An outstanding supervising staff consisting of Archibald Church, Sanger Brown, Richard Dewey, D. W. Lewis, and William Cuthbertson was also appointed in 1895.[77] Not until 1912, however, were the recommendations of the State Board of Charities with respect to turning the asylum over to the state carried out. On July 1, 1912, Cook County transferred to the State of Illinois all the lands, buildings, and equipment relating to the hospital; as the Chicago State Hospital, it continued to play an important role in the care of the mentally ill in Illinois. Located now at the city limits of Chicago in Norwood Park Township, the hospital embraces fifty buildings and one hundred and ten acres of land. The number of patients treated there rose from 2,218 in 1912 to 4,983 in 1949.[78]

The State of Illinois has developed a program of teaching and research in connection with the mental hospitals which it administers. A State Psychopathic Institute was established in 1907 to supervise and instruct physicians in the state hospital service and to conduct research on mental illness. This institute has been located successively on the grounds of the Kankakee, Chicago, Elgin, and again the Chicago state hospitals. An agreement was also reached with the University of Illinois in 1917 on a co-operative plan for research and teaching; a psychiatric service was added to the university's program in 1931 to facilitate this work. In 1942 a large Neuro-Psychiatric Institute was inaugurated under the joint auspices of the university and the Department of Public Welfare. The primary purpose of this project was the instruction of state hospital physicians, as well as students at the university, in mental illness. The institute also afforded excellent opportunities for original research; the care and treatment of patients was a third, but subsidiary, aim of the institute.[79]

After 1940 both city and state have faced the problem of increasing demand for psychiatric and hospital facilities for the mentally ill. There are too few public clinics to meet metropolitan needs. The Cook County Psychopathic Hospital, acting as a kind of clearinghouse for psychiatric cases, reported that most of its patients have received no psychiatric help of any kind prior to their admission. The shortage of trained psychiatrists made it impossible to establish the preventive clinics where incipient cases of mental illness might be halted short of disaster. In the state hospitals, too, there were long waiting lists by the late 1940's for those needing attention. The population of Illinois' nine mental hospitals had risen from 21,000 in 1930 to 32,200 in May, 1946, an increase of 50 per cent in only fifteen years. The increase was unfortunately not accompanied by anything resembling a proportionate expansion of housing facilities.[80]

The United States Public Health Service made a number of recommendations in 1946 designed to shift the emphasis in the state and county programs to prevention of mental illness. A comprehensive child guidance program in the public schools with attention to mental-hygiene problems was suggested, along with a fivefold increase in the psychiatric staff of the Institute for Juvenile Research, a pioneer enterprise in the field of adolescent delinquency.[81] The report called attention also to the pressing need for more inpatient and outpatient psychiatric facilities for Negroes, and for a general liberalizing of the eligibility rules for outpatient psychiatric care. The Cook County Psychopathic Hospital, it was felt, should be replaced with a new four- or five-hundred bed diagnostic and intensive treatment center. The purport of all these recommendations was to discover and treat mental disease before it became a full-blown psychopathic problem.[82]

The two great problems facing all Chicago hospitals today, whether government or voluntary, mental or general, are rising costs and the need for expansion to meet present or future needs. The financial question has been made more difficult by the great increase in necessary drugs, machines, and other costly equipment the expense of which must be passed on to the patient. Many hospitals are in danger of losing their historic function as shelters for the sick poor as they reduce the areas devoted to ward patients in response to the appeals of their business managers. A partial answer to the financial plight of contemporary hospitals has been found in group hospital insurance, financed by voluntary payroll deductions. As the cost of hospital care has shot up in the past fifteen years, enrollment in such plans as the Blue Cross has risen proportionately. The Chicago chapter of the Blue Cross numbered only 31,487 persons in 1938, but the figure jumped to 147,412 in 1940, to 729,671 in 1945, to 1,178,584 in 1947; the Cook County enrollment was estimated at 1,500,000 in January, 1952.[83]

But group insurance may not be the final answer to the problems of the hospitals. It seems doubtful whether existing plans will succeed in enrolling the entire self-supporting population. The greatest potential enemy of group insurance, however, is a failing economy. So long as employment is high, and prosperity is rife, there can be no question that existing plans are capable of caring for a major share of the country's hospitalization problem. But in the event of a severe business depression, the situation could again become acute. In 1934, a survey of Chicago's hospitals showed them to be floundering financially, with half of their beds unoccupied. Government-supported hospitals, at the same time, were overcrowded. Most of the beds in private institutions were reserved for paying patients, while most of their patients were unable to pay. In fact, those unable to make any payment accounted for more than half of the patients admitted to private hospitals in 1933.[84]

The other great problem facing Chicago hospitals at mid-century was the need for expansion. The greatest shortages were evident in the facilities for the care of chronic, mental, and tuberculosis patients. Hospital accommodations for Negroes, who were admitted to relatively few hospitals, even when they carried prepaid hospital insurance, was a special problem. The general situation was shown in the survey made by the United States Public Health Service in 1946, which pointed out that 17,200 beds were required in Chicago to meet the population's immediate need for institutional care, and found a deficiency of 1,700 beds for the care of patients with acute conditions in Cook County outside of Chicago.[85] Thus while hospital conditions had improved almost fantastically with the advent of modern medicine, they were yet far from perfect and, indeed, in terms of the possibilities offered by modern medicine, far from even adequate.

	Public Health Work
Chapter XI	
	in Chicago

The translation of the discoveries of modern medicine into practical results at the bedside is the most important medical problem facing human society today. The state of public health, one authority has suggested, is the "ultimate test of medical science." [1] One of the severest indictments of the contemporary world is the melancholy fact that millions of human beings continue to die from diseases which are remediable, if not preventable, by existing knowledge and techniques. The great masses of humanity in poverty-ridden Asia are the worst sufferers from man's inability to solve the technical, political, and socio-economic problems which keep at least half of the world's people in a semiprimitive bondage of superstition, ignorance, and deprivation. But the so-called "backward areas" of the globe are not the only regions suffering from preventable diseases. There are great inequities between areas of the United States in the matter of health services; for example, large areas in the South are still subject to high mortality and morbidity rates for the common communicable diseases. And even in Chicago, the medical center of the Middle West, an investigation in 1950 disclosed that more than a thousand persons with tuberculosis of infectious type were unhospitalized because of the lack of beds at the municipal sanitarium. [2]

The degree of public responsibility for the health of individual members of society has been raised considerably in the course of the last century. In 1850 public health measures were undertaken only during epidemics and other emergencies; even then they were suspect to some citizens and physicians. The care of the sick, it was felt, was the exclusive domain of the physician, and governmental interference was tolerated only when the profession could not or

175

would not act. The physician was usually willing to transfer the care of paupers and the insane to public authority because their treatment was a burdensome and normally unremunerated task; he welcomed too the co-operation of city officials in time of sharp epidemic since their power made possible an overall planning in meeting an attack; but he tended to view with suspicion, if not outright hostility, the provision by government of drugs and medical care to any but the most destitute. In view of decades of close-range experience with corrupt political mismanagement of local public health agencies, the reluctance of Chicago physicians to warmly endorse the expansion of government into medicine is not surprising. In the past hundred years, however, private physicians have consented to an increasing amount of community, state, and federal activity in the field of medicine. The federal government has assumed responsibility for the medical care of special classes of patients, notably veterans and certain federal workers; states have taken over almost completely the expense of hospitalization for tuberculosis and mental disease; and local communities have taken special interest in an increasing number of contagious diseases, in infant care, in the distribution of antitoxins and serums, as well as in the hospitalization and treatment of the poor.

In Chicago's early years, public action in health matters hinged upon the presence or absence of epidemic disease. An attack of smallpox or cholera was sufficient to launch a wave of sanitary and protective measures to guard the city's health, but with the passing of the epidemic, the old apathy returned. The town's first Board of Health was called into existence in 1834 to meet the threat of cholera. The board lasted long enough to witness the inauguration of Chicago's first sanitary regulation: every male over twenty-one years was required to work upon the streets and alleys under the supervision of the street commissioner. Failure to work or furnish a substitute was punished by a fine of five dollars. A permanent Board of Health of seven members was authorized in 1835 and given the power to inspect streets, alleys, and buildings. Where infractions of sanitary practices were found, the board could require owners "to remove all of the predisposing causes of disease." There is no record, however, that the board ever acted or existed in more than name at this time.[3]

When Chicago was incorporated in 1837, the city charter provided for a three-member Board of Health and a health officer authorized to visit persons suffering from infectious disease and board vessels suspected of harboring pestilence.[4] Daniel Brainard was chosen Chicago's first health officer but held the position only one year, when he was appointed to the Board of Health. The board was inactive for the most part until 1843 when a smallpox threat stirred up some enthusiasm. The city's first hospital was built in response to this attack.

Throughout the 1840's and 1850's the pendulum swung back and forth between feverish effort and lethargy. The smallpox epidemic of 1848 was met by the combined efforts of the board and the medical profession. A number of physicians volunteered to vaccinate the poor free of charge; the city marshal made their names public with the urgent request that the unprotected poor take advantage of the opportunity. A cholera epidemic the following year called forth more vigorous efforts. A thorough clean-up campaign was undertaken well in advance of the appearance of the disease. Once the contagion had spread, a cholera hospital was opened with Levi D. Boone, city health officer, in charge. Boone reported in August that the scourge was waning, and that the hospital could be closed in a few days. Fifty-nine patients, he wrote, had been admitted to the temporary hospital, while he had treated many more outside.[5]

During the middle fifties, Chicago was relatively free from smallpox and cholera—the only diseases which seemed to require municipal action—and the powers of the Board of Health were reduced accordingly. The financial depression of 1857 accentuated a growing feeling that the board was something of a luxury. It was therefore abolished altogether and its duties transferred to the Police Department. For a full decade, the city functioned without any health supervisory body and with no full-time health officer. An outbreak of smallpox in 1862 caused the City Council to appoint an acting health officer to work with the Police Department, but his tenure and duties were so severely circumscribed as to make the position virtually meaningless. Not until 1867, on the heels of another dreadful cholera epidemic, was the Board of Health re-created.[6]

A permanent city hospital, meanwhile, had been constructed in 1857 but the economic depression, coupled with the inability of the regular physicians to come to some agreement with the homeopaths as to its management, resulted, as stated before, in its abandonment even before the first patient was admitted. It was leased to a private group of physicians until military authorities commandeered it during the Civil War. Finally, in 1864, the hospital was reopened as a public enterprise, this time as the first Cook County Hospital. The institution fulfilled the obligation of county authorities to care for the sick poor of the whole county; the city was charged only with preventive measures against epidemics and the care of victims of contagious disease at this time.

Another important public health function, however, was assumed by the city in the 1850's, when the Board of Health began keeping a record of vital statistics. The early returns were far from satisfactory. They were, first of all, incomplete, since the ordinance governing the reporting of births and deaths was poorly enforced; and secondly, the nomenclature used by physicians in reporting deaths was exceedingly vague and unscientific. In 1851, for example, five people were reported dead of "decline," two died of "delirium," one of "cold," and one by "visit of Providence." [7] The following year fifteen persons perished from the "effect of traveling." Dr. N. S. Davis and others pleaded for stricter registration laws for burials and births. Davis took his fight to the Common Council in 1864; when told that the expense of his program would be too great, he volunteered the services of the Chicago Medical Society in tabulating the returns.[8] Gradually the system of recording was improved and Chicago's birth and mortality statistics became more reliable.

The city broadened its interest in medical matters to include a coroner's office in 1864. Ernst Schmidt, German liberal and friend of Rudolph Virchow, was elected the city's first coroner on the Republican ticket that year. He resigned the following year, claiming that political interference prevented him from making the dissections and post-mortem studies that he wished. Eventually, the position of coroner became a political plum and the real medical work was performed by the coroner's physician. The first such physician was Ludvig Hektoen, appointed in 1890. Hektoen made good use of his office, compiling many pathological reports of considerable importance. A number of other outstanding physicians, including E. R. LeCount, like Hektoen a student of Christian Fenger, held the office. LeCount collected during his lifetime ninety-nine fully indexed volumes of medico-legal problems with which he had dealt. A number of reforms in the work of the coroner's office have been introduced in the twentieth century. Dr. Herman Bundesen, for example, who held the office of coroner from 1928 to 1931, brought numerous changes to the routine of the office, and established an advisory committee of eminent pathologists.[9]

One of the most important aspects of public health work in a modern city is the assurance of general sanitary conditions, particularly with respect to water supply and the disposal of wastes. The growth of the public health movement in the nineteenth century was largely a matter of spreading the gospel of cleanliness and prophylaxis. Long before the germ theory was enunciated, sanitarians and health workers sought to convince communities of the preventive value of general cleanliness. Though public health work was given a tremendous boost by the demonstration of the pathogenic role of bacteria in disease, the empirically based health measures of the years before 1880 were not without effect. Attention was directed earlier to the effect of these measures on Chicago's mortality rate despite the disorder, confusion, and overcrowding attending the city's growth. The great value of the germ theory was the sharper direction it gave to health work, the increased public support for health programs which it inspired, and the immunization techniques which it made possible. The physician of 1900, however, even with his superior knowledge, could scarcely have improved on N. S. Davis' definition of the scope of "modern medicine" a half century earlier. Medicine, said Davis in 1853, included "the relations of man to the air he breathes, the earth he walks upon, and all the other elements around us. Hence the modern improvements in the construction of dwellings; the greater care to preserve pure air and good water; the reservation of ample parks, wide streets, and efficient sewers in all large cities, has not only prevented disease and lengthened the average duration of human life, but they have vastly enlarged the field of human happiness." [10]

Davis was active in sanitation work all through his long life. As early as 1854 he was appointed chairman of a Chicago Medical Society committee to investigate sanitary conditions in the city.[11] For many years the work of Davis and the Medical Society supplemented that of city authorities in erasing conditions prejudicial to health. The Society frequently criticized the city's water supply, which after 1853 was drawn from Lake Michigan by means of a wooden inlet six hundred feet long. Physicians and other critics complained that the sewage-filled Chicago River emptied into the lake in the vicinity of the crude inlet.[12] The city sought to solve the drainage problem by the use of canal pumps which, it was hoped, would create a backward current in the river and thus cause the stream to cleanse itself. But the pumps proved futile in combating the volume of sewage and refuse which an expanding city dumped daily into the river. The quality of the city's water grew worse. "At times," recalled several *Chicago Tribune* editors, "the stench in dwellings from the fearful water was intolerable. It was not only black, with a shocking odor, it was greasy to the touch." Finally, in 1864, ground was broken for an engineering venture which brought Chicago the attention of the scientific world. A tunnel, measuring five feet square, was laid two miles out into the lake. This project was brought to completion in 1867, and complaints about the city's water slackened off for a number of years.[13]

The problem of sewerage in the young city was first approached in 1855. Physicians had pointed for some time to the need for a system of sewers to handle the increasing volume of wastes being piled in alleys or dumped in the Chicago River. A Board of Sewerage Commissioners was created in 1855 and the city's first sewers were constructed the following year. The effectiveness of these early sewers was evidenced in the falling mortality rate after 1856. For the six years from 1849 through 1854 the death rate was more than double that of the six years following 1856. In the early sixties the duties of the sewerage commissioners were turned over to the Board of Public Works. With this change the construction of new sewers failed to keep pace with the growth of population and the death rate mounted. In 1867, with the creation of a new and more powerful Board of Health, interest in the disposal of wastes was revived and strengthened.[14]

It was the great cholera outbreak of 1866 which impressed members of the City Council with the need for a new Board of Health. The relative freedom of the city from epidemic disease, coupled with the general preoccupation with the Civil War, had engendered an attitude of indifference to public health problems. This indifference soon gave way to panic as reports of the impending cholera invasion reached the city. The council appointed a committee late in 1865 to investigate the sanitary condition of Chicago. The committee chairman, N. S. Davis, urged on the council the necessity of forcing landowners to connect their lots with city sewers; he recommended a scavenger service to remove all garbage and refuse, and a more vigilant patrol of the river to prevent the dumping of decomposable matter. A rigid inspection of the city's privies, slaughtering plants, and factories, he said, was a pressing necessity, along with regulations to prevent overcrowding in boarding and tenement houses. The city authorities took hasty steps to implement Davis' program; additional appropriations were made to finance a vigorous cleaning and inspection campaign under the joint supervision of the boards of Police and Public Works.[15]

But the campaign proved futile. Cholera struck in the summer of 1866. The numbers stricken by the disease mounted steadily until October, when the great fatality induced a near riot in the city. Many of the city officials lay dead of the disease; Professor Brainard of Rush Medical College perished a few hours after an onslaught of the dreaded scourge; the students of Rush held a protest meeting and decided to return to their homes; the hospitals were totally inadequate to house the sick and dying. The foolhardiness of the short-sighted economies of the preceding decade was now starkly clear. The City Council was anxious to make amends with all possible dispatch. A permanent Board of Health was established in 1867 with authority independent of the City Council and the police. It was consciously modeled along the lines of New York's Metropolitan Board of Health, which had enjoyed more success in staving off the epidemic. Of the seven members constituting the board, three were to be physicians; all appointments were made by the mayor and judges of the Superior Court. A corps of health officers including sixteen sanitary inspectors with police powers was made responsible to the board. The state of public excitement at this time was reflected in the petition which the board received shortly after its organization; signed by four thousand citizens, it requested the board to exercise its full powers to prevent the reappearance of cholera during the coming season.[16]

Within the year following its establishment, the new board went far to justify the public confidence which it inspired. By the end of 1868, 230,000 of the city's 241,000 inhabitants had been vaccinated against smallpox, the inspection of slaughterhouses and their products had been inaugurated, and the city's sewerage system was greatly extended. The following year attention was given to milk inspection for the first time. The board also improved the registration system for births and deaths, required the vaccination of all children, and undertook the forcible removal of epidemic victims to the contagious disease hospital. When the Great Fire leveled the city in 1871, the board had thrust upon it the herculean task of guarding the health of the sick and homeless. Ninety-three thousand persons were without homes in the months following the fire; the crowded, temporary barracks were subjected to daily inspections by sanitary officers. The sick and injured were cared for in hospitals, churches, and schoolhouses; ambulatory patients were requested to report to dispensaries established at convenient points about the city. Only physicians who served gratuitously were allowed to give treatment at these stations. Vaccination against smallpox was made a condition upon which relief supplies were issued to the needy. But despite these measures, the death rate rose ominously in the aftermath of the fire. Over two thousand persons contracted smallpox in 1872, and more than a fourth of these died. The fatality among children under five was the highest ever recorded. Only gradually was the health of the city re-established.[17]

The man most responsible for the successes of the restored Board of Health was John H. Rauch. Born in Lebanon, Pennsylvania, in 1828, Rauch graduated in medicine from the University of Pennsylvania at the age of twenty-one, and received an appointment to the faculty of Rush Medical College in 1857. An amateur geologist, Rauch made a valuable ichthyologic collection from the Upper Mississippi Valley for Louis Agassiz in the years before the Civil War. During the war, Rauch served as a volunteer on Gen. David Hunter's staff at Bull Run, and later as a camp sanitarian. His war experience confirmed his impressions of the value of sanitation to health and gave him excellent training in administration. Upon his return to Chicago, he immediately threw himself into the battle for better sanitation. He waged a partly successful campaign against intramural interments. At the same time he urged the establishment of a system of parks, which he called "the people's gardens,—the places to which the overtasked laborer and mechanic of the overcrowded city can . . . resort to breathe the breath of God's pure air, inhale the odors of fresh, blooming flowers, and enjoy the pleasures of a rural retreat." [18] His efforts were primarily responsible for spacious Lincoln Park in Chicago. When the city re-created its health board in 1867, Rauch was appointed sanitary superintendent. It was during his regime that the advances discussed above occurred.

With the creation of a state board of health in 1877, Rauch was chosen its first president. As president and later as secretary, this pioneer sanitarian accomplished much in improving the health of his adopted state. During his fourteen-year association with the state board, nearly every child in the state was vaccinated, exhaustive studies in stream pollution were made, physical examinations of immigrants were sporadically undertaken, rules and regulations regarding quarantine and sanitation were laid down, vital statistics were collected and published for the first time, and the state was virtually cleansed of unqualified practitioners of medicine. The regulation of medical practice was one of the important functions assigned to the board in 1877, and Rauch acquired a reputation as the "John the Baptist of education reform" in the Middle West.[19] Through Rauch the influence of the country's foremost sanitarians was felt in the West, for he was very active in the national public health movement. He participated in the formation of the American Public Health Association in 1872, and four years later became its president. With Rauch's resignation from the board in 1891, Illinois lost its most important figure in the development of the public health movement in the state.[20]

Rauch's association with public health work in Illinois coincided with the high tide of empirical sanitation in the United States. During this prebacteriological period, the origin of disease in filth was widely held to be the basis for sanitary action. This was the time when the teachings of the German sanitarian, Max von Pettenkofer, and his English counterparts, Chadwick, Simon, and Murchison, reached their largest audience in America. The "sanitary awakening" in the United States first found concrete expression in Samuel Shattuck's *Report of the Massachusetts Sanitary Commission* in 1850, but was not long confined to the Massachusetts area.[21] Shattuck and his contemporaries gave great attention to general cleanliness as a preventive of disease. In cases where no visible filth was apparent, they suspected sewer gas or other effluvia as causative agents. Public support for proposed sanitary projects was requested on the strength of an observed cause and effect relationship between dirt, faulty drainage or plumbing, on the one hand, and communicable disease on the other.[22] When Rauch sought municipal backing for a sewerage extension program in 1873, he wisely pointed to the statistical relationship between the prevalence of illness in certain wards and the amount of sewerage in those areas.[23] While knowing nothing of the germ theory—his writings reveal no acquaintance with it at this time—his observations carried sufficient truth to be practicable. The germ theory served only to make communities more exacting in their cleanliness; dirt, one writer has pointed out, "is the nurse, if not the mother, of disease." [24]

The health functions of the city government in Chicago were reorganized in 1876 under a department of health. The position of commissioner of health was created and tendered to Brockholst McVickar, one of the city's pioneer physicians. McVickar accepted the post, but retained it only a few months. He was succeeded by another important figure in the development of Chicago's public health program, Oscar Coleman De Wolf. De Wolf was given the appointment at the suggestion of Dr. Henry I. Bowditch, a famous Boston physician. A native of Massachusetts, De Wolf had first studied medicine at the Berkshire Medical College. After two years of further study in Paris, he had returned to the United States in 1860, just in time to enter the Union army. With his Chicago appointment following the war, De Wolf was free to give trial to certain ideas on health and sanitation which he had long entertained. One of his first steps was to attack the problem of scarlet fever and diphtheria control by requiring the use of warning cards on infected houses. He also gained some enemies among the medical profession in Chicago by his vigorous enforcement of regulations governing the reporting of communicable diseases. His administration was marked by a progressive attitude toward new developments in medicine and sanitation; the first laboratory in connection with the health department was opened under his direction in 1880. [25]

But De Wolf's most significant reforms were directed at the abuses of the health of Chicago's citizens by the manufactories springing up all over the city. Workshop and factory inspection was undertaken for the first time during his tenure in office; attempts were made to demonstrate the link between mortality rates and unhealthful working and living conditions. His biggest battle was with the packing houses which sought to thwart necessary sanitary regulations by every means at their disposal, fair and foul. The menace to health from the offal dumped in river and lake, quite apart from working conditions within the plants, was a serious health problem. Against determined opposition and legal reverses, De Wolf succeeded in forcing the packers beyond 39th Street, then the southern boundary of the city. [26] For political reasons, De Wolf was removed from office after the municipal elections of 1889, despite a strong recommendation from the Chicago Medical Society that he be retained by the incoming administration. [27]

The relations of city health officers with the public and with the medical profession were not consistently good during this period. Although the Board of Health had been resuscitated in response to popular demand in 1867, the public did not forfeit its right to criticize what it thought to be unnecessary or extravagant expenditures. When the board sought funds to combat an expected invasion of cholera in 1871, the short-memoried City Council was reluctant to provide them.[28] Supported by a section of the city's press, the council claimed that the board was squandering the monies already assigned for its use. On numerous occasions the worth of the board was questioned by local editors. It was less than an ornament, commented the *Chicago Times* in 1876; it was a nuisance. Ridicule was heaped on health officers who "POUNCE DOWN UPON A GROCERY once in a while and condemn a dozen rotten eggs,—only that, and nothing more." The budget for health activities, the editor continued, could be cut in half by disposing of all but the sanitary superintendent, smallpox hospital, and scavenger work. It was even suggested that the work of the board be turned back to the Police Department.[29]

The board was under fire also from the city's physicians who felt that swift action should be taken well in advance of expected epidemics. Medical critics seldom took cognizance of the financial dependence of the board on an unpredictable, economy-minded City Council. The editors of the *Chicago Medical Journal* charged health officers with inefficiency on several occasions during the 1870's for failing to ready the city for cholera attacks which did not materialize. In 1873 they called for the abolition altogether of the Board of Health.[30] Criticism from doctors, like that from the general public, reached a peak of indignation just before the board's reorganization in 1876. But even after the reorganization, the new Department of Health was called "little more than a bureau of registration of births and deaths." [31]

Greater public confidence in the work of the health department had to await the fuller realization of its value which came in the wake of the microbe-hunting excitement of the closing decades of the century. The germ theory, despite considerable opposition, gained steadily in favor among laymen as well as doctors in the 1880's. With the solution of the two riddles left by Pasteur—the occurrence of infectious disease among those who had no direct contact with the sick, and the failure of all persons in contact with disease germs to contract infection—support for the bacterial origin of disease became virtually universal.[32] The application of bacteriology to public health work in the United States began in Boston and New York. In the former city, the Massachusetts Institute of Technology developed a school of scientific sanitation, making use of recent discoveries in bacteriology, which maintained close relations with the Massachusetts State Board of Health. The board was reorganized in 1886 and an experiment station established the following year at Lawrence, where much of the fundamental knowledge underlying modern methods of sewage treatment was subsequently gained.

In New York the public health movement was given tremendous impetus by the work of Herman M. Biggs, who joined the staff of the recently founded Carnegie Laboratory in 1885. With T. Mitchell Prudden, he worked out the basis for a practical application of the new knowledge of bacteriology to health work. In 1892, at the insistence of Biggs and Prudden, New York established a division of pathology, bacteriology, and disinfection in its health department. From this point on, the medical laboratory became the fountainhead for much of the progress in public health work in America.[33]

The year after New York established its new division, the Chicago Department of Health took its first important step in coordinating knowledge of bacteriology with its health protection program. A deputy commissioner of health was authorized in 1893 to take charge of a new Bureau of Milk Inspection. Drs. E. B. Stuart and Adolph Gehrmann, two pioneer Chicago bacteriologists, made the first microscopical examinations of milk samples in the city.[34] In September, 1893, the bureau was placed under direct supervision of the Department of Health and a few months later, Gehrmann was made its director. As the only municipal laboratory, the bureau was soon expanded to take on new tasks. Routine examinations of throat cultures for diphtheria were begun in 1894 and the production of antitoxin was undertaken on a small scale the following year. By 1896 the laboratory was also examining ice samples and smallpox vaccines, conducting the Widal test for typhoid fever, and diagnosing suspected cases of rabies.[35] The health department, meanwhile, had been expanding its work in other directions. An effective "boil the water" crusade against typhoid was waged in 1893–1894; the public was circularized on the hot-weather care of babies in 1894; and a campaign against infant mortality in the summer of 1899 enlisted the support of a voluntary corps of seventy-three physicians.[36]

But the general sanitary condition of the city in the 1890's was still poor by modern standards. In the suburbs and outlying districts, unsanitary pumps and wells were still in service; the city's milk supply was at best adulterated, at worst contaminated; many streets were still unpaved; refuse and garbage were still dumped into alleys in many sections, and rarely was a garbage can found to be covered.[37] The city's water supply, moreover, was frequently impure. The new drainage canal was not opened until 1900; citizens were still pouring sewage into Lake Michigan in the 1890's and then drinking the lake water. The editor of the *British Medical Journal*, while visiting the Columbian Exposition in 1893, condemned the city for its lack of concern about its drinking water: [38]

I will say . . . that if it be the policy of your rulers to persist in fouling this magnificent source of water supply by continuing to pour this mass of sewage into it, in the vain belief that they can rely upon currents or reversing engines, or winds, which always go wrong. . . . If they are determined to do that; if they won't carry all their water cribs out four miles, insist upon their having subsidence and filtration . . . [then] it is criminal to give [it] to the poor, who cannot buy artificial water and who cannot always boil their water.

It may be more than coincidence that later that same year the health commissioner admitted the close causal relation between Chicago's water supply and the high typhoid incidence, suggesting filtration as possibly a better remedy than extension of the intakes any farther into the lake.[39]

Popular reaction to the changing scientific view of the origin of typhoid fever was destined to force city authorities into a reconsideration of the city's needs with regard to sewage disposal and a pure water supply. Before Eberth's discovery of the typhoid bacillus in 1880, it had been the common practice everywhere to empty filthy privy vaults and overflowing cesspools into common sewers which discharged into the nearest body of water. But after 1880 increased attention was given to complete separation of sewage outlets from water intakes, and treatment of sewage to render it innocuous before emptying it into lakes or streams.[40] In 1893 the first open filter of the slow sand type in the United States was put into operation at Lawrence, Massachusetts; the first mechanical filter was demonstrated later that same year before the International Congress of Hygiene. The treatment of water by chlorination, which antedated the germ theory, was employed more extensively than filters, however, because of the relatively small expense involved. The first commercial use of chlorine in sewage treatment was made at the Union Stock Yards in Chicago in 1908.[41]

Chicago's new drainage canal, which was to divert all sewage from the lake, was put into operation in 1900. Since the canal now emptied into the Illinois and Mississippi rivers, a number of states, especially Missouri, objected to the project. "Chicago's great open sewer," charged a member of the Missouri State Board of Health, would bring disease and epidemic to St. Louis and other cities.[42] Extensive preliminary studies had been made, however, by E. O. Jordan, professor of bacteriology at the University of Chicago and F. R. Zeit, professor of pathology and bacteriology at Northwestern University Medical School, which showed that all pollution caused by Chicago's sewage disappeared from the river system completely before reaching Peoria. Missouri, nevertheless, took the whole matter to the federal courts, where a decision was ultimately made in favor of the Chicago and Illinois defendants.[43]

Further steps were taken in the second decade of the new century to ensure a safe water supply. In 1913 sterilization of Chicago's water was begun, and four years later the entire supply was being sterilized. The effect of these measures on the city's typhoid fever rate was dramatic; from second highest rating among twenty of the nation's largest cities in 1881, Chicago fell to lowest by 1917. For the five-year period, from 1917 to 1922, Chicago's rate was far below that of any of the other nineteen cities.[44]

The reporting of communicable diseases in Chicago, while keeping pace with new developments in sanitation and public health work, was still far from satisfactory. There were numerous complaints concerning the inadequacy and lack of completeness of Chicago's records. In an address before the Chicago Medical Society in 1893, the editor of the *British Medical Journal* assailed the woefully incomplete statistics he had found in the city. The instability of political appointments, he conjectured, was responsible for the unreliability and lack of uniformity of the records. He accused city officials of manipulating the figures so as to show Chicago's mortality as "delightfully low." By announcing only the death rate, and failing to provide information on the birth rate and mean age in the city, these officials were giving outsiders the erroneous impression that Chicago was unusually healthy. "Then all we can say of the health of Chicago," he concluded, "is that in a population of unknown age and undoubtedly recruited from persons in the fullness and strength of life, the mortality is only seventeen per 1,000." [45]

The main obstacle in the path of a more dependable system of reporting contagious disease was a long dispute between the Department of Health and the city's physicians. Laws existed requiring all doctors to report immediately all cases of certain classes of communicable illness, but for this service doctors felt they should receive twenty-five cents for each report, as the state law provided with respect to the reporting of births. But the City Council did not see fit to appropriate funds to reimburse physicians for their trouble. The health department, saddled with the duty of compiling statistics with regard to contagious disease, was forced to seek the co-operation of physicians, even though they were not paid. Many refused to assist in the program. Commissioner John D. Ware prosecuted physicians who did not comply with the law. The Chicago Medical Society protested this action in 1892, emphasizing that "the principle at issue is whether our services can be extracted without pay." Ware reproached the recalcitrant physicians in his report the following year. The justification that they were not paid a fee he termed "an excuse unworthy of any physician." The department, he asserted, printed the postal blanks and distributed them free to any doctor requesting them. Ware's successor, Arthur R. Reynolds, vetoed the principle of prosecuting physicians for failure to co-operate with the department; he tried instead persuasion and appeal. But the results were equally unsatisfactory. New regulations were finally drawn up in 1904 which made the immediate reporting of certain diseases compulsory; no mention was made of compensation. This move was roundly condemned by many medical groups in the city. One journal used the epithet "slave labor" to describe the physician's new status.[46] The controversy dragged on for a few more years but gradually disappeared.

About the time the physicians gave up their fight, the Department of Health was winning new prestige and public confidence under the administration of William A. Evans (1907–1911). The most notable advance registered under Evans' leadership was a milk pasteurization program which became the basis for Chicago's compulsory pasteurization ordinance in 1909, the first such law in the

United States. Milk inspection had begun in 1877, but the search for disease germs was not inaugurated until 1893. The presence of formaldehyde poison to prevent souring was first detected in 1900 and soon eliminated. Evans, however, was first to consider the prohibition of nonpasteurized milk from the city. In this he met considerable opposition from the medical profession, notably from the Chicago Medical Society. The argument of this group, as expressed by an editorial in the *Medical Standard*, was that pasteurization would discourage cleanliness and prophylaxis in the production of milk and reduce all milk to the "dead-level standard of Pasteurization." The Medical Society established its own milk commission in 1909 precisely to assure a clean and wholesome milk supply, without pasteurization, to the city's invalids, infants, and others in need of pure milk.[47] Instead of pasteurizing milk, the commission undertook the certification of certain sources as pure after a rigid inspection of the milk, dairies, and cows of producers who wished the Society's endorsement. Pasteurization, supporters of the certification program claimed, had still other objectionable features. It did not destroy the tuberculosis and certain other bacilli. The consumer, moreover, had a right to "live" rather than "cooked" milk if such was his choice. Later, the health department steadily expanded its supervisory activity over the production and distribution of milk. A milk ordinance was passed in 1935 which greatly strengthened the hand of the department; the sanitation rating of Chicago's milk has shot up from 59 per cent in 1935 to well over 90 per cent in recent years. The main problem facing milk sanitarians in the late 1940's, according to a United States Public Health Service survey, was the raising of standards in certain Cook County communities—Evanston, Oak Park, and La Grange—where the milk rating was still less than the recommended 90 per cent.[48]

Commissioner Evans was responsible for a number of other innovations in Chicago's health program. He was especially interested in tuberculosis. The first tuberculin testing of dairy cows was introduced at his suggestion, and the Municipal Tuberculosis Sanitarium was opened during his administration. School health and nursing services were also inaugurated during Evans' years as health commissioner. His was the initiative, too, behind the first real enforcement of existing regulations regarding food-handling establishments; the basement bakeries which had flourished under his predecessors were at last ordered closed. A baby welfare campaign was commenced in 1908; one hundred physicians were dispatched to the poorer, congested areas of the city to instruct mothers in the care of their infants. A short-lived municipal venereal disease clinic was opened in 1910, and the department began making Wassermann tests the following year. It was Evans, finally, who was responsible for the organization of a School of Sanitary Instruction, whose weekly bulletin provided valuable information on health matters to the general public.[49]

The work of the Chicago health department was supplemented during these years by the state public health program. For a number of decades after its creation in 1877, the chief efforts of the Illinois Board of Health were concentrated on the regulation of medical practice. It was widely believed before 1900 that the most important step in raising the level of health in the state was the elevation of standards of medical education and practice. This has been characterized as the "good doctors theory" of public health; well-trained doctors, according to this view, meant a healthy population. But by 1900 James Egan, secretary of the board, was championing the separation of sanitary work from the regulation of medical practice. More of the board's time was now given to water supplies, milk, stream pollution, and the control of infectious diseases. In 1907, provision was made for the free distribution of diphtheria antitoxin in Illinois.[50] A survey made by the United States Public Health Service in 1915 resulted in strong recommendations that the health functions of the board be grouped together in one department, and that legislation be passed requiring fuller co-operation by the public and medical profession in the gathering of vital statistics.[51] These recommendations were carried out within two years following the report. A State Department of Public Health was created in 1917, devoted exclusively to sanitary and disease control work, while the registration and licensing of physicians was made the responsibility of a new State Department of Registration and Education. The health department was provided with a greatly enlarged budget and immediately became an important buttress to Illinois communities in their fight to raise the general level of health.[52]

A remarkable change in the nature of state and local health activities became apparent as the twentieth century wore on. During the preceding century, departments of health had been concerned almost exclusively with the acute epidemic diseases, typhoid fever, smallpox, cholera, and, toward the end of the century, diphtheria.

After 1900 the attention of health officers was directed more and more against the last strongholds of disease which might yield to sanitary and hygienic measures. Pneumonia, tuberculosis, venereal disease, and the care of infants and children were the subjects of increasing concern as the mortality from the more acute infectious ailments dropped lower and lower. The Chicago Department of Health, as early as 1894, noted the decline of croup, diarrhea, diphtheria, dysentery, malaria, measles, typhoid fever, and whooping cough in the city, while warning of the rising fatality from heart disease, cancer, Bright's disease, pneumonia, and cholera infantum. Commissioner Reynolds claimed credit for sanitary improvements in reducing the mortality from the first group, but pleaded the helplessness of the department to combat the rise in degenerative diseases. The mortality rate from cancer alone had risen 812 per cent in forty-four years, according to his computations, though he doubtless failed to allow for increasingly accurate diagnosis as a factor in the increase. Typhoid fever, smallpox, and cholera had all but disappeared by 1910, while the discoveries of von Behring and Schick made possible an all but perfect system of diphtheria control. The influenza outbreak of 1918 was Chicago's last experience with a large-scale epidemic of an acute infectious disease.[53]

While sanitary prophylaxis and immunization were scoring the last of their spectacular triumphs over the communicable diseases, new attacks against other unsolved health problems were organized. The control of tuberculosis and the acute respiratory diseases, and the reduction of infant mortality, were the greatest problems facing health officers in the first decade of the new century. An antituberculosis crusade was begun in the middle of the decade. The disease was made reportable in 1908, an antispitting campaign was prosecuted with vigor, a state law was passed in 1908 providing for the establishment by municipalities of sanitaria, and the Municipal Tuberculosis Sanitarium was authorized by a Chicago referendum the following year. The problem of tuberculosis was slow to yield to systematic control. The attack on pneumonia yielded even less satisfactory results; this disease continued to exact a heavy toll of life despite fresh-air campaigns, warnings against chilling, and advice on proper clothing.

The first serious attempt at the control of venereal disease was made in 1911, when the city's segregated vice district was abolished. Up to that time, syphilis, gonorrhea, and other "social diseases" had been considered beyond the pale of proper conversation, let alone public discussion or action. As late as 1884 the city officially regarded syphilis as more crime than illness, refusing to admit indigent cases of primary syphilis to County Hospital or any other charitable institution.[54] The first permanent municipal clinic treating venereal afflictions was not opened until the close of the First World War, when the city could no longer ignore the marked increase in these diseases engendered by the moral laxity of wartime. No important inroads were made against this class of diseases, however, until Herman Bundesen convinced the city in the 1920's and 1930's of the necessity of treating them as urgent public health problems.

Bundesen was made commissioner of health in 1922 and promptly began a campaign against venereal disease. His bold and unprecedented program envisioned a combination of prevention, through education, and the distribution of prophylactic outfits in brothels, public rest rooms, and drug stores, with intensive treatment at municipal clinics. His conception of the problem was totally practical and hygienic, amoral rather than cynical. But his suggestions met, nevertheless, a storm of public disapproval. He was opposed by virtually every newspaper and medical journal in Chicago. The *Illinois Medical Journal* called his plan "revolting," while the *Chicago Medical Recorder* quoted with approval the following *non sequitur*: "God forbid that above the Stars and Stripes any misguided, theoretical radical shall ever place the flag of Priapus and the bar sinister of the Phallic Symbol." The *Medical Standard* decried this "outrageous and unlicensed" exercise of the health commissioner's power.[55] The opposition of the medical profession, curiously enough, was based on moral rather than medical grounds. No one seemed interested to inquire whether the health department program would actually stamp out the scourge of syphilis. Bundesen answered his critics with the observation that attacks on venereal disease had traditionally been carried out along moral and educational lines, but had failed; why not try another method? If personal morality had failed, why not try personal hygiene?[56] But Bundesen was forced to retreat before the combined force of public and professional indignation; more than a decade was to pass before he had an opportunity to renew the fight. The unrealistic light in which the whole question was debated reflected the bewildered and confused reaction of an older generation to the loosening of moral and religious ties, with

the accompanying revolt against social restraint, which characterized the "jazz age" of the 1920's. Realism, Bundesen learned, was not
the order of the day.

Bundesen found the public reception of his infant welfare
program more sympathetic. An intensive parental education campaign was undertaken in the 1920's, resulting in a marked decrease
in infant deaths. The death rate dropped from 89.3 per thousand in
1921 to 76.9 in 1924 and 62.8 in 1927, the year of Bundesen's dismissal from the department.[57] Another important factor in the decline, probably, was the drive to detect all tuberculous cows in the
Chicago area and destroy them. Over 400,000 such cows were killed
during the drive. Bundesen's forced resignation in 1927 came as an
indirect result of his infant health program. When Mayor "Big Bill"
Thompson demanded that the health department include political
literature with the information about baby care which it distributed
to all Chicago mothers, Bundesen refused to comply and subsequently tendered his resignation. The *Chicago Daily News*, struck by
the injustice of Thompson's action, immediately presented the ex-
health commissioner one thousand dollars as the "city's most valuable citizen." Even the City Council presented him with a scroll
expressing its appreciation of his work.[58] The editors of the official
organ of the American Public Health Association protested Thompson's action bitterly.[59] Political corruption, however, was at its postwar heyday, and protests were little availing. Following Bundesen's
retirement, the Sanitary District became involved in one of the
worst scandals of municipal history when the grossest misuse of funds
was conclusively proved.[60]

Bundesen's career was far from ended by Thompson's ill-con-
sidered action. He ran for coroner shortly after his dismissal and was
elected by a majority of over one million votes. In 1930, with Anton
Cermak as mayor, Bundesen was reappointed to his old job of
health commissioner. An intensive campaign to eradicate diphtheria
completely through immunization was soon begun, and the drive
against needless infant deaths was taken up with renewed vigor. In
1936 Chicago registered the lowest infant mortality rate of any large
city in the United States. Commissioner Bundesen suffered some
diminution of his prestige in this period by his handling of a brief
but sharp outbreak of amoebic dysentery in 1933. The infection was
carried to other regions by visitors in the city, thus bringing the
whole affair to national prominence. Medical groups, especially the

Chicago Medical Society, criticized Bundesen for hesitating too long before publicizing the outbreak and seeking the co-operation of physicians.[61]

In 1937 a new attack was made on venereal disease with the co-operation of the United States Public Health Service. The Chicago Syphilis Control Project was established in January, 1937, with three main objectives: to determine the number of cases of venereal disease in the city, to place every case discovered under competent medical care, and to search for new educational and legal measures to prevent further infection. The entire emphasis in the campaign was on breaking the chain of infection. A public opinion survey was made in the summer of 1937 to determine whether the public would co-operate in a large-scale case-finding program. The response proved overwhelmingly favorable and a mass blood-testing drive was begun. Physicians were asked to give free tests to those requesting them, and Wassermann blood examinations were given to thousands. At the close of the campaign, it was discovered that over 450,000 serologic tests for syphilis has been made; an increase of 34 per cent in reported cases of syphilis and 19 per cent in gonorrhea appeared in the health records for 1937. The drive was not as complete a success as had been hoped, however. Many physicians, according to the United States Public Health Service, failed to co-operate, though the council of the Chicago Medical Society approved the plan. Some doctors refused to take specimens, while others charged applicants a fee; a few co-operated enthusiastically, according to the summary report released in 1938.[62]

The Chicago Venereal Disease Project (as it was renamed) did everything in its power to encourage physicians in the treatment of sufferers from syphilis and gonorrhea. Free laboratory service was provided for doctors treating venereal patients; free drugs were distributed to those handling syphilitics; generous use was made of the federal La Follette-Bulwinkle Act, which made funds available for instructing physicians and health officers in the latest principles of venereal control. In 1942 another pioneering step was taken in the opening of the Chicago Intensive Treatment Center, where rapid inpatient treatment of syphilis and other venereal afflictions was undertaken. The outstanding success of the whole venereal control program was sufficiently evident by 1943 to win a War Department commendation. The remarkable statistics on venereal disease since World War II have made the value of the program even more striking.[63] *Newsweek* reported in 1947 that while other large cities were faced with soaring venereal rates following demobilization, Chicago's rate was actually decreasing.[64]

Other important milestones in the long struggle to raise Chicago's health level have been passed during Bundesen's long tenure as health commissioner and later as president of the Board of Health. The Commissioner became greatly interested, for example, in the fight for life of babies born prematurely. The Board of Health inaugurated a twenty-four-hour incubator service and provided special medical care for these premature infants. Chicago in 1949 was the only city in the world providing stations where mother's milk was provided free to all babies who needed it. At the other end of the age scale, Chicago had taken the lead among large cities in establishing a functioning geriatrics program, and measures were being readied to give help to the aged in their fight against cancer, heart disease, nephritis, and other degenerative diseases. The aging of Chicago's population, along with that of the nation as a whole, has made this problem increasingly urgent, and it is certain that geriatrics will occupy a prominent part in the public health work of the future.[65]

One glaring defect of Chicago's health program has been the failure to control tuberculosis. Although knowledge of the method of its transmission and propagation has long been available, tuberculosis continues to exact a frightful toll of life and suffering in Chicago. As previously observed, the solution of this problem has been complicated and delayed by the racial factor involved. Pneumothorax and sanitarium treatment have been given to hundreds of thousands of patients, but shortages of hospital and medical facilities have prevented health authorities from delivering a decisive blow to this pestilence. Infection continues to take place at a faster rate than authorities can effectively care for new patients. There was in 1950 a waiting list of 1,385 patients for admission to the Municipal Tuberculosis Sanitarium, all of whom were potentially capable of infecting others.[66] The circle of infection must be decisively broken before the disease can be controlled. Great hope was placed in the late 1940's in the antituberculosis vaccine, BCG, which Dr. Sol R. Rosenthal announced as perfected in 1947. Plans for a mass immunization program were halted, however, when the Council on Pharmacy and Chemistry of the American Medical Association reported in 1950 that "the general use of BCG vaccine for all infants, children, and tuberculin-negative persons . . . does not appear to be warranted and should not be encouraged." [67]

Other health problems were uncovered by the Chicago-Cook County health survey undertaken in 1946 by the United States Public Health Service. This survey was a unique audit conducted by experts of all health facilities in the city and county. No other city had authorized a project comparable in size and scope. The auditors provided suggestions in their final report for improving various aspects of the city's health services. With regard to eating and drinking establishments, they recommended a sizeable increase in the number and salaries of the inspecting staff. The low sanitary rating of the city's restaurants—31.5 out of a possible 100 points—could be vastly improved by adding sufficient competent personnel. The city's water supply, the investigators found, would benefit greatly from a complete change-over to the filtration system and an increase in the chlorine dosage capacities of the pumping stations. An integrated water supply for the whole metropolitan area was also recommended as an answer to diminishing water supplies and inefficient administration of water systems by communities in the Chicago area. School health services, the experts reported, were inadequate, particularly with respect to health examinations. They urged that these examinations be extended promptly to all public schools in the county, and that they be administered under the jurisdiction of the health departments. Regarding refuse disposal, the report advised that the sanitary landfill method be substituted for existing techniques. All privately owned pay dumps, it was suggested, should be replaced with municipal dumps in view of the exorbitant rents charged the city. [68]

The Board of Health, the survey showed, would better serve the city if it were decentralized. The board had replaced the old health department in 1932 and was reorganized along modern lines. [69] But in view of the continued growth and increasing complexity of public health services, a number of persons and organizations have called for a regrouping of health services into local, subordinate health centers spread around the city. The Chicago Medical Society gave approval in 1938 to the district health center plan on the ground of increased efficiency. [70] The United States Public Health Service report of 1946 recommended a seven-member board of health with an executive director, and deputy directors in charge of engineering, preventive medicine, and district health services.

Bureaus would be organized under each branch; the preventive medicine branch, for example, would be divided into such bureaus as tuberculosis control, geriatrics, and venereal disease control. The proposed plan would ensure a greater delegation of power, while preserving an administrative echelon. It would provide the city, moreover, with a more flexible organization in the interim before the district health centers, probably twenty in number, became a functioning reality.[71]

Chapter XII | # Social and Political

Attitudes of Chicago Physicians

The relationship of the physician to the social and political environment in which he lives is influenced by a wide variety of cultural, economic, and professional considerations. In the case of the pioneer practitioner traveling the wilderness roads of the undeveloped American West, the struggle to push back the forest and fashion a new community did most to shape his social views. A sense of common purpose and common destiny inspired a general feeling of human equality which the doctor shared. The struggle for success in the West, however, was individual as well as social; a man sought to carve out for himself the largest possible stake even while he co-operated with his neighbors in necessary communal undertakings. Thus, while the early western doctor soon saw the need for local legislatures, courts, and constabularies, he was suspicious of interference from outside, especially from a strong central government at Washington.

As the nineteenth century wore on and the cultural isolation of the West was broken, economic and professional factors became more and more important in shaping the attitudes of physicians toward society and government. The rapid industrialization of the country, accompanied by a sharper division of society into the propertied and the propertyless, forced the physician to choose politically between the forces of conservatism, which rallied to the support of a laissez-faire economy, and the army of industrial and agricultural workers, many of them his neighbors, which protested its subjugation to the will of profit-driven producers. Increased professional competence was still another factor which had a bearing on the political thinking of the physician. The medical discoveries of Pasteur, Koch, and their followers armed the practitioner with knowledge and skills which inspired increased public confidence, and gave him a new position in the social order.

The doctor's attention became more and more fixed on strictly professional matters, with the result that his views on political and social topics became little more, in most cases, than reflections of those of the leaders of professional organizations or the editors of professional journals.

One of the results of the cultural isolation of the West during the nineteenth century was the development of a strong feeling of sectionalism which often expressed itself in antagonism toward the East and its institutions. Western medicine, like western literature and science, had a sharp inferiority complex with respect to the better-equipped hospitals and better-trained physicians of the East. Westerners were self-conscious about the cultural lag between East and West and often sought to conceal their feeling beneath a mask of boastful arrogance or sarcasm. Evidence of this western self-consciousness can be discovered as early as 1827 when Daniel Drake inaugurated the first medical journal published west of the Appalachians. "We trust," Drake wrote, "that our senior brethren of the East will not regard a journal in the Backwoods, as altogether unworthy of their more experienced pens."[1] When the Rush Medical College opened its doors in Chicago in 1843, a special plea was made to "Western Students" to attend. Aside from offering facilities equal to those of the best eastern schools, the Rush catalogue boasted, this school had the additional advantages accruing to a location in the heart of the West, where the endemic diseases which western physicians would meet in practice could be studied at length.[2] By 1859 the growth of western medical schools had reached the point where the president of the Illinois State Medical Society could refer to the sending of students to eastern schools as a "hindrance to medical progress." This practice, he said, might have been justified at an earlier period when colleges were scarce, but could no longer be defended "for we can boast of a sufficient number of medical schools, supplied with every material necessity to impart instruction, hospitals included."[3]

Western sensitivity to criticism was severely tested by Oliver Wendell Holmes in 1848, when he referred disparagingly to the proliferation of low-grade medical schools in the West. The wounded vanity of western professors found some solace in composing stinging rebuttals to Holmes' charges. Austin Flint, who taught at Rush in the 1840's, attacked Holmes' complacency with regard to the medical schools in his native New England. The problem of medical education, Flint insisted with considerable justification, was national, not sectional. There were a number of schools in small, provincial towns west of the mountains, it was true, but what of schools like Woodstock, Castleton, Hanover, and Bowdoin in Holmes' New England?[4] Daniel Brainard, president of Rush, also vented his spleen at Holmes' charges:[5]

The statement has recently been made by a Dr. Holmes, professor in a not very flourishing medical school at Boston, that the multiplication of medical schools at the West is doing great mischief in the profession. . . . For a country possessing all the advantages for containing a large population, calculated from extent and situation to be the center of the republic . . . to be dependent on some villages a thousand miles off for its physicians, would certainly present an anomaly in the general order of things.

Not only was the West prone to resent eastern superiority and criticism, but that section shared with the country as a whole an intense feeling of inferiority with regard to European science and culture. This sense of cultural and scientific backwardness was transformed into burning hostility whenever a European, usually an Englishman, chose to taunt Americans with the unimportance of American contributions to art, literature, or medicine. "In the four quarters of the globe," wrote Sydney Smith in his famous article in the *Edinburgh Review,* "who reads an American book? or goes to an American play? or looks at an American picture or statue? What does the world yet owe to American physicians or surgeons?"[6] It was the last question which greatly irked the American physician of 1820. The *Philadelphia Journal of the Medical and Physical Sciences* immediately fixed this hated phrase upon its masthead and kept it there for seven years as a prod to American medical men.[7] American medicine, like American science and art generally, was striving for independence from European influences during most of the nineteenth century; by 1900 the condescending attitude of Europeans toward the New World had all but disappeared. A marked deference to European medicine remained, however, as the result of the birth and growth of bacteriology in the Old World.[8] When Northwestern University constructed a new laboratory building for its medical school in 1893, no greater boast could be made than it had "been inspected and praised by Professors from eastern and even European universities."[9]

Western journals and medical men resented American subservience to foreign science even more strongly than their eastern colleagues. The nationalistic feeling of the country ran higher on the frontier, and the Westerner's strong pride in himself and his independence was injured when he saw American medical men pouncing upon the scraps of information which fell from European tables. The noted Chicago and Civil War surgeon, Edmund Andrews, complained in 1856 that after seventy-five years the United States possessed no original nor independent medical literature; the writing of Americans was confined to illustrating and commenting upon European texts. He censured his colleagues for ignoring the important work of Professor Brainard at Rush; he reminded them that Brainard had been warmly received in Paris. He recalled for American physicians, too, the investigations of Daniel Drake and Benjamin Dudley, and Benjamin Rush's doctrine of the unity of fevers.[10]

Brainard himself was vociferous in his denunciation of American servility to Old World ideas. This servility, he charged, was responsible for the uncritical adoption by American physicians of such stultifying European doctrines as universal purgation and heroic medication, as well as the sectarian teachings of homeopathy, hydropathy, and other "pathies." He attacked the therapeutic nihilism of European medicine: "All Louis' boasted researches on phthisis did not enable him to do more than pronounce the disease incurable, and are even less serviceable than the discovery of the use of cod liver oil." It was the West, said Brainard in 1852, which would deliver the country from its bondage to European medicine: "Held subservient . . . to the East, as the East to Europe, for its books and doctrines . . . it will soon have opinions of its own."[11] Three years later, all the physicians of Illinois were urged by the retiring president of the state society to assist in felling the "European monster:"[12]

We must do our own thinking and investigating, and we must be guided by our own philosophy. So long as we are satisfied with merely imbibing the froth and scum of medical science, which floats to us through the medical press from the other side of the Atlantic, so long will our native energies remain to a great extent inactive; so long will we remain without a literature characteristic of ourselves, or which will represent in a favorable light the medical mind and talent of the nation; and so long shall we remain comparatively destitute of ample medical libraries.

But Western antipathy to European science began to fade in the last quarter of the nineteenth century. The development of better American schools, hospitals, and doctors, coupled with the accomplishment of Europeans in bacteriology and medicine, promoted a spirit more akin to respect than envy. The triumph of American surgical appliances at the Paris Exposition of 1868, moreover, did much to soothe hostile feelings in this country.[13] When the English surgeon, John Erichsen, came to the United States in 1875, he received such a warm reception that he refused to accept it as a personal tribute, professing to think of it as an American compliment to the surgical profession of Great Britain.[14]

Only a lingering sensitivity to English and continental criticism marred the relations of the American profession with its foreign counterparts in the closing years of the century.[15]

Western resentment at the condescension and exclusiveness of eastern journals and societies, however, remained strong into the twentieth century and was indeed still a factor in any sociological analysis of the profession at mid-century. An interminable row between doctors east and west was begun in the early 1880's when the New York State Medical Society voted to permit consultations with homeopaths. Western physicians were strongly opposed, especially in Chicago where most of the country's homeopaths were congregated. The American Medical Association voted in 1882 to refuse delegates from New York on the ground that their action had violated the Association's code of ethics. *The New York Times* cauterized the injury to East-West relations by declaring that there was "probably more medical skill and scientific knowledge among the members of the New York Medical Society than . . . among all the members of the American Medical Association. If the latter can do without the New York doctors, most assuredly the New York doctors can do without the eminent medical practitioners of Oshkosh and Okolona."[16]

The American Medical Association established its journal in Chicago the year following these events with a Chicagoan, N. S. Davis, as its first editor. Scarcely had the first issue of the new journal reached the doctors of the country when a number of eastern journals began publishing caustic criticisms of the enterprise and particularly of Davis' editorship. The *New York Medical Journal* went so far as to publish lists of the typographical errors found in the Association's journal. Davis, himself an Easterner by birth and training, could not long endure these critical onslaughts without replying in kind. He culled a few mistakes from eastern journals and printed them in the Association journal with this accompanying remark: "Had either of these blunders occurred in The Journal or any other outside of 'one of the great *Eastern* cities' it would have been held up as a sample of incompetent provincial work for the next six months."[17] As an educator, Davis frequently found himself in sharp disagreement with the attacks made by spokesmen for eastern schools against the proprietary schools of the West. He was forced to remind these critics that the East had some low-grade, proprietary institutions, and that the West was passing through a different stage of physical and cultural development than the East. When several of New York's schools withdrew from the American Medical College Association in 1880, Davis confessed that "we are a little out of patience with this persistent Pecksniffian assumption that there is nothing of value or importance in the medical institutions of this country outside of that circumscribed strip of territory lying between the eastern part of the Alleghenies and Plymouth Rock."[18]

The Association of American Physicians was organized in 1886 largely by eastern medical men, many of whom had withdrawn from the American Medical Association in protest at its action against the New York delegation. This body was immediately characterized by one Chicago editor as a "mutual admiration society of medical mugwumps and man-milliners."[19] Steps were soon taken to build up an exclusively western society which became known as the Mississippi Valley Medical Association. The split between East and West spread also to specialty societies. A Western Ophthalmological, Otological, Laryngological and Rhinological Association, for example, was founded in 1896 as a protest against the exclusiveness of eastern-dominated national societies. Such western societies tended to be open to all qualified applicants, unlike many of the eastern groups, where membership was limited to a certain number.[20]

The rapid industrialization and urbanization of the United States after the Civil War had an important bearing on medical thinking regarding political and social questions. In Chicago, physicians were poorly organized before this time and tended to share the attitudes of their neighbors and other townspeople on political and social problems. The factors which affected the political beliefs of doctors were those which touched citizens everywhere: family political connections, economic status, social position, and personal feelings; there was no recognizable "medical opinion" on other than scientific topics until the closing decades of the century. But the economic expansion and growth in population of the city meant that the profession had to become more differentiated and better organized to meet increasingly complex medical needs. Medicine became more and more specialized, regimented, and compartmentalized in response to the demands of the industrial order. Physicians tended gradually to make up a distinct economic and social group with attitudes which could be identified as those of the profession as a whole. In a word, physicians, like bankers, industrialists, clerks, and laborers, now had a definite stake in certain political questions.

The political orientation of Chicago's physicians in the final quarter of the nineteenth century was definitely in the direction of the conservative elements in the community. As a strong middle-income group, they saw their interests coinciding with those of the commercial and industrial leaders of Chicago. With several notable exceptions, the articulate voice of medicine was raised against the use of tax funds for the amelioration of the plight of the lower classes through slum clearance, expansion of public health work, and unemployment relief. Medical writers were more addicted than most to a Spencerian fatalism regarding the welfare of destitute persons. The works of Herbert Spencer and Thomas Huxley were quoted as veritable Bibles of moral behavior when the ethical aspect of leaving the unemployed to the vagaries of private charity was questioned. The work of the Illinois Board of Health was challenged frequently on the ground of Huxley's dictum that it was better for people to learn to care for themselves than to depend on the state for protection. An example of the type of ridicule heaped on the state board in the 1880's was the following characterization of its work by a Chicago medical journal:[21]

Mousing after irregular practitioners, "steering" medical students, nursing their pet medical colleges, and stuffing the newspaper reporters with Falstaffian narratives of their combats with the quacks— these seem to be the favorite pursuits.

Not until the last decade of the century did Chicago's doctors first become aware of their political power. They found that representatives of organized medicine could exert considerable pressure at Springfield on behalf of legislation favorable to the profession and against bills inimical to their economic or professional welfare. Medical politicians, who sensed the power inherent in an organized profession, fought for office in the Chicago Medical Society and in the specialty societies. In some instances, they made themselves obnoxious to their colleagues, as was evidently the case with the editor of the *Weekly Medical Review:* "The medical politician is one who for self-aggrandizement pushes himself and friends to the front, captures all the offices of the medical societies, courts the notoriety of the newspapers, and is about as reliable as the average ward bummer in municipal politics."[22] By 1896, Dr. Arthur Reynolds saw political potential beyond mere medical questions in a tight organization of physicians:[23]

There are nearly 4,000 medical practitioners in Chicago who could, if they would, control votes enough to turn any election that is held to whatever ticket they choose. In that way they could demand and dictate not only the administration of medical institutions, but all institutions and all offices.

Chicago's physicians tended in the closing years of the century to adopt conservative views on national political questions. The feeling against labor organizations was very intense in the city, especially after the Haymarket Riot of 1886, when a number of policemen were killed by a bomb of unknown origin while attempting to break up a labor protest meeting in Haymarket Square. Medical men shared in this general antipathy and a number of their journals called for the suppression of all unions. The abolition of trade-unions, argued the *Medical Standard*, would not militate against basic American rights, because no punishment was too severe for those who "defy all principles of free labor."[24] The enormity of strikers' outrages was cited whenever the struggle between capital and labor was discussed. When a Chicago doctor was brutally murdered on the third anniversary of the Haymarket Massacre, the coincidence was not lost on physicians.[25] Several medical journals asked for a halt to immigration because, it was felt, foreigners were responsible for all the labor agitation and violence of these turbulent years. Physicians tended, too, to support high tariffs during this period as part of their general adherence to the conservative program. One Chicago homeopathic journal went so far as to oppose the importation of surgical instruments duty-free because[26]

America already contains too many undesirable exotics; too many demanding foreign flags on public buildings; too many anarchists, whose mission it is to destroy; too many socialists, to disturb established order; too many "strikers" to urge to violent methods; too many alien paupers, unsound of mind and diseased of body. These gangrenous ulcers came into our country duty-free. And now we are asked to put American labor into competition with the source of all this evil.

Not all medical men, of course, agreed with what seemed to be the dominant view of the profession regarding political matters. There were a number of physicians, particularly those in public health work, who espoused the cause of the workers in their fight against capital, and of the poor in their struggle for relief. Health commissioners, such as John Rauch and Oscar De Wolf, recognized the legitimate nature of most of labor's complaints. They knew at first hand the high mortality rates among the families of poorly paid workers, forced to live under abominable conditions in slums, lacking proper food, clothing, shelter, and medical care. It was as much the responsibility of government, De Wolf told the Chicago Medical Society in 1879, to protect these unfortunates from disease as from crime. The only property of the laborer was his health and ability to work; these, De Wolf insisted, society was bound to protect.[27] A city statistician named Gruenhut went even further in a report on labor statistics in 1889. This remarkably humane and enlightened document revealed a sympathy for the oppressed and a grasp of the economic and moral aspects of the whole problem which were out of keeping with Gruenhut's humble position. The capitalists who were responsible for making over the face of Chicago and for bringing the human misery, deprivation, and sorrow that went with that transformation, were, in his view, responsible for solving the great problems of industrial civilization. Gruenhut summed up brilliantly the humanitarian, moral, and economic justification for such reforms as the eight-hour day, abolition of child labor, and closing of work-places on Sunday.[28] He challenged leaders of public opinion to support this program; the alternative, he asserted elsewhere, was "legal and social interference with the present established order of business arrangements." The way to halt the march of socialism, he warned, was not to crush labor unions but to grant the legitimate and necessary reforms for which labor was crying.[29]

One of the most remarkable rebels against the conservative sympathies of organized medicine at the close of the nineteenth century was a private physician, Bayard T. Holmes. He had come to Chicago in 1871 after a farm boyhood in Vermont and a pioneer's existence on the Minnesota prairie. His rural background did not prepare him for what he was to find in the great metropolis of the Midwest. As a boy of nineteen, Holmes was entranced by the hustle, the impatience, the shrillness of life in the roaring city. His impressions proved to be indelible; he never forgot his own experience when he later observed the plight of persons caught and confused in the relentless and impersonal process of industrialization. Holmes attended the Chicago Homeopathic Medical College, and later the Chicago Medical College, receiving degrees from both institutions. He won an internship at the Cook County Hospital in 1884 at the age of thirty-two, then established a private medical practice of his own a few years later. Aside from an abiding interest in politics, Holmes made important contributions to medical education, the science of bacteriology, and the establishment of medical libraries in Chicago.[30]

Holmes was keenly sensitive to the newest currents in political and social thought. His delicate nature rebelled at accepting the social *status quo* as a desideratum for all time. During his internship at the County Hospital, he was moved to compassion by the poverty and helplessness of the jobless and the underpaid. While yet an interne, he met and befriended a scholarly Russian Jew, a patient at the hospital, who introduced him to the social thought of Karl Marx. He subsequently fell under the benevolent influence of Florence Kelly of Hull House, who worked with him in investigating health conditions in the sweating industry in Chicago. Holmes conducted a clinic for the homeless and unemployed during the terrible depression winter following the Columbian Exposition of 1893 and did everything in his power to induce the public authorities to act. He worked hard for reform; he undertook the organization of interested Christians in a reform group known as the National Christian Citizenship League.[31]

Spurred on by humanitarian sympathy, Christian altruism, and the writings of Marx and Henry George, this gentle and humane physician worked out his own social and economic philosophy. The limit of man's productiveness, he reasoned, had not yet been reached, yet mankind was confronted with the phenomenon of overproduction with its attendant depressions and human misery. "There is too much wheat, too much flour and too much bread, therefore, the economists say, women and children must starve. There is too much coal and too much oil, therefore they must freeze." The answer to this riddle, Holmes felt, was that there was, in reality, enough and more than enough for every man to live in decency, if not in comfort; but the great problem of distribution had yet to be solved. His personal experience informed him that not just the drunken and the shiftless starved, as defenders of the *status quo* charged; he had seen the half-starved bodies of the slum children and treated them for dietary diseases. It was the unemployed who were driven to crime and delinquency and their salvation should be the first goal of political action. Public ownership of the means of production and distribution, he concluded with the socialists, was the only effective answer to the indifference of owners of industry to the well-being of the employed and unemployed alike.[32]

In 1895 Holmes was persuaded to run as the People's Party candidate for mayor of Chicago. All the forces of discontent which were to erupt in the tumultuous campaign of William Jennings Bryan the following year were evident in the Holmes campaign. The liberal lawyer, Clarence Darrow, was chairman of the convention which nominated Holmes, the socialist supporters of Eugene Debs rallied to Holmes' candidacy, and Henry Demarest Lloyd took an important part in the campaign. Populists, socialists, single-taxers, progressives, and liberals of all shades supported the mild physician, but all to no avail. He was defeated; he never ran again for public office.[33]

The closing years of this unusual doctor's life were spent in another humanitarian cause. His son was stricken with dementia praecox in 1906; his death affected Holmes deeply, and he resolved to quit medical practice and devote the remainder of his life to study of the mysterious affliction which claimed his son's life. With characteristic energy he undertook basic studies in the field of mental disease, established a journal devoted to dementia praecox, and secured a floor of the Psychopathic Hospital of Chicago for his investigations. His death in 1924 attracted little attention but it brought from Graham Taylor, the noted social worker, the following tribute:[34]

On one occasion, when we were together on a western Chautauqua platform, he was so deeply moved with the sorrow of the East London poor, which he was describing that he ceased speaking, left the platform, and went out into the open to be by himself until he could control his voice. . . .

Dr. Holmes had the courage not only of his convictions but also of his sympathies. He was unafraid and not ashamed to think ahead of his time, to feel deeply and to express his feeling freely, to stand with and for the mute many against the dominant few, or to stand alone and dare to fail. . . .

Skillful surgeon and spirited citizen, he ministered to the public health at any cost to private practice, to "the mind diseased," and to the welfare of the body politic. He served his generation by seeking the coming of the better day, and died not until he saw its early dawning.

The impact of industrialism was one important factor which helped to shape the thinking of physicians in the late nineteenth century; the Darwinian theory of evolution was another. Promulgated as a strictly scientific hypothesis in 1859, the moral and religious implications of Darwin's theory stirred up a maelstrom of controversy in the years following the Civil War. Even scientists were at first unable to examine the question dispassionately because of deep prejudices and feelings. The theory of evolution collided head-on with the religious doctrine of the special creation of man in God's own image; few public figures dared embrace evolutionism openly. By the middle 1870's, however, the hypothesis was generally accepted by biologists and other scientists, while the struggle for acceptance had shifted to a more popular level. A number of popularizers of the Darwinian theory, such as the Englishman Huxley, undertook extensive writing and lecture campaigns during these years. More significantly, some writers sought to apply the evolutionary hypothesis to social as well as scientific phenomena. Herbert Spencer, for example, created an elaborate social philosophy which had as its co-ordinates the superiority of existing economic arrangements and the futility of resisting a deterministic evolution. Why palliate the hunger and misery of the lowly when that was nature's salutary method of eliminating those no longer able to compete? Such a philosophy provided the perfect rationale for the business community which found the laissez-faire economic doctrines of Adam Smith and John Stuart Mill beginning to wear thin.

Evolutionism found little support from Chicago's medical men even in the 1870's. Physicians, despite their closeness to the struggle, outrivaled clergymen in their denunciations of the Darwinian hypothesis. Their opposition was based not on scientific but on religious grounds, a curious anomaly in an age supposedly nursed on the independence of the scientific mentality. The Rush Medical College valedictorian declared in 1872 that he preferred the theology of revelation to the "theology of man." He was gratified to know, he continued, that the Rush faculty was virtually unanimous in asserting "that they do not regard men as baboons, nor the descendants of baboons." [35] The medical journals, too, were slow to accept evolution. The *Chicago Medical Journal* compared Darwin's theory with "infinitesimals, animal magnetism, womb burning, Newtonism, and hobby-riding in general." [36] The first recorded mention of Darwin at a Chicago Medical Society meeting came in 1874, when reference was made to "his slanderous theory of human origin." [37]

The Chicago Academy of Science was divided on the question throughout the 1870's. Dr. James S. Jewell, a pioneer neurologist, sided with the majority who were anti-Darwin and even wrote a book to disprove the theory. [38] Bayard Holmes, though not yet a physician, was one of the few to accept evolution in the early 1870's; he was considerably confused, however, by the opposition of Louis Agassiz, with whom he had spent a summer in study. [39] Many physicians found themselves in the position of De Laskie Miller, a professor of obstetrics at Rush, who leaned toward evolution, yet could not acccept it at the sacrifice of religious principle. With his minister beside him on the platform, Miller sought some compromise in 1874 between the revelations of theology and the demands of science. To be true, he argued, Darwin's theory "must and will be found in accord with religion and revelation." He tried to harmonize evolutionism with separate creation by citing the biblical assertion that in God's view a "day is a thousand years." Only the Bible, he concluded, could provide the answer to the ultimate origin of life; only revelation provided a satisfactory explanation of the existence of such a marvelous work as man.[40]

It was on the basis of just such a compromise that most of Chicago's doctors accepted the theory of evolution in the 1880's. A number of physicians continued to speak out against it, but no longer with the noisy confidence of membership in a majority. When Amos Sawyer, a Hillsboro, Illinois, practitioner, attacked Darwinism at a meeting in 1884, he tried to show that the evolutionary hypothesis was "contrary to the evidence," rather than attempting to shout it down. His conclusion, however—that it was unreasonable "to suppose that God would bestow His Divine Essence (the soul) on so repulsive a being as an ape"—was no more scientific than that of earlier adversaries.[41] Opposition faded rapidly in the latter 1880's. In 1890 an Evolution Club was formed in Chicago with medical men constituting a high proportion of the membership.[42]

The acceptance of medical men of the evolution theory gave them further arguments against the extension of public health work. The "survival of the fittest" concept, when applied to modern industrial life, gave a theoretical justification for refusing to render free medical and other aid to the poor; for by salvaging those whom nature intended to eliminate, the strength of the entire race would be weakened. Health Commissioner De Wolf found it necessary to protest to the Chicago Medical Society in 1879 against "the doctrine of the survival of the fittest as applied to sanitary matters."[43] The *Chicago Medical Journal and Examiner*, whose editors included some of the city's leading doctors, explained its position at length the same year:[44]

It is frequently stated that the poor should be protected by the government against the causes of disease which are said to infest the habitation of the lower classes. It is true that certain diseases are more often encountered among the poor than among the rich, but the reverse of the proposition is also true. Every class of people has to contend with its own peculiar difficulties; and if it is right for the government to assume the protection of any one class, there is no reason why it should not equally assume the protection of all. It is the lazy people and their sentimental friends who are always calling for government aid. If now you undertake to protect this fraction of the community, you have to protect it against the consequences of idleness, luxury, intemperance and vice—thus interfering with the operation of the wholesome monitory laws of nature; and you do it at the expense of the meritorious classes of society. Having accustomed such worthless people to rely upon government for protection against small-pox, and scarlet fever, and syphilis, and diphtheria, and sewer-gas, and scabies, it will not need the passage of many generations before they will demand protection by the government against the cold and hunger and nakedness for which they should themselves make provision. . . . This is the way in which Communists are produced; and a government which adopts the protective policy may thank itself alone for the growth of Communism and Socialism among its citizens.

It was not long after the advent of the germ theory of disease until it was related to the Darwinian struggle for existence. Ottomar Rosenbach in Germany had declared that disease was a special case of the struggle for existence, and was one of the means by which the natural selection process operated.[45] In Chicago, Henry Gradle stated in 1882 that "In the light of the germ theory, disease is a *struggle for existence between the parts of the organism and some parasite invading it.* From this point of view, diseases become a part of the Darwinian programme of nature."[46] Why then, argued the opponents of public health measures, should large sums of money belonging to the healthy classes of the community be spent in prolonging the lives of those whose bodies unfitted them to overcome the normal hazards of life?

These concepts borrowed from Darwin and his imitators served, nevertheless, as the basis for a considerable amount of speculation concerning the rôle of disease in natural selection. The *Medical Review*, noting the increase in cancer in the closing years of the nineteenth century, suggested that it was due to the successful attack on the infectious diseases, which allowed many persons "with weak constitutions" to survive childhood and middle life only to face an attack of carcinoma in their later years.[47] Henry Favill, noted Chicago internist, examined the Darwinian struggle with respect to disease in 1905 and concluded that illness was not completely selective. He was convinced of the "power of nature to breed out weakness and viciousness," but recognized that it was not always the weak who were weeded out by disease in the human struggle for existence.[48] In 1907 another Chicago journal signified its acceptance of the "social Darwinist" principle with respect to disease. By aiding the unfit to survive and reproduce their kind, wrote the editor of the *Medical Standard*, the average resisting power of the race would be lowered.[49] In the first quarter of the twentieth century, a few Chicago medical men continued to use the doctrine of the survival of the fittest as an argument against extending further medical and economic aid to the destitute. As late as 1924, William Allen Pusey, famed Chicago dermatologist, declared in his presidential address to the American Medical Association:[50]

It is clear that our civilization is committed to a sort of socialism, to the effect that the economically fit and competent shall take care of the weak and inefficient. It is an unconscious endeavor to set aside the law of natural selection and to counteract nature's cruel but salutary process of eliminating the unfit.

More than one authority has reminded men of Pusey's persuasion that the medical profession itself has no reason for existence other than counteracting nature's "cruel but salutary process."[51]

In the early years of the twentieth century, most physicians and their publications became more conscious of politics and social problems than they had been since the pioneer era. During the Progressive Era, medical men shared in the general enthusiasm for constitutional and legislative reforms aimed at making the American social system more equitable and the American democracy more responsive to the people. In sharp contrast to their earlier views, Chicago's medical publications now espoused such reforms as workmen's compensation, slum-clearing, and abolition of child labor. The Progressive interest in constitutionalism was reflected in the concern of physicians for making their societies more representative and in the democratic movement within the American Medical Association. Everywhere there was evidence that the medical profession had joined with other middle-class, normally conservative, groups in providing the impetus by which the liberal reforms of the first decade and a half of the twentieth century were achieved. "There is a progressive movement," intoned the new president of the Chicago Medical Society in 1912, "which is extending over the entire land today in all activities of society for the betterment of everything, and I hope that it will come to your honorable body and inspire you all for good work and friendly gatherings at all of the meetings."[52]

The *Medical Recorder*, under the editorship of a representative board of Chicago physicians, illustrated medicine's new social consciousness in the Progressive period. Numerous editorials were written dealing with the problems of capital and labor, slum housing, women's suffrage, workmen's compensation, and malnutrition among the poor. Even more space was devoted to political problems at the local level; a surprising proportion of the contents of this periodical was devoted to political and social topics not immediately connected with medicine. Never before or since have medical journals exhibited such a deep concern for civic and national problems. When workmen's compensation was widely debated in the first decade of the century, the *Recorder* published a series of scholarly articles on the subject. Editorials followed, outlining the advantages of compensation laws as a practical, as well as a humanitarian, means of averting social upheaval. Among many other social reforms backed by the *Recorder* at this time was an inheritance tax to eliminate "swollen fortunes."[53]

Other journals participated in the reform campaigns. The *Medical Standard, Illinois Medical Journal, Clinique,* and *Journal of the American Medical Association* all devoted some space to the pressing questions of the day. Several of these periodicals attacked the clergy for their failure to join with them in the fight for reform. One of them criticized sharply the continued clerical references to ignorance and drunkenness as the sole causes of poverty, while another applauded the decreased popular interest in otherworldliness.[54] The attention of mankind, declared the editors of *Clinique,* can not be "averted from present wrongs by glowing pictures of a better world to come." The *Medical Standard* was concerned especially with the conditions of the slum-dwellers. In 1913, this journal compared Chicago's slums to those of Europe to the disadvantage of the former:[55]

All through northern Europe the poor are better provided for than they are in America, which is becoming more and more a land of contrasts. The able man finds ready opportunity to get ahead in this country, and there are [sic] an abundance of "big prizes" for the brilliant; but the average person is finding it harder and harder to keep his head out of water, and the mediocre . . . soon learn that the United States has little of the "milk and honey" for them. Our great cities are filled with dirt, squalor and wretchedness in a degree only rivalled abroad by places like Cairo and Naples.

The Chicago Medical Society also felt the spur of liberal thought in the first decade of the twentieth century. In 1902, a committee was formed to assist and co-operate with the Civil Service Reform League.[56] The following year it was unanimously resolved that "the members of this Society will use their influence collectively and individually to secure the passage of the child labor law."[57] Other discussions favorable to slum clearance and workmen's compensation were held. The Society's council became angry in 1910 at slanderous references in a report of the state medical society to the "women, negroes and foreigners" who attended Chicago's medical schools. A faculty member of one of the schools arose in the council meeting to admit that "we have had Japs . . . Egyptians, Indians and representatives of various other races and I must oppose any report of any committee that seeks to gain weight . . . by drawing upon the very lowest prejudice in the human body—the race prejudice."[58]

Many of Chicago's leading physicians came to look with increasing favor during these years on a larger rôle for government in medical affairs. When the Chicago Medical Society censured Health Commissioner Evans in 1909 for making certain vaccines and drugs freely available to victims of epidemic disease, the *Medical Standard* came to Evans' support. An editorial compared the society's attitude with the panic which possessed workingmen at the introduction of machinery; some members of the profession, the editor asserted, were afraid that the march of preventive and state medicine would gradually put them out of business. The medical profession, advised the *Standard*, should adjust to change, rather than whine vainly against it.[59]

A number of the city's physicians joined the American Association for Labor Legislation, a liberal organization which espoused the cause of state-operated health insurance during the First World War. Henry B. Favill, the internist, was an influential member of this group.[60] Other of the city's doctors called for governmental aid to medical schools to supplement the undependable financial support which came from private sources. Arthur Dean Bevan, Chicago surgeon and Chairman of the American Medical Association's Council on Medical Education and Hospitals, saw the future of medicine as tied inextricably to constantly increasing support from the state. He warned on the eve of the First World War that medical men should recognize the inevitable trend toward federal participation in medical education, public health, and medical care for the people; doctors, he wrote, should adopt insurance schemes for the care of the less fortunate classes in society and direct them themselves. His views were summarized in the following sentences:[61]

Medicine has become not only a function of the state, but also one of the most important functions of the state. . . . In the interest of the people we should demand adequate state support for medicine in order that medicine in return may properly perform its great function to the state and the people may benefit from the great possibilities offered by preventive medicine, intelligent medical practice and medical research.

Dr. Bevan, like many other of the city's physicians, joined the Progressive Party in 1912 in an effort to keep alive the spirit of reform.

He took an active part in the political campaign of that year, as did ex-health commissioner Evans and George Kreider, editor of the *Illinois Medical Journal*, the official publication of the state medical society.[62] Dr. S. V. Clevenger, a psychiatrist who had won fame by his exposure of conditions at the County Insane Asylum in the 1880's, was a founder of the Progressive Medical League, which purported to be the medical branch of the party. Clevenger wrote a number of pamphlets during the campaign supporting the party of Roosevelt and condemning both old parties as "bought by Big Business Interests." He related his struggle for non-political treatment of the insane to the aspirations of the Progressive Party, whose creators, he assured his readers, were "vastly more honest and intelligent than old party demagogues, who fill positions in public hospitals and insane asylums with cruel, brawling incompetents."[63]

In the realm of medical politics, the impact of this reform era was equally sharp. On the local, state, and national levels of medical organization, individuals and groups arose to protest abuses of democracy in their professional societies. The Chicago Medical Society, as a result of strong protests against the concentration of power in the hands of a few specialists, was decentralized into branch groups in 1903. A strong fight developed between those who wished to abolish all multiple voting for council members by specialists belonging to constituencies in both branch and specialty organizations, and the defenders of the *status quo*. Former health commissioner Evans led the insurgents here as he did physicians within the Progressive Party. In 1910 victory came to the Evans faction and representation of specialty societies on the council of the Chicago Medical Society was discontinued. During this first decade of the century, politics played an increasingly important rôle in the Society's activities; definite parties became discernible, political platforms were drawn up, and great controversy centered around the appointment and duties of the election commission. There was, moreover, a great deal of bickering on points of order and constitutional changes, reflecting the national penchant for "constitution-tinkering."[64]

The American Medical Association, whose headquarters were in Chicago, also felt the pressure for reform. A number of undemocratic features in the constitution and practice of the Association were severely censured by individual members and constituent societies. Criticism was directed particularly at the practice of assigning several executive positions to the same person; the lack of provision in the Association's journal for free discussion of policies and methods was also scored; and some Chicago doctors, in the best tradition of Progressivism, called for a system of initiative and referendum to make the organization more responsible to its members. The Chicago Medical Society at one point adopted a resolution, later rescinded, condemning the absence of democracy in the management of the Association.[65] Several of the city's medical journals joined the Society in the attack. The *Medical Standard*, for example, accused the "bureaucracy" at the helm of the Association of seeking to destroy the nation's independent medical press through deprecating journals which relied on the advertising of proprietary remedies for their support.[66] By 1909 the *Standard* was criticizing the whole structure of the American Medical Association. The entire organization, it was charged, was controlled by a small group of powerful trustees, who were only nominally elected by the house of delegates. The rank and file were completely without voice in the transactions, policies, and deliberations of the Association; "the pyramid," the editor accused, "hangs by its apex instead of resting on its base." What was most needed, according to the *Standard*, was some constitutional provision for a direct channel of communication between the members and the executive departments. There must be an opportunity for delegates to deliberate on important questions of policy, instead of rubber-stamping the decisions of the officers; what passed for debates in the annual conventions were in reality only "prayer and mutual admiration speeches."[67]

Soon after the armistice of 1918, however, the movement to democratize medical societies, along with the other political and social reforms with which physicians had busied themselves, began to fail in interest. From the peak of idealism to which Woodrow Wilson had led them, Americans now plunged to a new low of pessimism and disillusionment. The national mood changed from one of concern over social and political justice at home and abroad to one of indifference to social problems in America and rejection of American commitments in Europe. The revelation of the secret treaties, the cynicism of the Paris negotiators, and the uproar over communist successes in Russia and Eastern Europe, all combined to create a climate of despair and distrust in the United States. Everything European became suspect, whether it was French literature, the Weimar Republic, or social welfare legislation. All Europeans were scheming and designing, ready to despoil innocent and beguiled Americans; the nation retreated into a new isolation motivated by suspicion of foreigners and a defensive adulation of American institutions. One positive factor in the national outlook following World War I was the widespread confidence in business and business techniques. The American economic system was heralded as incomparably superior to anything the Old World had been able to produce; the difference, some people began to suggest, was that business in the United States was not saddled with all sorts of restrictive laws governing employment, compensation, and social insurance. The decade following the return of peace to the United States, in summary, was characterized by an anti-social individualism, an opposition to reforms, reformers, and foreign ideas, and a glorification of American business.

Chicago's medical press reflected faithfully this change in the national temperament. A number of medical journals became quickly involved in the Great Red Scare of the 1920's. Articles on such subjects as "The Three Internationals," "The Red Menace," and "Random Shots at Pacifists" appeared with increasing regularity. A typical edition warned in 1923 against the combined danger of "pacifists and reds." The pacifists, declared the writer, were weakening the United States Army by their "unholy stand" against universal military training; an army was urgently needed "for protection against the friends and co-workers of the pacifists, the 'reds,' the Soviets, the Bolsheviks, all blood-thirsty anarchists." The remedy for this situation, suggested the editorial, was "a dictatorship which would promptly deport to Russia all these imbecile pacifists . . . and their progeny, the conscientious objectors, and all the cursed anarchists."[68]

Other journals concerned themselves with health fads, the latest dance crazes and their effect on health, birth control, Couéism, immigration, or psychoanalysis. During most of the 1920's, Freud's theories failed to receive a scientific hearing in any of the city's journals, but were subjected instead to ridicule and derision on the editorial pages. As late as 1933, the *Illinois Medical Journal* unleashed a savage attack on psychoanalysis to prevent its being taught in American colleges. Typically, a heavy weapon in the *Journal's* assault was the fact that psychoanalysis had been "imported" from Europe; American psychiatrists, the editor boasted, would never hand out such "pabulum." Freud's work was characterized by the editorial as "pseudo-analysis" and "sexoanalysis," while Freud's world was declared to be "an open sewer and men and women merely floating blobs of pestilence." The conclusion was a curious one for a scientific periodical: "In the final analysis it all reminds you of bad little boys writing dirty words upon the barn."[69]

The anti-reformism of the 1920's was also clearly visible in the writings of Chicago's medical men. Charles J. Whalen, editor of the *Illinois Medical Journal* throughout this period, expressed at least the official attitude of the state's physicians in his frequent attacks on reforms and reformers. Whalen's vitriolic pen assailed the curse of reform as "UPLIFTUS PUTRIFACIENS" and reformers within the profession were dismissed as "medical bolsheviks."[70] A leading editorial appeared in 1921 under the revealing banner, "Professional Reformer a PERVERT." The *Journal* at various times opposed the eight-hour-day for women, a national child labor law, workmen's compensation, free clinics, the Sheppard-Towner Act for maternal benefits, and compulsory health insurance. The reasons which Whalen advanced for opposing these measures were sometimes comfortably free of logic. The child labor amendment, for example, was opposed on the ground that "it is sponsored and supported by every red and communist in the United States."[71] Whalen also found communists and bolsheviks behind compulsory health insurance and the Sheppard-Towner Act.

As the possibility of national health insurance waned in the 1920's, Whalen's attacks on reform increased rather than decreased in acerbity. Scarcely an issue passed during 1922 and 1923 without a petulant rehearsal of the dangers of "revolution." Socialists were seen to be lurking in every corner, ready to impose socialized medicine on the unsuspecting physician. Women's clubs were viewed with particular suspicion by Whalen; they were often infiltrated, he warned, with bolshevists. All pretense of detachment vanished from the editorial columns in the course of the decade. Where he had earlier stressed the suffering of the public under government medicine, he now wrote more of the suffering doctor. All federal legislation respecting medicine was rejected as imposing on the prerogatives of the medical profession; for a number of months in 1924 the editorial page of the *Journal* was headed as follows: "DOCTOR WRITE YOUR SENATORS AND CONGRESSMEN AT ONCE OPPOSING THE SHEPPARD-TOWNER BILL NOW IN CONGRESS." Another favorite caption read "Medicine must shake off its false leadership or be bolshevized."[72] In 1932 Whalen saw the fulfillment of his prediction of ultimate bureaucracy and socialism in the use of government monies by President Hoover to stimulate business recovery. In the "stifling blanket of over-legislation . . . [and] the murderous burden of taxation" of 1932, editor Whalen felt the closeness of the end of republican government in America.[73]

Other of Chicago's medical leaders shared Whalen's keen distrust of government. William Allen Pusey, in his presidential address before the American Medical Association in 1924, also discerned a sharp trend toward socialism in the increase of governmental power. But there were certain influences, in Pusey's view, which would in time bring to a halt the march of socialism; nature could not forever be denied in her efforts to cut down the unfit, for example, and the machinery of governmental bureaucracy would eventually become so large and cumbersome that it would simply fall apart. The power of an "enlightened minority" to shape events was also a factor in the equation. Pusey believed that medical men must take their place among those followers of Spencer who refused to compromise with the uplifters on even such measures as the Sheppard-Towner Act.[74] As late as 1929, with the American economy at an all-time peak of unregulated expansion, another well-known physician was arguing that the federal government was trying to dominate both labor and capital. It was government, not capitalism, which medicine had to fear; the only menace from capitalism, he suggested, came from its support of unethical foundations which operated clinics and laboratories, and supported research on socio-medical problems.[75]

Doctors, like everyone else, were absorbed in the fascinating process of making money during the 1920's. Since medical men possessed a legendary lack of acumen in financial matters, they were bombarded from every corner with advice on how to invest and speculate on the stock market. In a single issue of one medical journal in 1920, there appeared the following articles: "The Physician from the Banker's Point of View," "The Business of Medicine," "Education the Cure [for physicians' economic problems]," "The Doctor and His Money," "Therapeutic Exigencies Having an Economic Bearing," and "Economic Phases of Medicine."[76] Physicians were keenly aware of the respect accorded business and financial leaders in this era; they were advised by their own leaders and journals to pay greater heed to the business aspects of medicine, to emulate the philosophy and example of the business world. An editorial in the *Medical Standard* in 1925, for example, advised the doctor to "sell himself" to his clientele for "in the last analysis the doctor sells his services just as the merchant does his goods, and the patient buys them just as he does the merchant's goods."[77] The *Standard* would have deplored such a comparison as odious a decade earlier. Another typical article in 1929 defined medicine frankly as the "business of selling health service." The medical businessman, doctors were advised, could no more afford to await passively buyer demand than his commercial counterpart; he should encourage employers to pay their workers higher wages so that the latter might be able to buy more health services.[78]

The depression years after 1932 brought some change in the social and political thinking of Chicago's physicians, but the alterations were dictated more by expediency than conviction. Franklin Roosevelt's bold program in 1933 brought a ray of optimism and hope into the deepening abyss of lethargy and gloom in America; his early efforts, therefore, met with the approval of the medical profession. "The Council of the Chicago Medical Society," wired the Society's secretary in March, 1933, "wish to voice their enthusiastic approval of the President in his entire economic program from first to last."[79] The Chicago Roentgen Society displayed a new attitude toward positive government in its plea in 1934 that the United States restrict the immigration of doctors because of the competition they brought to an already suffering profession.[80] Chicago's doctors were enthusiastic, too, about the medical relief program which furnished not only medical care to the unemployed, but financial salvation to many physicians. The chairman of the Chicago Medical Society's advisory committee declared in 1936 that[81]

Your Committee believes that in this project these people have been furnished the best type of medical care that they have ever had in this State. We hope that plans may be maintained whereby each individual physician may still be privileged to render medical service to his client and to receive compensation for claim.

But many of the articulate spokesmen for the city's physicians did not conceal their continued opposition to any and all plans for using the resources of government to aid the more unfortunate persons in the community. Dr. Whalen fought every social welfare measure debated in the 1930's and the *Illinois Medical Journal* became almost a personal vehicle in his campaign. He told a group of manufacturers in 1934 that they should cease "gagging on chocolate coated communism . . . [and] discard . . . all of these 'workmen's welfare' schemes that are only socialistic and paternalistic passing of the buck from the individual to industry at large."[82] He pleaded with industry to make common cause with medicine against the common foe—socialism. In 1935 this official journal of the state's doctors professed to find communism in the Social Security Act of that year:[83]

Finding a joker in the new Social Security Act is as easy as seeing the water in Lake Michigan. This new law is a horse laugh on scientific medicine and American patriotism. Tentacles of this octopodan law will entwine the medical profession more securely than has been managed by any other communistic traps or socialistic twiddle-dee-dees emanating from the patriotically-paralytic bureaucracy bossing the country. . . . Even the dullest economist discerns readily the fist of politics clutched in the cash box of appropriations. . . . Surely the scarlet stain far more than tinges that provision of the Act where the nefariously non-patriotic Children's Bureau, sponsor of the Shepherd-Towner [sic] and other bilge of like ilk, get a chance to manipulate still another appropriation of about seven million dollars.

Although it was scarcely possible that Whalen reflected the point of view of the average physician during the 1930's, there was little evidence to show that he did not. The membership of the Illinois State Medical Society continued to approve, tacitly if not openly, his edi- - torship. Perhaps only men who felt as strongly as Dr. Whalen about social welfare measures took the trouble to set down their views, while other Chicago physicians lacked the courage or the interest to answer his tirades. In the council debates of the Chicago Medical Society, at any rate, a number of delegates did display strong social consciences at various times, though the arguments were usually dominated by those who were antagonistic to all welfare plans. Certainly no Bayard Holmes appeared in the 1930's to champion the cause of the underprivileged and the underfed; and there was no N. S. Davis to insist that human dignity take precedence over property rights in every debate.

Virtually all of Chicago's doctors agreed that some kind of "means test" was necessary for the admission of charity patients to hospitals and clinics. A dispute arose in 1937, however, over the method of weighing income against responsibilities in evaluating a patient's ability to pay. The committee of the Chicago Medical Society which was charged with drawing up a schedule advocated some sort of flexible yardstick of measurement because of the delicate nature of the problems involved. But when this report was laid before the whole council, considerable opposition developed because the standards had not been set fast and hard at the minimal estimates of the amount necessary to sustain life without charity. Dr. Edward Ochsner, a well-known surgeon, took the leadership in denouncing the committee's budget. The flexible standard, he charged, played "into the hands of the up-lifters and the emotionalists. In my opinion the up-lifters are a bigger handicap to humanity's progress than our gangsters and our criminals."[84] Three years earlier, Ochsner had written a book which strenuously opposed all social insurance schemes, public and private, industrial and medical. His outlook on social problems was reminiscent of the early nineteenth century liberal who saw complete economic freedom as the most desirable state this side of paradise; all economic and social ills he blamed on deviation from the laissez-faire policy. All forms of social insurance he characterized as "economic disease"—which was true in a sense since insurance palliated the illnesses of an unregulated capitalistic order—but for Ochsner the insurance itself was the disease, making a mockery of the rugged virtues of free enterprise. So marked was his prejudice against all measures of social amelioration that he confessed to presenting only one side of the question since "there is only one side."[85]

Looking back over a century of medical thought on social and political matters in Chicago, what may be said of the over-all pattern? In general, Chicago's physicians have been identified with the *status quo* and with the dominant political and social ideas of any given period. There has been little originality, little heterodoxy; there have been few political leaders and few reformers among them. Though always wont to remind critics of their private medical philanthropy, physicians have seldom been identified with leadership in movements for social amelioration. A doctor like Bayard Holmes is so rare as to be an anomaly. In periods of reform, doctors often supported the reformers; when liberalism was under attack, they tended to ally themselves more closely with the conservative groups in the community. In the pioneer era, Chicago doctors followed the libertarian lead of their freedom-loving neighbors; and in the wake of industrialism they aligned themselves with those who had an economic stake in society and politics. When the city felt the sting of liberal thought in the 'Progressive Era,' Chicago's doctors once again raised high the banner of reform; but when conservatism and reaction ruled the city in the 1920's, the banner was deeply buried.

With respect to participation in politics, the city's doctors have seemed to swing back and forth between two poles of thought, one regarding politics as an unprofessional and undignified activity for a physician, the other stressing the realistic necessity for medical men to organize and work together politically to achieve certain ends. During those periods when the relations between the medical profession and the city administration were reasonably good, there was little talk of politics. But when the reform spirit prevailed, when physicians were moved by accounts of political usurpation of medical functions in public institutions, then physicians organized (or spoke of organizing) to remedy the situation. In their social thought and in their politics, physicians tended, under pressure of work and the expansion of medical knowledge, to rely increasingly on a few spokesmen to express the "medical point-of-view." Whether these leaders of opinion represented the thinking of the profession is at best an open question. The absence of any vocal criticism, however, leads one to conclude that, for all practical purposes, a small number of men formed the opinions which the economic and social prepossession of the vast majority re-enforced.

Chapter XIII	The Profession and
	the Public

The public attitude toward medicine and medical men has undergone a series of marked changes in the past hundred years. Medicine has been transformed from a practical, poorly paid occupation, to which little prestige or publicity attached, to a highly skilled and respected profession, claiming the allegiance of some of America's best minds. The Chicago physician of 1850 had far less training and education than today's doctor; he was likely to be engaged in sharp economic competition with his colleagues; his qualifications for practice were not reviewed by any public body; he was apt to be interested only in the practical aspects of medicine; and he was largely helpless in the presence of most diseases.

The manner of establishing a practice in the West in 1850 bore little resemblance to a modern initiation into medicine. A young man finishing his apprenticeship to some local physician or just graduating from medical school set out to find a practice with some older doctor or else sought a new community on the frontier. John Hollister, one of the early professors at Rush Medical College, recalled that after graduation from Berkshire Medical College, he had gone to Michigan where he "hired a good saddle horse and visited six county sites while crossing the State of Michigan, but in not one of these did I find an acceptable opening." Hollister was fortunate in finding a friend who had preceded him into the West; together they established a partnership in medicine.[1] Hollister's experience was not atypical; the slowness of transportation and communication, joined to the isolation of western settlements, made a personal canvass of possibilities almost imperative.

The coming of the railroad made possible a more rapid communication between certain points, but by no means eliminated the need for the doctor's horse and buggy. Throughout the nineteenth century, the doctor depended on horse-drawn vehicles to reach his patients; when a call came from a considerable distance he might travel via railroad to the nearest junction, but a long trip by carriage usually awaited him at the station. Dr. Carl E. Black recalled his own experiences before the coming of the automobile and hard-surface roads: [2]

When the doctor depended on horse and dirt roads, often poorly drained and graded, the problems of travel were important factors in his life. . . . He spent one half of his life in the mud and the other half in the dust. The local doctor did not often go more than 10 miles from his home, but the consultant and surgeon was called on to make much longer trips. My own work took me into ten or twelve counties, and therefore many of the trips were long. Thirty to 50 miles was a common distance. Often, too, the consultant or surgeon had to make a trip to see the patient, confirm the diagnosis and arrange for the patient to be removed to the hospital.

Travel, then, occupied a large part of the physician's life, and he was always on the alert for any means of reducing the time spent on the road. In 1866 physicians were accorded special consideration by the Chicago Police Department, when an order was issued giving them precedence in crossing bridges over the Chicago River.[3] Before this time it was not uncommon for a doctor to find himself detained for a half hour at the end of a long line of carriages while the drawbridge was up. When bicycles and tricycles came into prominence in the 1880's, medical men were quick to see the possibilities for their profession. One journal editorialized on the advantages of the tricycle to "medical men traveling over a level country, [who] have not only a rapid means of locomotion, but a beast that does not tire, and which is not subject to the various ills to which horse flesh is heir." [4]

But as the century came to a close, the country stood on the threshold of a mechanical revolution in transportation which would immensely facilitate the physician's ministrations to the sick. Physicians were among the first to own automobiles; the medical journals of the first decade of the new century were full of advice regarding the treatment of automobiles as well as patients. Communities generally gave doctors on sick calls exemption from the provisions of speed laws; physicians, for example, were not subject to the ten to two hundred dollar fine which Evanston levied on those who exceeded eight miles per hour.[5] The advent of the hard road was just as important as the automobile in revolutionizing conditions of medical practice. There was now no place in the county or state which could not be reached swiftly, and the sick person could easily be transferred, if necessary, to a well-equipped hospital. The advantage to rural areas was incalculable; one thoughtful downstate medical man opined that "If it were not for the hard roads, we would still be doing many operations in the home. From my point of view, the hard road has been the greatest single contribution toward the improvement of the practice of medicine in central Illinois. It has had much to do in lifting it from the crude pioneer level to the high level of modern medicine." [6]

The doctor labored under other difficulties than transportation during the second half of the nineteenth century. Economically, he faced the competition not only of his colleagues—regular, homeopathic, and quack—but of druggists who freely dispensed all types of medicine. He suffered, too, from a widespread reluctance to render payment to physicians either promptly or in full; in the grocery and dry goods stores he was himself forced to surrender the full price for his food and clothing, yet his patients felt no such obligation toward him.[7] The doctor sometimes had to cope also with the interference of politicians; he was not infrequently the victim of the political intrigue of city officials in places like County Hospital and the insane asylum. In his professional work the physician met with additional hazards and obstacles, especially in the private home, where most of his medical and surgical work was done. An intubation for diphtheria in a crowded kitchen with the mother holding her loved one as best she could was to say the least a serious and difficult matter.[8]

In periods of epidemic and crisis the doctor had additional burdens thrust upon him. Following the Great Fire the city's physicians worked frenziedly to aid victims of the catastrophe, though many of them had themselves lost everything they owned. According to one account, they could be seen "wildly rushing from shelter to shelter, attending to sickness brought on mostly by hardships and exposure immediately after the fire." Work in the burned district was difficult and dangerous; there were no lights, no street or alley markings, ditches were filled with debris, patients were often hostile, and the whole scene was dominated by the terrible filth and disorder.

Sanitation, of course, was completely disrupted; the city's water supply was polluted, sewers were few, and almost all residences had privies in the yards.[9] The medical task was herculean, yet the worst for some physicians was yet to come. A number of them had lost their practices almost completely; for a long time after the Fire, moreover, many doctors had formerly prosperous families on their lists who were never able to pay again for medical service. About a fourth of the city's doctors applied for a share of the physicians' relief fund which had been collected by their colleagues all over the country.[10]

Chicago's doctors, too, played their part in the political and reform movements of the middle years of the nineteenth century. These were years of reform everywhere, of extension of the democratic franchise, of abolition of imprisonment for debt, of striving after that perfection which seemed attainable to the optimistic Americans of this era. Reforms and reformers held the center of the stage; antislavery, temperance, common schools, women's rights, and health fads all found the nation in a listening mood. In Chicago, Drs. Levi D. Boone, Charles V. Dyer, N. S. Davis, and William B. Egan all played important roles in the antislavery and Negro colonization campaigns. Dr. Dyer, indeed, was assaulted in 1848 for aiding the escape of a runaway slave.[11] Six years later, John Evans rallied the Democratic opposition to the Kansas-Nebraska bill; he subsequently left the Democrats for the newly formed Republican Party, where he worked for Lincoln's nomination and election in 1860.[12] Evans was active in other reform movements during his fifteen years in Chicago; his humanitarian efforts on behalf of the insane attracted the attention and praise of Dorothea Dix.

A number of the city's doctors were active in the temperance campaign. Serving on the strategic Reclaiming Committee of the Washingtonians (as the temperance advocates called themselves) in 1842 were Drs. Dyer, Freer, and Egan.[13] In the 4th of July celebration of that year, Dr. E. S. Kimberly acted as marshal of the Cold Water Army, while Dr. Levi D. Boone was active on the committee to select badges. But Dr. N. S. Davis was the most prominent physician engaged in temperance work in Chicago. His opposition to the use of alcohol, even medicinally, was so well known that it was the butt of a number of jokes among medical men. Davis eventually organized a group of interested physicians into the American Medical Temperance Society; this project occupied much of his time during the closing years of his life. Davis was one of the few men of that boisterous era to achieve the dual distinction of belonging to the Democratic Party and espousing the cause of teetotalism at the same time. No lesser man, suggested his biographer, could have risked such an inconsistency.[14]

In the common school movement in Chicago, another physician, James C. Goodhue, was especially active. His was the initiative behind the establishment of the city's first public schools. John Evans was also greatly interested in the city schools. Elected in 1852 to the City Council, Evans was appointed chairman of the committee on public schools. In that position he fought hard against the prevailing trend of selling valuable school property. When confronted with a proposed sale of more school land, he advised his colleagues that "unless they were satisfied that Chicago was done growing they were doing a foolish thing in selling any more property." Many a public official has since regretted the haste with which school lands were sold, but Evans was virtually alone at the time in opposing the trend.[15]

But the medical profession, despite its moments of heroism and public service, did not enjoy a large measure of public confidence in the last half of the nineteenth century. People were skeptical of physicians and their ministrations; they were suspicious of medical students who irreverently cut up the human body; they were easily diverted to homeopathy and other sects which did not employ bitter medicines and debilitating measures; they accepted naïvely the vaunted powers of patent and quack remedies, especially when the drugs of the regular physician seemed no more efficacious; and they were greatly disturbed by the attachment of leading medical men for laboratories and theoretical work and their seeming indifference to the welfare of actual sufferers from disease.

The public was continually outraged during much of the period from 1840 to 1880 by the nocturnal activities of Chicago's medical students in local graveyards. On several occasions, the offending students were caught and fined, but the public had no conception, fortunately, of the complete dependence of the city's schools on local sources of supply. The demonstrator of anatomy was forced to seek out venal coroners and superintendents of hospitals and poor houses in order to assure a supply of bodies sufficient to warrant carrying on a course in his specialty.[16] Great scandals were usually inspired by the discovery of the destination of persons dying in county institutions; each time the County Board would dutifully shut off this source of material for a few months.[17] "Well," wrote D. W. Graham of the Woman's Medical College to another staff member in 1883, "they have cut off the supply of all material for dissection in so far as it came from county institutions and county employees which of course were almost the entire reliance. Next winter we will all have to confine ourselves to the bones, I guess, in anatomy. Suppose you bring your trunk full of material and show our friends of the Board we are not dependent on home produce." [18]

The drift of patients from the regulars to the homeopaths, botanics, and other sectarians was another indication of the feeling of the public with regard to the regular profession. The stubborn addiction of most physicians to mercury, bleeding, and calomel was responsible for a widespread fear of medical men and their medicines. Professor Brainard, as early as 1846, understood perfectly the reason for the success of homeopathy: "It is impossible . . . not to see . . . that homeopathy is but a reaction against the excessive use of drugs." A quarter of a century later, the therapeutic repertory of the regular physician was still largely unchanged, and the homeopaths enjoyed a peak of popularity. A member of the Chicago Medical Society declared without opposition in 1869 that "the people of these days prefer quacks to the regular members of the profession." [19] Many physicians seemed unable to understand that patients were loath to have their bodies used as an impersonal battleground between doctor and disease. The following dramatic description of a doctor's fight against illness in 1868, though doubtless overdrawn, illustrates the prevailing indifference to the patient's welfare at that time: [20]

The battle is now raging furiously between the doctor and the disease, each firmly fixed in his purpose, the latter to destroy the patient, the former to destroy the disease. Each organ in the body of the now prostrated patient bows submissively to the tremendous efforts of the physician to overcome his inveterate opponent. Finally, to make quick work of it, the doctor turns his heaviest pieces upon the strongholds of the disease, and accordingly fifteen grains each of *calomel* and *jalap* are sent rumbling along the alimentary canal to drive it out, a huge blister is applied over the spinal column or chest to draw it out, powerful diuretics or diaphoretics are administered to wash it out through the urinary apparatus or the pores of the skin, a pint or two of blood is withdrawn from the arm in hopes to capture it alive, and, while this bombardment is going on, the devoted doctor keeps his line of skirmish well advanced, and maintains a continuous fire of small arms in the form of *Dover's powders, Sweet spirits of nitre, Paregoric, Rhubarb,* and tinctures and infusions of various kinds.

Toward the end of the century, osteopathy, chiropractic, and Christian Science replaced the earlier cults in competition with the regular physician. But by 1900 far fewer persons were ready to forsake scientific medicine for sectarian treatment. The popularization of recent medical advances, the dramatic results achieved with serums and antitoxins, and the borrowing from the homeopaths of such lessons as drug palatability and small dosage made the regular profession far more appealing. The success of Christian Science was due partly to a new failure on the part of medical men: their indifference to mental influence in the genesis and cure of physical ailments. Christian Science exploited the vacuum left by medicine's rejection of functional disorders in the wake of the germ theory.[21] Mr. Dooley of the *Chicago Daily News* showed, as usual, an astute insight into the problem when he wrote:[22]

Father Kelley says th' styles iv medicine changes like the styles iv hats. . . . He says they ought to enforce th' law iv assault with a deadly weapin' again th' doctors. He says that if they knew less about pizen and more about gruel an' opened fewer patients and more windows, they'd not be so many Christyan Scientists. He says th' diff'rence between Christyan Scientists an' doctors is that Christyan Scientists thinks they'se no such thing as disease an' doctors thinks there ain't anything else. An' there ye ar're.

Patent and proprietary remedies, though known as the "poor man's medicines," were widely used by all classes of society throughout the nineteenth century. The therapeutic nihilism of the medical profession caused many persons who should have known better to seek cure through some widely advertised panacea. Patent medicines were extolled in every newspaper, almanac, and magazine which fell into the hands of the nineteenth-century American, and in terms which would cause even present vendors of these cure-alls to blush. A survey of the advertising pages of the *Chicago Tribune* from 1860 to 1875 reveals a bewildering variety of these concoctions, all with miraculous properties. Lawyers, clergymen, and politicians were advised of the soothing laryngeal effects of Dr. Foord's Pectoral Syrup; Dr. Sweet's Infallible Liniment was compounded from a secret recipe of the great bonesetter, Stephen Sweet; there was no better tonic than Greeley's Bourbon Bitters; tuberculosis could be avoided by imbibing Dr. Jayne's Expectorant; for problems connected with infant teething there was the efficacious Mrs. Winslow's Soothing Syrup; old people whose blood was sour or thin (as well as young folk with adolescent humour in their veins) were importuned to cleanse their systems with Wishart's Pine Tree Tar Cordial; an expenditure of one dollar would bring one the wonderful metallic alloy, Oriede, which was used extensively in this country as a substitute for gold; all and every kind of lameness would succumb to the ministration of Dr. Plumleigh's Indiana Botanic Plaster; this last would also cure cancer and old ulcers, failing which one might still turn to Kennedy's Medical Discovery, noted for its rapid cures of these afflictions; the noted Professor Silliman of Yale College was advertised as endorsing the curative powers of Old Sachem Bitters and Wigwam Tonic.[23] These remedies were in most cases harmless and possibly beneficial in view of the psychological effect they might have in inspiring hope and confidence; but such a medicine as Mrs. Winslow's Soothing Syrup, found to obtain one grain of morphine per ounce of liquid, might, when given according to directions on the bottle, cause very serious illness.[24]

Despite the quacks, irregulars, and patent medicine vendors, the Chicago physician opposed the regulation of medicine by law until well into the 1850's. Long after the last Conestoga wagon had disappeared, his thinking was still colored by the experience of the early years and the belief that government should provide maximum protection with a minimum amount of interference with the individual. He sincerely believed the liberal dictum that only by granting liberty to his irregular competitors would he himself be assured of freedom. The remedy for charlatanry, one journal declared, should not be sought in government decree, for "Man can't be cured of ignorance or insanity, nor endowed with common sense and understanding, by the force of law." Chicago's first medical journal, almost in its first issue, declared that it was unalterably opposed to restrictive laws governing the practice of medicine. Such laws, declared the editor, only gave undeserved popularity to those against whom they were directed. A discussion by the city's leading physicians in 1858 revealed only a few favoring regulation; most of those taking part saw the improvement of medical schools and public education as the only answers to quackery.[25]

Similarly, quarantine was regarded by most physicians before

1880 as an unwarranted infringement on personal liberty and commercial intercourse. Despite the speeches and writings of John Evans, who became convinced during the cholera epidemic of 1849 that quarantine was necessary, the majority opinion held that cholera was not contagious and should not be subject to quarantine. It was doubtless more than coincidence that Evans' logical arguments were rejected at a time when Chicago was undergoing tremendous commercial expansion. The force of middle-class liberalism, with its emphasis on freedom, collided with Evans' theory of contagion with its unwelcome corollary of regulation and disruption of commerce. Chicago's physicians read the German and British authors on epidemic diseases; it was not strange that they accepted them over Evans' observations and statistics when they coincided so well with their own prepossessions. Many of the city's leading doctors—Brainard, Boone, Egan, Kimberly—were heavily engaged in large-scale commercial and real estate activity and thus tended naturally to oppose quarantine, so long at least as any reasonable doubt of the validity of the contagion theory remained. Evans himself was engaged in several business ventures, but for him all doubt about the contagiousness of cholera had now vanished.

Further evidence that opposition to the theory of contagion was linked with general devotion to freedom may be gleaned from the fact that Evans, who was the only outspoken advocate of quarantine, was also the only physician of importance to call for public regulation of medicine in the 1840's.[26] The political atmosphere continued to be unhealthy for both quarantine and the regulation of medicine until well after the Civil War. As late as 1879 the editors of the *Chicago Medical Journal and Examiner*—N. S. Davis, D. R. Brower, J. N. Hyde, and W. H. Byford—were still warning that quarantine placards were an unjustifiable attack on personal liberty: ". . . even if the profession were unanimous in their approval of warning cards, that would not make it right for the government to intrude them into the private abode of private citizens. The warning card, as a notice of sickness, is in itself harmless enough, but as the symbol of an officious intrusion by the government, it is thoroughly outrageous."[27] With the firmer establishment of the germ theory in the course of the 1880's, this journal, like other opponents of quarantine, was forced to reverse itself. Where the injury to commerce had been put forward as an argument against quarantine heretofore, it was now argued that only immigrants, and not goods, were likely to be infected; cargoes therefore need not be delayed.[28]

Public regulation of the practice of medicine was finally undertaken in 1877. The Medical Practice Act of that year provided that all physicians in the state must register, those with diplomas from approved medical schools to be licensed immediately, those lacking them to be examined by a state medical board. Physicians who had been in practice ten years were exempted from the examination. The beneficial effect of the law was immediately evident: of thirty-six hundred nongraduates practicing medicine in Illinois in 1877, fourteen hundred left the state within the year. The board moved against dishonest advertising by physicians and began laying down regulations for medical colleges in 1878; no medical school, the board ruled, would be considered in good standing while graduating two classes of students in one year or failing to require two full terms of lectures for graduation.[29] Curriculum standards for all of the state's medical schools were adopted in 1884. Six years later Illinois schools were required to give three courses of lectures for graduation. In its first decade, the board was successful in ridding the state of over three thousand unqualified practitioners, as well as preventing countless others from settling in Illinois.[30] The regulation of medical practice was a function of the State Board of Health until 1917 when, as mentioned earlier, a Department of Registration and Education, separate from the new Department of Public Health, was created to handle licensing and related tasks. By providing that the director of this department should not be a physician, the new law sought to assure impartiality and justice to all of the state's doctors, regardless of their school or medical experience.[31]

The question of fees for medical service was one which greatly disturbed the relations between public and profession in the second half of the nineteenth century. Before 1850 the western practitioner was content to receive produce and local services in exchange for his work; rarely was he paid in money. But a rapid rise in the cost of living after 1850—one estimate put the increase at 50 per cent for the years from 1843 to 1870—made it necessary for him to charge larger fees.[32] He also began to demand that payments be made in cash, since barter was becoming an increasingly cumbersome and unsatisfactory means of exchange. In 1855, therefore, the Chicago Medical Society adopted a fee table representing an advance of about 50 per cent over previous charges; but Chicago fees were still low in comparison with other sections of the country. The new schedule recommended the following fees: [33]

Ordinary visits	$1.50
Night visits	3.00 (10:00 P.M. to daylight)
First consultative visit	5.00-10.00
Subsequent consultative visits	2.00- 3.00
Examination of chest	3.00- 5.00
Office prescriptions	1.00
Obstetrical attendance	10.00-20.00 ($5.00 to $20.00 additional for instrumental delivery)

These charges were gradually increased in the following years. In 1869, the city's doctors were charging a minimum price of two to three dollars for a day visit and from five to ten dollars for a night call. Other factors combined by 1880 to push the cost of medical care even higher; improvements in training and medical education, the advent of specialization on a large scale, and mounting hospital costs all had to be paid for by the consumer of medical service. When coupled with the growing public consciousness of the advances made by medical science and the consequently increased demand for professional care, a situation was created in which medical costs became a subject of widespread social concern.[34] Few critics recognized that doctors' services were subject to the same inflationary pressures as the sellers of groceries and clothing, of coal and other services. The physician, pressed by economic necessity and a feeling, in some cases, that he was not receiving his just due, began to temper his dedicated view of his calling with an increased consciousness of his economic self-interest, while the public, confronted with rapidly rising medical fees, adopted a more critical view of the doctor. This rupture was aggravated by the growing impersonality of medical practice in Chicago. The continued expansion of the city, combined with the mushrooming of specialists and consultants, brought to an end the friendly personal relations which had existed between patient and doctor; the family doctor, as A. Reeves Jackson commented in 1881, was rapidly passing from the scene.[35]

Even the medical journals were ready to co-operate in the general denigration of the high fees of the specialist. The average practitioner, like the public in general, was out of sympathy with the rising power, prestige, and wealth of the city's specialists. The *Medical*

Standard likened their fees to highway robbery in 1896, accusing them of taking advantage of life-or-death situations to extort money from helpless victims.[36] It had become a rather common practice for specialists to divide their fees with the physicians who referred patients to them; this promoted a kind of commercial competition for patients which the profession as a whole deplored. Doctors might, and some did, send patients to the specialist who offered them the most, rather than the one most competent to deal with a particular case. The Chicago Medical Society condemned fee splitting in 1901 as reducing medicine to the lowest commercial basis. It was, in actuality, the resolution read, "the practicing of a confidence game upon the patient." The *Chicago Tribune*, a decade later, sought to determine the extent to which the practice prevailed in the city, but came to no definite conclusions. Reporters did discover that a large minority of surgeons were willing to consider fictitious propositions for dividing a fee. Most doctors at this time admitted that the practice existed, though denying it was widespread.[37]

The Chicago Medical Society had a code of ethics to serve as a guide to physicians in their relations with each other and the public. Identical with the code of the national association, it had as its objectives the upholding of the dignity of the profession, the protection of physician and public against unscientific doctrines and ideas, and the prevention of a commercial-type competition among doctors. The weapons which the Chicago Medical Society might use to enforce standards of professional behavior were those of similar groups everywhere: social pressure and the power of expulsion from organized medicine.[38] The hostility of the local profession was a hazard to professional reputation and success which few physicians would dare to risk. During the first thirty years of its existence, the Chicago Society used its power of excommunication sparingly, usually against the heresy of homeopathy. Occasionally a member was dropped for advertising or for deprecating some member or members of the local profession in public, but this type of offender normally expiated his offense short of the extreme penalty. In 1865 the Society heard a report that "no physician that has ever advertised should be admitted to membership," but again this pronouncement was honored more in the breach than in the observance.[39]

In the last two decades of the century, however, the Society became aware of its power to combat economic heresy: free clinics, contract medical schemes, and voluntary health insurance plans. The growth of public medical clinics, in particular, was an important source of friction between the doctors and citizens of Chicago. By 1880, the expansion of the medical colleges and an increase in the number of teaching hospitals had greatly enlarged the need for clinical material. A number of free clinics were created to meet this need. Though ostensibly providing care only for the poor, many of them doubtless admitted also a number of marginal and undeserving cases. The Chicago Medical Society charged these clinics with abusing medical charity; they were operated, according to a committee report in 1880, by medical schools interested only in increasing the number of clinical cases at their disposal. A "ring" of older professors was accused by the Society of responsibility for this maladministration of medical charity. The *Chicago Tribune* joined in the attack on the clinics, while one medical journal came to their support. The *Chicago Medical Journal and Examiner* denied the Society's charges; some of the offending dispensaries, the editor pointed out, were not connected with medical colleges, while it was in any case difficult to distinguish those able to pay for care. If a fee were charged, as some physicians suggested, the result would be only the exclusion of the most destitute.[40]

The abuse of medical charity became a frequent topic of discussion among medical men and societies during the 1880's. Though the economic competition of the clinics was clearly the basic reason for the profession's interest in the problem, other considerations influenced the thinking of some. Medical spokesmen expressed a great concern for those who had been getting free care without deserving it; the fear was repeatedly voiced that this group was being "pauperized" by having free medical care thrust upon it by the clinics. A more realistic statement of the profession's position, however, was made by I. N. Love in his presidential address to the Mississippi Valley Medical Association in 1887; the time had arrived, declared Love, "to call a halt in these efforts to . . . diminish the proper compensation of . . . the profession by reckless and misdirected benevolence." [41]

The question of clinics and their abuse increased, rather than decreased, in importance in the early years of the twentieth century. By 1907 there were fifty-five dispensaries in Chicago, sixteen of them connected with hospitals, nine with medical schools, and thirty unattached. In six of these clinics, all treatment and medicines were free; eighteen made a charge for medicines; in twenty-six, attempts were made to collect as much as possible. The Chicago Medical Society discovered that only half of these dispensaries claimed to make any investigation of the patient's ability to pay, and these efforts consisted of a few perfunctory questions from the physician in charge. Members of the Society were further antagonized by the efforts of clinics to attract patients via newspaper advertising and handbills. In 1909, therefore, the Society co-operated with the homeopathic, eclectic, and physio-medical societies in establishing a bureau of investigation which would compile information on dispensary patients and their financial status. This project was not viable, apparently, since three years later the Society was considering a scheme to force all applicants for dispensary or hospital charity to present a statement from a physician stating that they could not pay. Again, in 1913, another plan was devised—that all hospitals and clinics be asked to send to the Society each week the names, addresses, and occupations of all persons receiving free treatment—but this proved as impracticable as the others.[42]

The number of clinics in Chicago increased rapidly during the years following the First World War. Clinics caring for certain classes or types of patients appeared; existing clinics were subdivided into more specialized sections; all clinics expanded steadily the scope of their operations. Among the new dispensaries which opened their doors after 1918 was the Public Health Institute, an organization which was to become the center of a vast controversy involving the Chicago Medical Society, the public, the press, and a number of doctors.

The Public Health Institute was organized as a venereal disease clinic in 1920 with Joseph G. Berkowitz as medical director. Under the guidance of a board of prominent laymen, serving without compensation, the institute opened with facilities for treating three patients at one time. The response to the first announcement in the Chicago papers was tremendous; 1955 examinations and treatments were given during the first month. As a nonprofit institution, the clinic charged very low fees: three dollars for an examination, six gonorrhea treatments for four dollars, injections of antisyphilis drugs for one to three dollars. Many patients, unable to pay anything, were treated free of charge or with charity funds. Private specialists at this time were charging considerably more for treating venereal patients. The institute quickly expanded its facilities to care for the huge demand; clinics for women and Negroes were added in 1923.[43]

From the outset the Chicago Medical Society resented the competition afforded private physicians by the institute. The Society was particularly incensed by the widespread advertising used by the clinic to attract reluctant sufferers. Newspaper advertisements, streetcar bulletins, booklets, and large-scale posters were all used by the publicity department of the institute. This publicity, the clinic felt, was necessary because of the delicacy and urgency of the medical problem involved, but the medical society was deeply concerned with the professional ethics involved. The Society repeatedly warned doctors connected with the enterprise that such advertising must be discontinued.

The controversy came to a rapid climax in 1929 when Dr. Louis E. Schmidt was dropped from membership in the Chicago Medical Society because of his association with the Public Health Institute through the Illinois Social Hygiene League, which Dr. Schmidt had aided in founding twelve years previously. Schmidt and the Illinois Social Hygiene League signed a contract with the Public Health Institute, under which (1) the League would aid in caring for indigent cases applying to the Public Health Institute, for which the Institute would pay the League one thousand dollars per month; and (2) the Public Health Institute would, through its representatives, "assume full control over the management of all the Clinic's property and personnel." Although this latter provision of the contract was not actually carried out in practice, its existence indicated the close association between Schmidt and the Public Health Institute.

Schmidt appealed the verdict of the Society, charging that the real issue was not advertising, but the high cost of medical care; he warned the profession that it must act to bring down medical costs. By providing medical service to those who would not otherwise be able to afford it, Schmidt declared, the Institute was not competing with private physicians, but only rendering a public service. The Society, however, insisted that Schmidt had flagrantly violated that section of the Code of Ethics which forbade members to co-operate with any organization that advertised medical services. Schmidt, like all members of the Chicago Medical Society, had signed a pledge that he would govern his conduct by the official Code of Medical Ethics. He violated this pledge by his co-operation with the Public Health Institute. The state and national medical organizations upheld Schmidt's ouster; the vote in the Judicial Council of the American Medical Association was 3-2 against Schmidt, with the Chairman and J. B. Herrick of Chicago dissenting.[44]

Schmidt's expulsion attracted tremendous newspaper interest. The drama was heightened by the action of Health Commissioner Bundesen in resigning from the Society as a gesture of protest; in a public statement he declared he would stand "shoulder to shoulder with Dr. Schmidt in his efforts to bring down the cost of being sick." [45] The press, paying no heed to the Society's declaration that Schmidt's ouster was solely on the grounds of advertising, attacked the Society and its leaders as a group of self-seeking men who sought to obstruct the expansion of low-cost clinics that would aid the masses.[46]

Although the Society succeeded partially in getting its point of view recognized in the following months, the damage to public relations was serious. The lack of public confidence in medical men was admitted by the Society in its bulletin the year following the incident; an article in the bulletin attributed this public mistrust to the profession's firm refusal to support "all the schemes of philanthropists and sociologists for lowering the cost of illness." [47] Most of Chicago's medical leaders continued the fight against abuses of charity. The attitude of the profession regarding medical charity in 1929 was summed up by Dr. Charles B. Reed: [48]

The practice of charity is one of the most ancient and glorious traditions of the medical profession and only recently the Chicago Medical Society reaffirmed . . . the ethical ideal that it is ready and willing at all times to serve the citizens of Cook County irrespective of their economic status. The profession feels, however, that only too frequently its desire to serve the public is misunderstood or taken advantage of by the unworthy. That charity is pernicious which takes from independence its proper pride and from mendicity its proper shame.

This has continued to be the view of a large part of organized medicine. Doctors will take care of all deserving charity cases; all others should pay all or part of their medical fees through arrangement with their own physicians. Critics of organized medicine have pointed out that many persons have no family doctor, that such agreements in practice are hard to arrange, that sickness brings additional burdens including loss of income, that serious illness can be catastrophic in its effect on a family's fortunes. As for the recipients of charity, critics have insisted that all human beings have a right to the benefits of modern medical science without stigma or feelings of "proper shame." But defenders of the profession have questioned whether this right extends to the very best and most expensive type of medical care. If the charity patient deserves the very best medical care, why not the very best food, clothing, and shelter?

During the depression years following 1929, the Chicago profession became increasingly alarmed at the multiplication of clinics. Medical agencies were established during the 1930's to guard the health of a wide variety of ethnic, religious, racial, and economic groups. A survey of thirty-four clinics in 1934 revealed that 50 per cent of the patients treated were recipients of unemployment relief. More than two million patient visits were recorded at these clinics the year preceding the survey, yet Chicago ranked fifteenth in a list of twenty-two large cities in its clinic service to the poor.[49] The plight of the unemployed with respect to medical care was considerably eased by the adoption in 1934 of a federal program of free medical service for the recipients of unemployment relief, to be administered by the Illinois Emergency Relief Commission. The Chicago and Illinois medical societies appointed advisory committees to co-operate with the commission in working out satisfactory fees and administering the project. By 1940, Cook County physicians had been paid about two and a quarter million dollars from public funds for their services to the indigent.[50] The sum paid to individual doctors was not at all large, when one considers that it was spread over six years and divided among many hundreds of physicians. Whatever the sum, however, participation was a reversal of organized medicine's stand on government aid; the Sheppard-Towner Act was vehemently denounced a decade earlier. The profession's explanation was that the emergency medical program was an undesirable, yet necessary, expedient, and in no way altered the honest conviction of most doctors that "state medicine" is poor medicine. The Judicial Council of the American Medical Association expressed its reluctant approval as follows: "This is a complete and undisguised example of 'state medicine.' The avidity with which in general the government's offer was received can be explained only on the basis of an acute economic situation in the profession itself. The occurrence must be considered as a temporary expedient only, due to the unparalleled stress of the time, and must be discontinued as rapidly as the stress on the profession is relieved." [51]

To combat clinical abuses in the 1930's, the Chicago Medical Society itself undertook a survey of medical charity. According to the budget standard adopted by the investigating committee, described as a "rather liberal one," the proportion of actual cases of abuse of clinic facilities was set at 13 per cent.[52] The Society then established in 1935 a committee on hospitals and clinics to work out some criteria of clinic eligibility. The report of this committee recommended a flexible standard of measurement based on such intangibles as the nature of the disease, the cost of treatment, the patient's family responsibilities, the length of his employment, the financial strain under which he lived, and the cost of living. These recommendations were sharply challenged in the council, however, notably by Dr. Edward Ochsner, who felt that a flexible standard played into the hands of impractical reformers and social workers. Ochsner submitted a budget geared only to income and size of family. A single man or woman earning forty dollars a month in 1936 was able, in his view, to pay a private physician; for a man, wife, and three children, he set the minimum figure at one hundred dollars. The council threw over both sets of recommendations and resolved that doubtful cases should be admitted pending receipt of a letter from the family doctor outlining the family's economic status. It was further recommended that physicians should be detailed to police the dispensaries, since the profession lacked confidence in social workers.[53] These resolutions were never carried out, probably because of their impracticability.

Concomitant with the growth of the clinic problem there had come increasing pressure for a readjustment in the method of paying for medical care. The great medical and technological advances after 1880 aroused a greater demand for medical and hospital service; the practice of medicine rapidly became more complex and more specialized; and the number of medical men and resources employed in combating an individual illness mounted. These changes usually reduced the duration of illness, saved many persons from permanent or long-term disability, and greatly increased the chances of survival in case of illness, and as a result the overall, average cost to society of sickness dropped tremendously. At the same time, the unit cost of treatment of individual patients mounted steadily. Where the services of one family practitioner might have constituted the entire financial obligation in sickness heretofore, the added expense of specialists, consultants and nurses, as well as fees for routine and special laboratory tests, medicines, and hospital beds, had now to be borne by the victim of illness. Obviously, the most costly care was infinitely less expensive than death, which was a virtual certainty in many kinds of cases before this array of technological and scientific assistance existed. Nonetheless, if disease attacked the breadwinner in a family, or if the illness were of long duration, the effect on the family's finances and independence could be disastrous.

The Chicago Medical Society's recommended fee table was adjusted upward regularly after 1880. By 1913 patients were being charged from three to five dollars for a general office consultation, from five to fifteen dollars for a house visit, and from five to twenty-five dollars for a night call.[54] The Society recommended in connection with this schedule that no fee for a major surgical operation be less than 10 per cent of a patient's annual income, but set no upper limit on surgeons' fees.

A number of proposals for meeting the problem of rising medical costs began to appear in the last decade or so of the nineteenth century. Several plans were put into actual operation in Chicago. As early as 1889 a proposal for contract service was laid before the Illinois State Medical Society. Citing the scientific and social changes which had occurred recently in the United States, this plan had as its premises the importance of preventive medicine and the need for physicians to adapt to changing conditions. The proponents of this plan urged the State Society to encourage families to enter into contracts for annual medical service, the fees to be paid quarterly or monthly.[55] The following year a prepaid medical program was inaugurated in Chicago by Dr. J. K. Crawford and former Health Commissioner Oscar De Wolf. Under the title of "The Mutual Medical Aid Association of Chicago," this organization proposed to "secure to those of limited means prompt and efficient medical & surgical treatment and medicines in cases of sickness or accident, by a corps of competent physicians & surgeons, at nominal cost." The dues payed by members of the association ranged from three dollars per quarter for a single person to five dollars for a family of five or more. This fee was to cover all professional services except obstetrical attendance, for which an extra ten dollars was charged. Physicians hired by the association were paid monthly salaries.

Both Crawford and De Wolf were tried by the Chicago Medical Society for "unprofessional conduct" for their role in originating and administering the plan. They were charged specifically with advertising, contract practice, and cheapening professional skill "by teaching the public to regard it as being of small pecuniary value." In their own defense the two doctors claimed that their plan was in accordance with "the best lines of modern thought," that it was "encouraged by enlightened and humane employers of labor almost without exception," and that it was the first real attempt to put the principles of preventive medicine into operation in Chicago. The association would, they promised, confine its activities to the employees of large corporations and manufacturing plants where adequate medical care was sorely lacking. The insurance principle behind the organization was heavily stressed—"those who do *not* require medical aid help to pay for those who *do*"—but to no avail. The two doctors were convicted on all charges but were not expelled from the Society.[56]

During the following two decades, much of the Society's time was taken up with consideration of contract schemes. All such plans were still condemned on the ground that they destroyed the personal relationship between doctor and patient, but there was a general reluctance to expel members guilty of association with them. The feeling grew that though contract medical practice was unethical, it was at least an attempt to meet a very real and pressing problem.[57] The committee appointed to study the subject admitted in 1907 "that many of the men working under these various contracts are desirous of improving the conditions of things, that they are not wanton violators of the ethical codes and that they are willing to co-operate in any amicable solution of the question." [58]

The movement for public health insurance did not gain momentum until just before World War I when the question of workmen's compensation for injury or sickness suffered on the job was widely debated. The success of the compensation program in virtually all states during the following decade lent encouragement to those who advocated a system of governmental health insurance for the United States. The successful campaign for health insurance in Great Britain in 1911 stirred up considerable interest among liberals and progressives in America. The American Association for Labor Legislation became interested in the question in 1912 and created a committee to study all types of health insurance. This committee, with the assistance of the American Medical Association, drew up a draft for a model health insurance act in 1915. In the next three years, health insurance bills were introduced in fifteen state legislatures, including Illinois, but none of them was passed. In the disillusionment and return to conservatism which marked the postwar period, support for government health insurance began to melt away. The American Medical Association, which had not previously formally committed itself, went on record as opposed to compulsory health insurance in 1920. The principle of state-sponsored insurance had been endorsed during the war by a number of local and state medical societies, as well as the American Hospital Association and the American Association of Industrial Physicians and Surgeons; but the larger urban societies, notably in New York and Chicago, actively opposed health insurance from the outset.[59]

The bill which went before the Illinois legislature in 1917 was designed to cover all persons earning less than one hundred dollars per month. The cost of the plan was to be divided equally between the employer and his employee, with the state contributing 20 per cent of all costs. Benefits included complete medical, dental, surgical, nursing, and hospital service for the employee and his dependents, in addition to cash payments up to two-thirds of his earnings for a period of twenty-six weeks. This proposal was strongly criticized by the Chicago Medical Society, which argued that it was premature and unnecessary. Health insurance in Europe, opponents of the bill charged, had not improved the level of public health and had, in fact, produced a great deal of malingering. From the standpoint of the profession, said a spokesman for the Society, compulsory insurance might mean a greater equalization of income, but only through subsidizing the less efficient. Personal relations between physician and patient would be destroyed; the incentive for medical research would be eliminated; professional competence would decrease since the largest rewards would go to those who made the most calls. Finally, the spokesman claimed, compulsory health insurance was "Un-American and Subversive of American Ideals of Democratic Government." [60]

A considerable minority in the Chicago Society, as in the American Medical Association, favored compulsory health insurance. Such well-known doctors as Arthur Dean Bevan and Malcolm L. Harris were at this time sympathetic to the idea. Harris was a leader in the fight to give health insurance a fair hearing in the American Medical Association; he saw sickness insurance as the only alternative to state medicine and argued that the American people, not the medical profession, should be allowed to make the decision.[61] Dr.

Frank Billings, though he did not actively support the program, kept his mind open on the question.[62] But by 1920 most Chicago and Illinois physicians were convinced of the dangers of compulsory medical insurance; the State Society instructed its delegates to the American Medical Association that year to "oppose state medicine, compulsory health insurance, county and state health agencies, and 'allied dangerous Bolsheviki schemes.' "[63]

Though the possibility of enacting any sickness insurance legislation in Illinois was clearly lost, the state's medical leaders kept up an almost constant barrage against the idea throughout the twenties. The state journal hammered away incessantly at the evils of state medicine, the horrors of the panel system in Germany, the dissatisfaction of the British doctors with their lot, and the peril that threatened the American profession. As late as 1931 the official organ of the state's doctors still contained numerous editorials and articles on "Socialization of Obstetrics," "Socialism a Failure in Medicine," "Physicians Give One-Eighth of Time to Charity," "Menace to Medicine from Economic Sins," "Maternity Act a Flop," "Lay Public Taking Advantage of Medicine," and "Why More Dispensaries in Chicago?"

On the national scene, there was created in the late 1920's a National Committee on the Costs of Medical Care composed of leaders in medicine, public health, and the social sciences to study the whole problem of medical economics. The group, headed by a physician, Ray Lyman Wilbur, who subsequently became secretary of the interior in the Hoover administration, was composed of twenty-four other doctors and twenty-three laymen. Seven Chicagoans served on the committee, four of them physicians. In the course of the next five years a series of twenty-eight comprehensive reports on sickness, medical costs, and the availability of health facilities was published under the direction of this body. The committee's final report, released in 1932, attracted a great deal of interest and comment because of the growing economic depression in the country.[64] The majority report, signed by the chairman and thirty-five of his associates, called for rapid extension of group practice by physicians in America and recommended that the cost of medical care "be placed on a group payment basis, through the use of insurance, through the use of taxation, or through the use of both these methods." This report was signed by Rollin T. Woodyatt, a Chicago physician, Herman Bundesen, health commissioner of the city, and by all three Chicago laymen on the committee.[65] The minority report, signed by eight physicians, including M. L. Harris of Chicago and Olin West representing the American Medical Association, asked for an end of governmental competition in medicine and a restoration of the "general practitioner to the central place in medical practice." Replying to the majority's endorsement of group clinics, the minority commented that medicine was a personal service, not amenable to mass production techniques.[66] Representatives of the Chicago and Illinois Medical societies strongly supported the stand of the minority group.

The political atmosphere of the 1930's, especially the overriding interest in relief and reform, brought a renewal of interest in the problem of medical costs and their payment. Health surveys, conferences, and community planning became increasingly common as the decade wore on; the American Hospital Association endorsed group hospitalization; the report of two doctors from the Michigan State Medical Society on British health insurance flatly challenged the version which the *Journal of the American Medical Association* had for years been implanting in its readers; the California Medical Association approved in 1934 the principle of compulsory insurance and drafted a suitable bill for the state; a group of liberal doctors formed a Committee of Physicians in opposition to the negative policies of the American Medical Association; a National Health Conference was held in 1938 at President Roosevelt's suggestion, following which the first national compulsory insurance bill was introduced into Congress.[67]

The first reaction of organized medicine to these developments was to deny the need for reform. "No one," declared Charles B. Reed of the Chicago Medical Society's Public Relations Committee in 1935, "has ever lacked adequate medical care in America except in remote unsettled districts." [68] But gradually the feeling grew that if health surveys and medical reforms were to be made, they had best be directed by members of the medical profession. When the Chicago Hospital Council approached the Society in 1936 with a group hospitalization plan, the council did not reject it, but instead insisted that control of the plan be vested in members of the Chicago Medical Society. Though the Hospital Council could not accept this amendment, the stand of the physicians did represent a liberalizing of attitude since the 1920's.[69] A survey of the available medical resources in Cook County, as against the amount required for good health, was conducted by the Society in 1938. Though the Society's report emphasized the adequacy of existing facilities and institutions, there was nevertheless considerable evidence of a new willingness to compromise. The most outstanding feature of the report was the sympathy it revealed for the marginal economic group, not eligible for free service, which could not afford the medical, surgical, and dental care it needed; this confirmed an observation of the Committee on the Costs of Medical Care which Chicago's medical spokesmen had heatedly denied only a few years earlier. The solution recommended in the Society's report was a nonprofit, voluntary insurance plan.[70] Following the presentation of this report to the council, N. S. Davis III proposed that lists of physicians who would treat this lower income group on the basis of its ability to pay be prepared. This, he urged, was the only way to save for the profession those borderline patients who were now forced to turn to the dispensaries and clinics. Davis' proposal, together with the recommendations in the report, constituted the first realistic attempt to deal with the medical charity problem which had so long plagued the relations between profession and public.

After 1940, the profession was constantly on the defensive against enactment of a national system of health insurance. By the close of the Second World War the campaign for federally subsidized medical care had gained considerable momentum. In November, 1945, the Murray-Wagner-Dingell health bill was introduced into the Congress following a plea from President Truman. This plan proposed a 4 per cent payroll tax on the incomes of all persons earning less than thirty-six hundred dollars annually to cover all costs of medical care; it called also for a rapid extension of public health services and federal aid to medical education and research, but these features of the bill were largely forgotten in the ensuing controversy over compulsory health insurance.[71] The fight against the medical insurance provision of the Wagner bill was led by spokesmen for the American Medical Association, who enjoyed the support of the American Bar Association, the American Hospital Association, and a number of insurance and drug firms. Backers of the program included organized labor, the American Public Health Association, some farm groups, and the Association of Internes and Medical Students.[72] The reaction of the Chicago Medical Society to the Wagner plan was expressed by Dr. Warren Furey, who termed the bill "a further extension, pure and simple, of outright collectivism." Illinois congressmen, in general, were also opposed to the bill. Senator Scott Lucas commented: "I have always been opposed to socialized medicine. I see no reason for changing my viewpoint at this time." [73]

The controversy dragged on for several years. The issue was thoroughly debated, pro and con, but most appeals were directed to the emotions rather than to the mind. Almost unnoticed was the cool, scholarly analysis of the whole problem undertaken by the New York Academy of Medicine. A Committee on Medicine and the Changing Order was created by the New York body in 1942 to study economic and social changes and their effect on the practice of medicine. Associated with the committee in this work were such distinguished medical historians and writers as Henry Sigerist, Richard Shryock, and Iago Galdston, social scientists like Max Lerner, Robert S. Lynd, Bernhard Stern, Edmund Day, and Leo Wolman, and the public health expert, Thomas Parran. After a number of preliminary studies, the final report of the committee was released in 1947. In substance, the committee recommended the continued development of voluntary, prepaid plans, adapted to the exigencies of local situations, and subsidized where necessary by government funds—local, state, and federal—in order to achieve a maximal use of existing medical resources at minimal cost. While the committee did not approve "compulsory health insurance *at the present time*, we also disapprove *at the present time* any other form of prepaid, full-coverage insurance to be applied as suitable for all sections of the country.[74] The conclusions thus reached were not in basic disagreement with the position of the Chicago Medical Society in the late 1940's.

Under the continued threat of a federal system of health insurance, the medical profession has grown increasingly liberal in its concessions to the trend of the age.[75] During the 1940's, the American Medical Association went on record in favor of extending medical care to the lower middle class (the "medically indigent" as they have been defined), and also endorsed group practice and voluntary health insurance, the two major recommendations of the earlier Committee on the Costs of Medical Care.[76] The Chicago Medical Society, while continuing to fight the national health program through the American Medical Association and its own Committee on Medical Service, instituted a voluntary medical insurance program co-ordinated with the local Blue Cross plan. As the Blue Shield Chicago

Medical Service Plan, operations were begun in June, 1948. The organization was subsequently amalgamated into the statewide Illinois Medical Service Plan, which eight years later had an enrollment of almost two and a half million persons, most of them residents of Cook County.[77]

There is still much to be done before supporters of the city's medical and hospital plans may claim that the problem of medical economics has been solved for Chicago's citizens. Essentially, however, Chicago medicine has moved and continues to move rapidly in the direction of providing more care for more persons. Certainly a revolution in medical practice has taken place in Chicago, as elsewhere, since 1900, and the impact on the health and welfare of Chicago's citizens has been as profound as it has been dramatic. In looking back to the 1890's, Arthur Hertzler, the famous Chicago-trained "horse and buggy doctor," remarked that "in the light of my present knowledge, I can scarcely think of a single disease that the doctors actually cured during those early years of my memory." [78] The main business of the doctor was to relieve suffering, set bones, sew up cuts and assist at childbirth. How much more effective is the modern doctor with his antitoxins, serums and vaccines, his knowledge of bacteriology and sanitation, his laboratories for chemical analysis and diagnosis, his mastery of new techniques in surgery and anesthesia, and his armamentorium of vitamins, insulin, liver extract, sulfa drugs, penicillin and other antibiotics.

The impact of twentieth-century medicine has been equally dramatic on the medical profession. The doctor beginning practice in 1900 had two or at most three short years of medical training behind him; his clinical and hospital experience had been all too brief; his instruction had been chiefly through lectures and demonstrations in anatomy; for post-graduate training he normally went to Europe. Sometimes the young graduate had never seen the delivery of a baby; this was changed by Joseph De Lee for graduates of Chicago medical schools. Some of the complicated equipment of today's hospital laboratory, from flame photometers to machines for determining the basal metabolic rate to electrocardiographs, would have been totally foreign to the young doctor of a short half-century ago. Medicine was then more art than science and a large measure of the increased respect for today's followers of Hippocrates springs from the knowledge that behind the doctor stands a mysterious world of scientific laboratories, clinics, and literature, which the layman only dimly understands. In the grim battle against sickness and death, the mid-twentieth century patient knows that he has a more worthy and resourceful ally in the modern doctor than any fellow sufferer in all of human history.

Notes

CHAPTER 1: PROLOGUE TO 1850

[1] *Biographical Sketches of Some of the Early Settlers of the City of Chicago: Part I* (Fergus' Historical Series, Chicago, 1876), 11–14.

[2] For information on the Fort Dearborn surgeons consult Milo M. Quaife, *Chicago as a Medical and Surgical Center: The Surgeons of Fort Dearborn* (n.p., [1913]); Francis B. Heitman, *Historical Register and Dictionary of the United States Army* (2 vols., Washington, 1903); and Alfred T. Andreas, *History of Chicago from the Earliest Period to the Present Time* (3 vols., Chicago, 1884), 1:457–459.

[3] Lloyd Lewis and Henry J. Smith, *Chicago: The History of Its Reputation* (New York, 1929), 33–34.

[4] Harriet Martineau, "Chicago in 1836," in *Annals of Chicago* (Fergus' Historical Series, Chicago, 1876), 37–38.

[5] Milo M. Quaife, *Chicago's Highways, Old and New* (Chicago, 1923), 12.

[6] In 1833 the pioneer physician, Edmund S. Kimberly, was still treating Indians in his office and submitting his bills to the federal government. E. S. Kimberly, Claim against the United States (Indian Department), September 27, 1833, in Edmund S. Kimberly Papers, Chicago Historical Society.

[7] The first druggist to reach Chicago in the 1830's did so in a canoe towed by two Indians. Albert E. Ebert, "Early History of the Drug Trade of Chicago," in *Illinois State Historical Society Transactions* (1903), 240.

[8] Quaife, *Chicago's Highways*, 165.

[9] Lewis and Smith, *Chicago*, 39ff.

[10] *Daily Chicago American*, June 25, 1840.

[11] Lewis and Smith, *Chicago*, 55–60; Mildred E. Chuchnut, Plank Roads as a Phase of Transportation History in Illinois, master's thesis, Northwestern University, 1947.

[12] *Gem of the Prairie* (Chicago), October 19, 1850.

[13] *North-western Medical and Surgical Journal*, N. S., 3:48 (Chicago, May, 1850).

[14] Daniel Drake, *A Systematic Treatise, Historical, Etiological, and Practical, on the Principal Diseases of the Interior Valley of North America*, 1:648 (Cincinnati, 1850).

[15] Isaac D. Rawlings and others, *The Rise and Fall of Disease in Illinois* (2 vols., Springfield, 1927), 1:30.

[16] John Reynolds, *My Own Times* (Belleville, Illinois, 1855), 72.

[17] Erwin H. Ackerknecht, *Malaria in the Upper Mississippi Valley 1760–*

1900 (supplements to the *Bulletin of the History of Medicine*, No. 4, Baltimore, 1945), 22–26.

[18] General Scott disclaimed responsibility for infecting the town, blaming the detachment commander who had ignored orders and entered Chicago for provisions. Scott to Lewis Cass, Secretary of War, reprinted in John B. Hamilton, "The Epidemics of Chicago," in *Bulletin of the Society of Medical History of Chicago*, 1:77–79 (October, 1911).

[19] *Chicago Democrat*, June 24, 1835; *Chicago American*, October 3, 1835.

[20] Lillian Foster, letter from Chicago, November 7, 1854, reprinted from *Way-Side Glances, North and South* (New York, 1859), in *Journal of the Illinois State Historical Society*, 5:391 (October, 1912). An immigrants' information book denied in 1857 that Illinois was an unhealthy state in which to live, declaring that, on the contrary, it was a "veritable paradise for those with tuberculous consumption." Fred. Gerhard, *Illinois as it Is . . .* (Chicago, 1857), 264.

[21] *Weekly Chicago Democrat*, October 12, 1850. The newspaper warmly endorsed Davis' plan.

[22] *Gem of the Prairie*, October 19, 1850.

[23] Richard H. Shryock, *The Development of Modern Medicine: An Interpretation of the Social and Scientific Factors Involved* (2d ed., New York, 1947), 151–169.

[24] Iago Galdston, *Progress in Medicine: A Critical Review of the Last Hundred Years . . .* (New York, 1940), 96–97; Henry E. Sigerist, *Civilization and Disease* (Ithaca, New York, 1943), 171–172; Richard H. Shryock, "Factors Affecting Medical Research in the United States, 1800–1900," in *Bulletin of the Society of Medical History of Chicago*, 5:9 (July, 1943). For the best account of the controversy over the discovery of anesthesia, see Howard R. Raper, *Man against Pain: The Epic of Anesthesia* (New York, 1945), 105–154.

[25] Quoted in Henry B. Shafer, *The American Medical Profession 1783 to 1850* (New York, 1936), 136.

[26] *Proceedings of the Medical Convention for the Purpose of Organizing the Illinois State Medical Society* (Chicago, 1850), 25.

[27] Henry B. Favill, "Early Medical Days in Wisconsin," in John B. Favill, comp., *Henry Baird Favill: A Memorial Volume* (Chicago, 1917), 604.

[28] Shryock, *Development of Modern Medicine*, 110.

[29] *North-western Medical and Surgical Journal*, N. S., 2:426 (October, 1853).

[30] *Western Medical and Physical Journal, Original and Eclectic*, 1:xii (Cincinnati, April, 1827).

[31] *North-western Medical and Surgical Journal*, N. S., 3:79 (May, 1850). The title of Drake's work was *A Systematic Treatise, Historical, Etiological, and Practical, on the Principal Diseases of the Interior Valley of North America.*

[32] "The Illinois State Medical Society: Archives Era," in *Illinois Medical Journal*, 77:391 (Springfield, May, 1940).

[33] Philip Maxwell, Prescription and Diet Book, 1832–36, Fort Dearborn, Hospital Dept., in Chicago Historical Society.

[34] Ackerknecht, *Malaria in the Upper Mississippi Valley*, 117–118.

[35] Most doctors considered themselves fortunate if they escaped infection themselves. Dr. E. S. Kimberly, who practiced in Alabama before coming to

Chicago, wrote in 1826 that "My health has as yet been remarkably good among a sick community indeed I have been one of 3 only who have escaped the fever." E. S. Kimberly to John Kimberly, October 8, 1826, in Edmund S. Kimberly Papers.

[36] Madge E. Pickard and R. Carlyle Buley, *The Midwest Pioneer: His Ills, Cures, & Doctors* (Crawfordsville, Indiana, 1945), 169.

[37] *Chicago American*, August 8, 1835.

[38] See Pickard and Buley, *The Midwest Pioneer*, 35–97, for a charming account of home remedies and domestic medicine on the midwestern frontier.

[39] Richard H. Shryock, "Public Relations of the Medical Profession in Great Britain and the United States: 1600–1870," in *Annals of Medical History*, N. S., 2:312 (New York, May, 1930).

[40] *Chicago Express*, January 11, 1843.

[41] Kimberly's partner wrote one drug firm in 1836 that a proposed specific for fever would be unsatisfactory because it would not appeal to sufferers from both intermittent and remittent fevers. The specific, he advised, should "be equally applicable to both diseases." "We would like," he continued, "the agency for the district of Illinois as wholesale agents & as such would use all the means in our power to enable your medicine to supersede withe the publick the use of all others of that class of medicines now before the Publick." P. Pruyne to drug firm, February 25, 1836, in Edmund S. Kimberly Papers.

[42] Ebert, "Early History of the Drug Trade of Chicago," in *Illinois State Historical Society Transactions* (1903), 245. A druggist, it should be noted, held a very respected position in early Chicago. He was usually a man of education and strong personality. Philo Carpenter, the first druggist to settle in the city, became a leader in civic and charitable enterprises.

[43] Lucius H. Zeuch, "Early Legislation and Organization in the Illinois Country," in *Bulletin of the Society of Medical History of Chicago*, 4:203–206 (July, 1930).

[44] Henry E. Sigerist, *American Medicine* (New York, 1934), 135–137.

[45] *North-western Medical and Surgical Journal*, N. S., 1:164 (August, 1852).

[46] Morris Fishbein, *A History of the American Medical Association 1847 to 1947* (Philadelphia, 1947), 22–31; Sigerist, *American Medicine*, 134–135.

[47] Robert Fergus, comp., *Fergus' Directory of the City of Chicago, 1839* (Fergus' Historical Series, Chicago, 1876), 5–36.

[48] J. W. Norris, *Norris' Business Directory and Statistics of the City of Chicago for 1846* (Fergus' Historical Series, Chicago, 1883), 49–50.

[49] *Illinois Medical and Surgical Journal*, 1:135–137 (Chicago, December, 1844).

[50] Of thirty-five prominent physicians listed in *Mosher's Centennial Historical Album* in 1876, fourteen were born in New York, while a number of others had lived there just prior to coming to Chicago.

[51] William G. Todd, "Early Medicine in Illinois: Founding of Rush Medical College, and Early Chicago," in *Bulletin of the Alumni Association of Rush Medical College*, 7:3 (Chicago, April, 1911).

[52] Fielding H. Garrison, "Contribution of the West to American Medicine," in *Lectures on the History of Medicine: A Series of Lectures at the Mayo Foundation* . . . (Philadelphia, 1933), 161.

[53] *Illinois and Indiana Medical and Surgical Journal*, 1:261 (Chicago, 1846).

[54] Obituary of William B. Egan, in *Chicago Weekly Democrat*, November 3, 1860.

[55] *Barrington* (Illinois) *Review*, September 18, 1903.

[56] *Chicago Democrat*, September 26, 1838.

[57] *Chicago American*, August 6, 1836, April 1, 1837, November 17, 1840; Andreas, *History of Chicago*, 1:459.

[58] George H. Weaver, "Beginnings of Medical Education in and near Chicago: The Institutions and the Men," in *Bulletin of the Society of Medical History of Chicago*, 3:342–343 (September, 1925).

[59] *Barrington Review*, September 18, 1903.

[60] *Chicago Weekly Democrat*, November 3, 1860.

[61] Lucius H. Zeuch, comp., *History of Medical Practice in Illinois Preceding 1850* (vol. 1, Chicago, 1927), 206–208.

[62] *Chicago Weekly Democrat*, February 13, 1858.

[63] *North-western Medical and Surgical Journal*, N. S., 2:297 (September, 1849).

[64] Edgar C. McMechen, *Life of Governor Evans* (Denver, 1924), *passim*.

[65] E. Fletcher Ingals, "The Life and Work of Dr. Daniel Brainard," in *Bulletin of the Alumni Association of Rush Medical College*, 8:1–13 (July, 1912). There has been some confusion about the spelling of Brainard's name. It seems clear that the family name was *Brainerd*, but that the doctor for some reason changed the spelling, possibly because a relative, Dr. Daniel Brainerd, was in practice contemporaneously. David D. Field, *The Genealogy of the Brainerd Family in the United States* (New York, 1857), 187–189.

[66] *Illinois Medical and Surgical Journal*, 1:57–60, 129–131, 146–147, 161–164, 177–178; 2:20–22, 33–34.

[67] *Illinois and Indiana Medical and Surgical Journal*, 1:206 (August, 1846). The first use of ether in Chicago was reported by Brainard in a case in January, 1847. He concluded that, with proper precautions, the anesthetic might be "generally administered with safety." Brainard, "On the Inhalation of Etherial Vapor for the Prevention of Pain during Surgical Operations," in *ibid.*, 1:544–549 (February, 1847).

[68] The wording in this quotation has been transposed.

[69] For a list of Brainard's more important articles, see the *Index to the Transactions of the American Medical Association* (Philadelphia, 1883), 18.

[70] *Daily Democratic Press* (Chicago), January 25, 1854.

[71] The *Daily Democratic Press*, March 1, 1858, said of Brainard's candidacy for mayor: "Every pimp, every shyster, every blackleg, base men and lewd women are working with fiendish energy to elect Dr. Brainard."

[72] *Chicago Medical Journal*, 23:530 (November, 1866).

CHAPTER II: MEDICINE AND THE EXPANDING CITY

[1] Lewis and Smith, *Chicago*, 92–95; Edith Abbott, *The Tenements of Chicago, 1908–1935* (Chicago, 1936), 26.

[2] Lewis and Smith, *Chicago*, 132–146, 202–214.

[3] Chicago Board of Health, *Report*, 1890 (Chicago, 1891), 91.

4 *Ibid.*, 1883–1884, p. 59; 1893, p. 99.

5 Abbott, *Tenements of Chicago*, 31–32. The study was made in 1894.

6 George Homan, "Public Health and the Land Question," in *Weekly Medical Review*, 22:362 (St. Louis, November 8, 1890).

7 Chicago Medical Society, Minutes, December 17, 1883, in Chicago Historical Society.

8 *Lakeside Annual Directory of the City of Chicago*, 1874–1875 (Chicago, 1875), 4.

9 Chicago Board of Health, *Report*, 1879–1880, pp. 14–16.

10 S. B. Grubbs, "Public Health Administration in Illinois," in United States Public Health Service, *Public Health Reports*, 30:1534 (May 21, 1915).

11 Chicago Board of Health, *Report*, 1890, p. 124.

12 *Ibid.*, 1870–1873, pp. 12–13.

13 *Ibid.*, 1878, pp. 13–18.

14 *Ibid.*, 1890, pp. 7–10.

15 *Chicago Medical Recorder*, 28:351 (June 15, 1906).

16 "First Report of the Committee on Public Hygiene of the American Medical Association," in American Medical Association, *Transactions*, 2:431–432 (Philadelphia, 1849).

17 Abbott, *Tenements of Chicago*, 8–25.

18 Chicago Board of Health, *Report*, 1881–1882, pp. 30–31.

19 *Ibid.*, 47.

20 *Ibid.*, 1883–1884, pp. 21–22; 1886, pp. 50–55; 1889, pp. 45–46.

21 Abbott, *Tenements of Chicago*, 63–64.

22 "Cities and Parks," in *Atlantic Monthly*, 7:416 (April, 1861). "The first murderer," intoned the critic, "was the first city-builder."

23 Bernhard J. Stern, *Society and Medical Progress* (Princeton, New Jersey, 1941), xiv–xv; New York Academy of Medicine, Committee on Medicine and the Changing Order, *Medicine in the Changing Order* (New York, 1947), 29.

24 Rawlings and others, *Rise and Fall of Disease in Illinois*, 1:107, table 11. The death rate fell below twenty per thousand in 1845. There was a sharp outbreak of cholera in 1873, but it overlapped smallpox and typhoid fever epidemics and failed to occasion the panic and alarm of the earlier attacks.

25 Galdston, *Progress in Medicine*, 14–30.

26 Erwin H. Ackerknecht, "Anticontagionism between 1821 and 1867," in *Bulletin of the History of Medicine*, 22:567 (Baltimore, September–October, 1948).

27 John H. Rauch, *A Sanitary History of Chicago from 1833 to 1870* (Chicago Board of Health, *Report*, 1867–1869), 22.

28 John Evans, "Observations upon the Spread of Asiatic Cholera, and Its Communicable Nature," in *North-western Medical and Surgical Journal*, N. S., 2:247, 285 (September, 1849).

29 *Ibid.*, 279.

30 See the *Chicago Tribune*, October 11, 1866.

31 John Evans, *Memorial of Doctor John Evans Praying the Establishment of a System of Quarantine Regulations for the Prevention of the Spread of Cholera* (39th Congress, 1 session, House Miscellaneous Document, No. 66, Washington, 1866).

[32] John H. Rauch, *Public Parks: Their Effects upon the Moral, Physical and Sanitary Condition of the Inhabitants of Large Cities* (Chicago, 1869), 57, 79n.

[33] Chicago Department of Health, *Report*, 1911–1918, p. 1432.

[34] Reynolds, *My Own Times*, 72.

[35] Ackerknecht, *Malaria in the Upper Mississippi Valley*, 27–30, 62–66.

[36] Rauch, *Sanitary History of Chicago*, 20.

[37] Hamilton, "The Epidemics of Chicago," in *Bulletin of the Society of Medical History of Chicago*, 1:82–84 (October, 1911); Chicago Board of Health, *Report*, 1870–1873, pp. 11–12, 14–17.

[38] Chicago Board of Health, *Report*, 1881–1882, p. 11.

[39] Bayard Holmes, "The Sweat-shops and Smallpox in Chicago," in *Journal of the American Medical Association*, 23:419–422 (Chicago, September 15, 1894).

[40] Although reports of the work of Semmelweis and of the Englishman Robert Storrs appeared in Chicago journals in 1844 and 1852, respectively, there was no more disposition on the part of physicians to believe in the contagiousness of puerperal fever than of any other fever. For Semmelweis, see the *North-western Medical and Surgical Journal*, N. S., 1:76–77 (June, 1852), and for Storrs, the *Illinois Medical and Surgical Journal*, 1:137–140 (December, 1844).

[41] Howard W. Haggard, *The Science of Health and Disease: A Textbook of Physiology and Hygiene* (New York, 1927), 491.

[42] Chicago Medical Society, Minutes, August 3, 1874.

[43] See Charles W. Earle, *Synopsis of Lectures on Obstetrics* (Chicago, 1885), lectures 38 and 39.

[44] Isaac A. Abt, "A Survey of Pediatrics during the Past 100 Years," in *Illinois Medical Journal*, 7:490 (May, 1940).

[45] John H. Rauch, *A Report to the Board of Health of the City of Chicago on the Necessity of an Extension of the Sewerage of the City* (Chicago, 1873), 8–9.

[46] *Ibid.*, 9.

[47] Chicago Hospital for Women and Children, *Annual Report*, 1884–1888, p. 16.

[48] *Chicago Medical Journal*, N. S. 1:402 (August, 1858). Holmes was a former member of the co-operative colony at Brook Farm, Massachusetts, and a future president of Rush Medical College.

[49] *Ibid.*, 404–406.

[50] *North-western Medical and Surgical Journal*, N. S., vols. 1 and 2 (1848–1850), *passim*.

[51] B. M. Randolph, "The Blood Letting Controversy in the Nineteenth Century," in *Annals of Medical History*, N. S., 7:180–187 (March, 1935).

[52] *Chicago Medical Journal*, N. S., 5:463 (July, 1862).

[53] Chicago Medical Society, Minutes, April 17, 1871.

[54] For Chicago notice of Gross's objection to the abandonment of general bloodletting, see the *Chicago Medical Journal*, 32:552 (July, 1875). See, too, Edward Montgomery, "A Plea for the Antiphlogistic Treatment of Disease," in *ibid.*, 29:474–488 (August, 1872). As late as 1883, surgeons at the American Surgical Association meeting in Cincinnati heard a paper deploring the "reckless abandonment" of bloodletting in combating inflammation; most of the doctors

present, including Moses Gunn of Chicago, tended to agree with this view. *Chicago Medical Journal and Examiner*, 47:152–153 (August, 1883). An editorial writer for the *Weekly Medical Review* was still recommending in 1888 the local application of leeches as one of the "most potent remedies at our command." *Weekly Medical Review*, 18:596 (St. Louis, December 1, 1888).

CHAPTER III: THE BIRTH OF MODERN MEDICAL SCIENCE

1 Shryock, *Development of Modern Medicine*, 273–303; Galdston, *Progress in Medicine*, 54–55.

2 *Chicago Medical Journal*, 28:650–666 (October–December, 1871).

3 Isaac N. Danforth, "Disease Germs," in *ibid.*, 29:167 (March, 1872).

4 Besides Andrews, those who have been given credit for priority are Christian Fenger, Edwin Powell, Henry Banga, and Charles T. Parkes. Andrews' article published in 1869, however, gives him priority over Fenger, who did not arrive in Chicago until 1877; over Powell, who did not publish until 1878; over Banga, who came to Chicago in 1876; and over Parkes, who did not see Lister operate until 1879. There is interesting testimony to show that Banga was directly responsible for the work on antisepsis in open fractures of the bones of the extremities, for which the noted German surgeon, Richard Volkmann, was given credit. See J. Holinger, "An Incident in the Development of Antisepsis," in *Bulletin of the Society of Medical History of Chicago*, 5:105–112 (January, 1937).

5 William E. Quine, "Edmund Andrews," in *Surgery, Gynecology and Obstetrics*, 35:825 (Chicago, December, 1922); Frank H. Davis, "Atmospheric Germs and Their Relation to Disease," in *Chicago Medical Examiner*, 12:195–196 (April, 1871).

6 Edmund Andrews, "The Sum and Substance of Antiseptic Surgery," in *Chicago Medical Examiner*, 10:732–739 (December, 1869).

7 Edmund Amdrews [*sic*], "The Present State of Opinion on Antiseptic Surgery in the United States," in *Chicago Medical Journal and Examiner*, 44:459 (May, 1882); *Chicago Medical Journal*, 27:358–360 (June, 1870); *Chicago Medical Journal and Examiner*, 39:50 (July, 1879). One former student of Gunn's recalled that the surgeon's views on infection changed during his own student days at Rush, 1885–1887. Ethan A. Gray to James P. Simonds, chairman, Chicago Medical Society Committee on Medical History, February 14, 1950, Chicago Medical Society.

8 *Chicago Medical Journal*, 32:349 (May, 1875); C. D. Haagensen and Wyndham E. B. Lloyd, *A Hundred Years of Medicine* (New York, 1943), 245; Robert F. Weir, "On the Antiseptic Treatment of Wounds, and Its Results," in *New York Medical Journal*, 26:561 (December, 1877).

9 *Chicago Medical Journal*, 32:350 (May, 1875).

10 Christian Fenger and Bayard Holmes, "Antisepsis in Abdominal Operations: Synopsis of a Series of Bacteriological Studies," in *Journal of the American Medical Association*, 9:444 (Chicago, October 1, 1887); Coleman G. Buford, "Rubber Gloves in Surgery," in *Bulletin of the Northwestern University Medical School*, 2:610–612 (Chicago, February 28, 1901). See, too, the account of the introduction of rubber gloves at St. Luke's Hospital in Chicago in William

C. Van Benschoten to James P. Simonds, August 31, 1949, Chicago Medical Society.

[11] H. R. M. Landis, "The Reception of Koch's Discovery in the United States," in *Annals of Medical History*, 4:531–537 (September, 1932). The *Chicago Medical Journal and Examiner*, 45:408 (October, 1882), said of the impact of Koch's work: "Koch's discovery of the bacillus of tuberculosis has . . . attracted an attention of the profession and the public which probably exceeds that directed to any similar subject during the past year."

[12] Chicago Medical Society, Minutes, April 16, 1883, February 16, September 7, 1885, October 18, 1886, October 4, 1886.

[13] William T. Belfield, *On the Relations of Micro-organisms to Disease . . .* (Chicago, 1883), 83. To see the relation of this to other early work on the subject in America, consult L. S. McClung, "Early American Publications Relating to Bacteriology," in *Bacteriological Review*, 8:119–160 (Baltimore, June, 1944).

[14] Henry Gradle, *Bacteria and the Germ Theory of Disease: Eight Lectures Delivered at the Chicago Medical College* (Chicago, 1883). When Gradle returned to Europe later to pursue his studies, he had the flattering experience of being advised that a good starting point for his research would be a survey of the subject by one Henry Gradle of Chicago. A. Gaebler to James P. Simonds, February 21, 1950, Chicago Medical Society. An address given by Gradle in November, 1882, outlining substantially the same views, may be found in *Popular Science Monthly*, 23:577–586 (September, 1883).

[15] Bayard T. Holmes, "Medical Education in Chicago in 1882 and After," in *Medical Life*, N. S., 28:409 (New York, 1921).

[16] Fenger and Holmes, "Antisepsis in Abdominal Operations: Synopsis of a Series of Bacteriological Studies," in *Journal of the American Medical Association*, 9:444 (October 1, 1887).

[17] Chicago Medical Society, *History of Medicine and Surgery and Physicians and Surgeons of Chicago* (Chicago, 1922), 95–96. Courses in bacteriology were given in universities before the medical schools added them to their curricula. Professor Thomas J. Burrill of the University of Illinois gave the first course in bacteriology in the United States in the 1870's. Frederic P. Gorham, "The History of Bacteriology and Its Contribution to Public Health Work," in Mazÿck P. Ravenel, ed., *A Half Century of Public Health* (New York, 1921), 72. Other early contributions by Chicagoans to medical bacteriology were the discovery by Belfield of actinomycosis in American cattle (1884); the report by Lester Curtis on micro-organisms found in the blood of a tetanus victim (1882); and the pioneer work of Nicholas Senn on spontaneous osteomyelitis in the long bones. Senn published his work on surgical bacteriology in 1889. Notice should also be taken of the remarkable researches of the Illinois dentist, Greene Vardiman Black, whose *Formation of Poisons by Micro-organisms* (Philadelphia, 1884) was an early indication of his interest in the bacteriological field. He won worldwide renown and the epithet "Father of Modern Dentistry" for his pioneer work in demonstrating the role of bacteria in dental caries.

[18] William A. Pusey, *A Doctor of the 1870's and 80's* (Springfield, Illinois, 1932), 78–79.

[19] The fullest account of Davis' life is the biography by Isaac N. Danforth, *The Life of Nathan Smith Davis* (Chicago, 1907). See, too, the sketch by H. T.

Byford in Howard A. Kelly and Walter L. Burrage, eds., *American Medical Biographies* (Baltimore, 1920), 290–293.

20 Nathan S. Davis, "Does Etiology Constitute a Proper Basis for the Classification and Diagnosis of Diseases?" in *American Practitioner*, 13:349–350 (Louisville, June, 1876).

21 For Pettenkofer, see Edgar E. Hume, "Max von Pettenkofer's Theory of the Etiology of Cholera, Typhoid Fever and Other Intestinal Diseases," in *Annals of Medical History*, 7:319–353 (December, 1925). A selective list of Davis' writings covering his views on this subject is the following: *Lectures on the Principles and Practice of Medicine* (Chicago, 1884), 77–85; "The History, Present Status, and Future Progress of Practical Medicine," in *Chicago Clinical Review*, 3:9–20 (Chicago, October, 1893); "On the Influence of the Ship Canal, Now Being Constructed . . . on the Sanitary Condition of Chicago and the State of Illinois," in Illinois State Medical Society, *Transactions* (1893), 463–477; Letter to Charles N. Shepard, May 28, 1894, Northwestern University Medical School; "The Present Status of Bacteriologic Investigations and Their Relations to Etiology and Therapeutics," in Illinois State Medical Society, *Transactions* (1895), 486–493.

22 Nathan S. Davis, "The Basis of Scientific Medicine and the Proper Methods of Investigation," in *Journal of the American Medical Association*, 16:114–120 (January 24, 1891). The reception of Davis' ideas by the more thoughtful of his contemporaries was illustrated by a comment on a paper he read in 1895: "The paper shows that we think the views we hold at the present day are the correct ones, and that those held in the past were wrong, and that we have now a cure for everything. This is a wrong view to entertain." Another agreed with Davis when he said: "That all diseases may be the result of germs I will not contend, but I think we have fallen far short of reaching them on this basis, and I think that some day our younger men will have to unlearn some of the things they are learning to-day." Illinois State Medical Society, *Transactions* (1895), 494–495.

23 See, for example, A. P. Ohlmacher, "The Parasite of Carcinoma," in *Scalpel*, 1:35–40 (November, 1892). The *Scalpel* was a student magazine at the College of Physicians and Surgeons of Chicago.

24 Nathan S. Davis, *What Are the Most Efficient and Practical Means for Limiting the Prevalence and Fatality of Pulmonary Tuberculosis?* (Chicago, 1899), 4–5. Many of the Davis articles listed above are available in reprint in Nathan S. Davis, Collected Papers, 1849–1904, John Crerar Library.

25 Nathan S. Davis, *History of Medicine* (Chicago, 1903), 171.

26 *Medical Visitor*, 1:290 (Chicago, August, 1885); William H. King, ed., *History of Homeopathy and Its Institutions in America* (4 vols., Chicago, 1905), 1:346–347.

27 *Medical Visitor*, vols. 9–14 (1893–1898), *passim; Medical Current*, 2:82–95 (Chicago, February, 1896).

28 Carter H. Downing, *Principles and Practice of Osteopathy* (Kansas City, 1923), 53.

29 Zeuch, comp., *History of Medical Practice in Illinois*, 1:244; David S. Smith, "Homoeopathy in Chicago 1838 to 1865," in *Medical Visitor*, 2:1–2 (January, 1886); King, ed., *History of Homeopathy*, 1:345.

[30] Smith, "Homoeopathy in Chicago 1838 to 1865," in *Medical Visitor*, 2:6–7.

[31] *North-western Journal of Homoeopathy*, 3:18–20 (Chicago, October, 1850).

[32] Quoted in C. S. Nelson, "Medicine in the Illinois Country," *Illinois State Historical Society Transactions* (1925), 93.

[33] George E. Shipman, *Homoeopathy, Allopathy, and the City Hospital: A Legend of the XIXth Century, Addressed in Form of a Letter to N. S. Davis, M.D.* (Chicago, 1857), 3–8; *Chicago Times*, July 15, 1857; *Chicago Daily Democratic Press*, July 16, 1857; *Chicago Medical Journal*, N. S., 1:88–94 (February, 1858).

[34] James Brown, *The History of Public Assistance in Chicago 1833 to 1893* (Chicago, 1941), 158. The eclectics claimed 102 practitioners in Chicago in 1884 and nearly a thousand in Illinois. *Chicago Medical Times*, 16:287 (September, 1884).

[35] John E. Gilman, "History of the Medical Profession and Medical Institutions of Chicago," in *Magazine of Western History*, 12:549 (New York, September, 1890).

[36] *Medical Visitor*, 19:226 (May, 1903).

[37] William K. Higley, *Historical Sketch of the Academy* (Chicago Academy of Sciences, *Special Publication No. 1*, 1902), 5, 32. It was not uncommon for men planning to do work in the natural sciences to take training in medicine, as, for example, did David Dale Owen. One graduate of the Chicago Medical College in 1866 became state entomologist in Illinois. For the very important connection between medical men and early work in geology, see William Browning, "The Relation of Physicians to Early American Geology," in *Annals of Medical History*, N. S., 3:547–562 (September, 1931).

[38] Arno B. Luckhardt, "Edmund Andrews, M.D., and His 'Oxygen Mixtures,'" in *Current Researches in Anesthesia & Analgesia*, 19:2–11 (Elmira, New York, January–February, 1940).

CHAPTER IV: MEDICAL SCHOOLS IN CHICAGO

[1] Fishbein, *History of the American Medical Association*, 21.

[2] Address delivered by Arthur D. Bevan, University of Illinois, in *Addresses Delivered upon the Reopening of the Medical Department of the University of Illinois* (n. p., [1913]), 6.

[3] William F. Norwood, *Medical Education in the United States before the Civil War* (Philadelphia, 1944), 384–385; William H. Welch, "Some of the Conditions Which Have Influenced the Development of American Medicine, Especially during the Last Century," in *Bulletin of the Johns Hopkins Hospital*, 19:38 (Baltimore, February, 1908); Henry E. Sigerist, in his foreword to Norwood's *Medical Education before the Civil War*, viii.

[4] "Report of the Committee on Medical Education," in American Medical Association, *Transactions*, 4:409 (1851).

[5] John B. McMaster, *A History of the People of the United States, from the Revolution to the Civil War*, 1:27–28 (New York, 1888).

[6] Norwood, *Medical Education before the Civil War*, 396.

7 John S. Graham to John McLean, March 12, 1844, in John Crerar Library.

8 Graham N. Fitch to John McLean, January 29, 1849.

9 Shafer, *The American Medical Profession*, 35, 88–91; Norwood, *Medical Education before the Civil War*, 400–402.

10 George H. Weaver, "Beginnings of Medical Education in and near Chicago," in *Bulletin of the Society of Medical History of Chicago*, 3:345, 368 (September, 1925).

11 *Proceedings of the National Medical Conventions Held in New York, May, 1846, and in Philadelphia, May, 1847* (Philadelphia, 1847), 79–80. The five schools were: the Medical Department of La Porte University (later Indiana Medical College), La Porte, Indiana, 1842–1850; Franklin Medical College, St. Charles, Illinois, 1842–1849; Illinois College Medical School, Jacksonville, Illinois, 1843–1848; Rush Medical College, Chicago, 1843–1941; and Rock Island Medical School, Rock Island, Illinois, founded in 1848. This last school moved from Rock Island to Davenport and then Keokuk, Iowa, and was finally absorbed by the State University of Iowa College of Medicine. Weaver, "Beginnings of Medical Education in and near Chicago," in *Bulletin of the Society of Medical History of Chicago*, 3:347–367.

12 It is noteworthy that all the men responsible for the founding of these first medical schools in Illinois received at least part of their medical training at the Fairfield school. This was true of Daniel Meeker of the Medical Department of La Porte University, George W. Richards of both the Franklin and Rock Island schools, David Prince of the Illinois College Medical School, as well as Daniel Brainard of Rush Medical College. Dr. N. S. Davis, who was to found the sixth medical college in Illinois, was also a graduate of this small but influential institution. By reviving somewhat the generally forgotten requirements of preliminary education, and with the help of an able, progressive faculty, this school at Fairfield attracted considerable attention during its brief existence. Weaver, "Beginnings of Medical Education in and near Chicago," in *Bulletin of the Society of Medical History of Chicago*, 3:341–342; Norwood, *Medical Education before the Civil War*, 150–153.

13 Chicago Medical Society, *History of Medicine and Surgery*, 189.

14 See the *Chicago American*, March 25, 1837. The editor wrote that "It is greatly to be desired that the young men of the West should be educated at home, in preference to being sent into other States: in medicine this is more particularly to be wished, since new varieties of disease, which of course require a modification of treatment, are here often met with."

15 *Chicago Daily American*, January 13, May 2, 1842; *Chicago Express*, January 25, 1843. The Board of Trustees of the nonexistent school apparently continued to meet in the interim. There is testimony at least of a meeting in 1840. *Daily Chicago American*, August 14, 1840.

16 *Chicago Democrat*, November 22, December 27, 1843.

17 James V. Z. Blaney to John McLean, July 17, 1844, in John Crerar Library; *Chicago Democrat*, August 28, October 2, 1844.

18 George H. Weaver, "The First Period in the History of Rush Medical College, 1843–1859," in *Bulletin of the Alumni Association of Rush Medical College*, 8:15–16 (July, 1912).

19 See, for example, *Chicago Democrat*, December 27, 1843, February 14,

1844; *Chicago Daily Journal,* January 6, 1846; Zeuch, comp., *History of Medical Practice in Illinois,* 1:210–211.

[20] *Illinois and Indiana Medical and Surgical Journal,* N. S., vols. 1 and 2 (1846–1847), *passim;* Zeuch, comp., *History of Medical Practice in Illinois,* 1:221–222.

[21] James V. Z. Blaney to John McLean, July 17, 1844, and John Evans to John McLean, March 9, 1847, both in John Crerar Library. Knapp subsequently became dean of the Rock Island Medical School. A. E. McEvers, "The Rock Island Medical College and the College of Physicians and Surgeons of the Upper Mississippi," in *Surgery, Gynecology and Obstetrics,* 55:252–253 (August, 1932).

[22] John Evans to David Evans, January 21, 1836, printed in *Bulletin of the Society of Medical History of Chicago,* 3:429 (September, 1925).

[23] Zeuch, comp., *History of Medical Practice in Illinois,* 1:211–214; Notes concerning Gov. John Evans, given by Mrs. Evans, Mrs. Dickinson, Gov. Sheldon, and John Evans [ca. 1889], photostatic copies of Bancroft Library MSS, Deering Library, Northwestern University. See, too, McMechen, *Life of Governor Evans,* 38–45, and Elizabeth F. Carr, "Dr. John Evans: The Medical Career of the Founder of Northwestern University," in *Quarterly Bulletin of Northwestern University Medical School,* 25:113–117 (Summer, 1951).

[24] McMechen, *Life of Governor Evans,* 74–91.

[25] Quoted in *ibid.,* 49.

[26] John Evans to John McLean, June 21, 1847, in John Crerar Library.

[27] Rush Medical College, Minutes of the Board of Trustees, December 4, 1875, January 5, 1898, in possession of Earl D. Hostetter, Chicago. Only the minutes for the years 1875–1941 are available, earlier records having been destroyed in the Great Fire.

[28] Rush Medical College, *Annual Announcements,* 1849–1850, 1856–1857. When Rush began with 22 students in 1843, the University of Pennsylvania could boast 424 students, and Jefferson Medical College 341. By 1850, Rush had an enrollment of 132, while Jefferson numbered 504 and the University of Pennsylvania 466. Rush ranked about tenth among American medical schools in 1850 in the size of her student body. *Illinois Medical and Surgical Journal,* 1:32 (May, 1844); *North-western Medical and Surgical Journal,* N. S., 4:84–85 (May, 1851).

[29] Rush Medical College, *Annual Announcements,* 1847–1848, p. 7; 1848–1849, p. 8.

[30] *North-western Medical and Surgical Journal,* N. S., 1:364–366 (October–November, 1848).

[31] Danforth, *Life of Nathan Smith Davis,* 25.

[32] Nathan S. Davis, *History of the American Medical Association from Its Organization up to January,* 1855 (Philadelphia, 1855), 23–30.

[33] The similarity of the ideas of the two men is emphasized by the similarity in language, even to the repetition of an occasional telling phrase. Davis himself sometimes admitted his debt to Drake when discussing medical education. On Drake's influence, compare Drake, "Practical Essays on Medical Education and the Medical Profession, in the United States," in *Western Journal of the Medical and Physical Sciences,* 5:9–23 (Cincinnati, June, 1831), and Davis,

"Introductory Address by Prof. N. S. Davis, on the Opening of the Medical Department of Lind University," in *Chicago Medical Examiner*, 1:1–22 (January, 1860).

[34] *North-western Medical and Surgical Journal*, N. S., 2:362–363 (November, 1849).

[35] Nathan S. Davis, "On the Intimate Relation of Medical Science to the Whole Field of Natural Sciences," in Illinois State Medical Society, *Transactions* (1853), 32–33.

[36] *North-western Medical and Surgical Journal*, N. S., 5:138–145 (March, 1856); H. A. Johnson, *History of the Chicago Medical College: An Introductory Lecture to the College Session of 1870–71* (Chicago, 1870), 8–9.

[37] Nathan S. Davis, "History of the Medical Profession and Medical Institutions of Chicago," in *Magazine of Western History*, 11:419–420 (February, 1890); Johnson, *History of the Chicago Medical College*, 10; Northwestern University Medical School, Minutes of Faculty Meetings 1859–1881, pp. 1–6.

[38] James Nevins Hyde, *Early Medical Chicago: An Historical Sketch of the First Practitioners of Medicine with the Present Faculties, and Graduates since Their Organization, of the Medical Colleges of Chicago* (Fergus' Historical Series, Chicago, 1879), 43.

[39] Nathan S. Davis, *Inaugural Address Delivered at the Opening of the Medical Department of Lind University* (Chicago, 1859), 11–12; *First Annual Announcement of the Medical Department of the Lind University*, 1859–1860, p. 9.

[40] Fielding H. Garrison, for example, wrote that "The first real reform in American medical education was made, in 1871, by President Charles W. Eliot, of Harvard, who raised the entrance requirements of the Harvard Medical School, lengthened its curriculum to three years, and graded it." *An Introduction to the History of Medicine* (3d ed., Philadelphia, 1922), 783. Most historians have followed Garrison, but see Stern, *Society and Medical Progress*, 92. Eliot himself wrote later that he had not been aware of the steps taken by the Chicago Medical College and had "mistakenly thought that the Harvard Medical School was the pioneer in these respects." Charles W. Eliot to Nathan S. Davis, Jr., August 24, 1896, in Church Library, Northwestern University.

Other schools that followed the Chicago Medical College in adopting the graded curriculum and still preceded Harvard were the New York Medical College and Hospital for Women and the St. Louis College of Physicians and Surgeons. Elizabeth F. Carr, "Northwestern University Medical School and the Graded Curriculum," in *Quarterly Bulletin of Northwestern University Medical School*, 15:56–61 (Spring, 1941).

[41] Titus De Ville, "Valedictory Address," in *Chicago Medical Examiner*, 1:706–707 (December, 1860). The faculty, it might be noted, had voted to "inform him [De Ville] freely of the condition of the college, its prospects and the arrangement of lecture fees" when it tendered him the appointment. Northwestern University Medical School, Minutes of Faculty Meetings, July 16, 1859.

[42] Nathan S. Davis, *Lecture Introductory to the Fifth Annual Course of Instruction in the Chicago Medical College* (Chicago, 1863), 9.

[43] Northwestern University Medical School, Minutes of Faculty Meetings, August 26, 1868; Harold E. Farmer, "An Account of the Earliest Colored Gen-

tlemen in Medical Science in the United States," in *Bulletin of the History of Medicine*, 8:607 (April, 1940). It is interesting that Davis voted to deny Negroes membership in the American Medical Association. M. O. Bousfield, "An Account of Physicians of Color in the United States," in *ibid.*, 17:69 (January, 1945).

⁴⁴ Samuel J. Jones, "History of Northwestern University Medical School," in H. G. Cutler, ed., *Medical and Dental Colleges of the West: Chicago* (Chicago, 1896), 163; Northwestern University Medical School, Minutes of Faculty Meetings, June 19, 1863.

⁴⁵ Northwestern University Medical School, Minutes of Faculty Meetings, June 4, 1865; Davis, "History of the Medical Profession and Medical Institutions of Chicago," in *Magazine of Western History*, 11:423.

⁴⁶ Jones, "History of Northwestern University Medical School," in Cutler, ed., *Medical and Dental Colleges of the West*, 163–164; Norwood, *Medical Education before the Civil War*, 382–383.

⁴⁷ *Chicago Medical Journal*, N. S., 2:185 (March, 1859).

⁴⁸ *Ibid.*, 252–255 (April, 1859).

⁴⁹ *Ibid.*, 383 (June, 1859).

⁵⁰ Rush Medical College, *Dedicatory Exercises of the New Building of Rush Medical College* (Chicago, 1876), 20–21.

⁵¹ See, for example, *Chicago Medical Journal*, 25:672 (October 15, 1868).

⁵² The Rush students were close to panic after their master had fallen victim to the great cholera epidemic of that year. About two hundred of the students met on the afternoon following Brainard's demise and voted almost unanimously to adjourn until December in view of the danger. The cooler judgment of the faculty and a sharp rebuke from the *Tribune* prevented any such disbandment, however. "One would think," scolded the *Tribune* editor, "that they of all men should not fly, as, if they be well enough to practice, their services are wanted here and if not yet skilled they have a good opportunity for study." *Chicago Tribune*, October 11, 1866.

⁵³ N. S. Davis, Basis of Union for the Rush and Chicago Medical Colleges, December 1, 1866, in Church Library, Northwestern University.

⁵⁴ Andreas, *History of Chicago*, 2:522, 531; N. Bridge and J. E. Rhodes, "History of Rush Medical College," in Cutler, ed., *Medical and Dental Colleges of the West*, 17; Rush Medical College, *Annual Announcement*, 1862–1863, pp. 5–6.

⁵⁵ *Chicago American* (weekly), July 17, 1840.

⁵⁶ Weaver, "Beginnings of Medical Education in and near Chicago," in *Bulletin of the Society of Medical History of Chicago*, 3:372.

⁵⁷ Zeuch, comp., *History of Medical Practice in Illinois*, 1:544–548.

⁵⁸ Quoted in Carl E. Black, "A Pioneer Medical School," in *Illinois Medical Journal*, 23:12n (January, 1913).

⁵⁹ *Chicago Daily Press*, January 12, 1858; *North-western Medical and Surgical Journal*, N. S., 6:525–528 (November, 1857).

⁶⁰ Quoted in *Chicago Medical Journal*, 24:215 (May, 1867).

⁶¹ *Chicago Medical Journal and Examiner*, 51:197–199 (August, 1885). In 1830 Massachusetts became the first state to pass a law giving bodies unclaimed by friends to medical institutions. The Pennsylvania law of 1883 served as a model for Illinois and many other states. Weaver, "Beginnings of Medical Edu-

cation in and near Chicago," in *Bulletin of the Society of Medical History of Chicago*, 3:373.

[62] *Chicago Medical Journal*, 27:353–356 (June, 1870).

[63] Bridge and Rhodes, "History of Rush Medical College," in Cutler, ed., *Medical and Dental Colleges of the West*, 42–45; James B. Herrick, *Memories of Eighty Years* (Chicago, 1949), 40.

[64] Drake, "Practical Essays on Medical Education and the Medical Profession, in the United States," in *Western Journal of the Medical and Physical Sciences*, 3:16.

[65] Rush Medical College, *Annual Announcement*, 1844, p. 5.

[66] James V. Z. Blaney to John McLean, February 16, October 21, 1845, in John Crerar Library. See, too, the large collection of certificates of indebtedness from students of Professor John McLean in the Society of Medical History of Chicago Collection at the John Crerar Library.

[67] *North-western Medical and Surgical Journal*, N. S., 4:228 (September, 1851), and 1:187–191 (August, 1852); *Chicago Medical Journal*, 26:447 (July 15, 1869); *Chicago Medical Journal and Examiner*, 39:205 (August, 1879).

[68] Fishbein, *History of the American Medical Association*, 82.

[69] Charles W. Earle, *The Demand for a Woman's Medical College in the West* (Waukegan, Illinois, 1879), 7–8. A Mrs. Brockway of Jonesville, Michigan, attended lectures during the Rush session of 1850–1851; *Gem of the Prairie*, November 10, 1850; Rush Medical College, *Annual Announcement*, 1851–1852.

[70] Northwestern University Medical School, Minutes of Faculty Meetings, September 16, 1869, June 10, 1870; *Bulletin of the Alumni Association of Rush Medical College*, 6:32 (July, 1910).

[71] Chicago Medical Society, Minutes, October 1, 1869; *Chicago Medical Journal*, 28:363 (June, 1871); Fishbein, *History of the American Medical Association*, 91; Chicago Medical Society, *History of Medicine and Surgery*, 118–119.

[72] Earle, *The Demand for a Woman's Medical College*, 8–10.

[73] Marie J. Mergler, "History of the Northwestern University Woman's Medical School," in Cutler, ed., *Medical and Dental Colleges of the West*, 258–259; *Chicago Daily Tribune*, April 20, 1881; S. D. Jacobsen, Recommendation of Dr. Mary E. Bates, October 1, 1882, in John Crerar Library.

[74] Eliza H. Root, "The Woman's Medical School," in Arthur H. Wilde, ed., *Northwestern University: A History 1855–1905* (3 vols., New York, 1905), 4:381–384; John M. Dodson, "The Affiliation of Rush Medical College with the University of Chicago," in *Bulletin of the Alumni Association of Rush Medical College*, 13:24 (September, 1917); *Medical Standard*, 25:98 (Chicago, February, 1902).

[75] John E. Gilman, "History of the Hahnemann Medical College and Hospital," in Cutler, ed., *Medical and Dental Colleges of the West*, 201; King, ed., *History of Homeopathy*, 2:341–349. Shipman's humane concern for the underprivileged caused him later to establish the famous Chicago Foundlings' Home. Francis E. Shipman, George E. Shipman, A.M., M.D., M.S., manuscript in the John Crerar Library.

[76] Francis R. Packard, *History of Medicine in the United States* (2 vols., New York, 1931), 2: appendix 1, pp. 1221–1222.

[77] *Chicago Medical Times*, 1:7–14 (January, 1869).

[78] E. R. Booth, *History of Osteopathy and Twentieth-Century Medical Practice* (memorial ed., Cincinnati, 1924), 546–547.

[79] Cutler, ed., *Medical and Dental Colleges of the West*, iii.

[80] "The Great Fire Medically Considered," in *United States Medical and Surgical Journal*, 7:208–209 (January, 1872); Jane A. Gunn, *Memorial Sketches of Doctor Moses Gunn by His Wife* (Chicago, 1889), 200; Ebert, "Early History of the Drug Trade of Chicago," in *Illinois State Historical Society Transactions* (1903), 257.

[81] *Chicago Medical Examiner*, 12:629–630 (October, 1871); *Chicago Medical Journal*, 28:671–672 (October–December, 1871).

[82]: *Chicago Medical Journal and Examiner*, 42:559 (May, 1881).

[83] Rush Medical College, Minutes of the Board of Trustees, May 10, 1875, June 17, 1887.

[84] Chicago Medical Society, *History of Medicine and Surgery*, 75–76; Chicago Medical Society, Minutes, March 28, 1900.

[85] Bridge and Rhodes, "History of Rush Medical College," in Cutler, ed., *Medical and Dental Colleges of the West*, 27.

[86] Northwestern University Medical School, Minutes of Faculty Meetings, June 23, 1884.

[87] John H. Long, "The Laboratories, the Museum and Library," in Wilde, ed., *Northwestern University*, 3:336–350.

[88] Henry W. Chaney to James P. Simonds, July 28, 1949, Chicago Medical Society; Isaac A. Abt, *Baby Doctor* (New York, 1944), 26.

[89] Joseph McFarland, "The Beginning of Bacteriology in Philadelphia," in *Bulletin of the Institute of the History of Medicine*, 5:160 (February, 1937).

[90] Holmes, "Medical Education in Chicago," in *Medical Life*, N. S., 28:11–12; Chicago Medical Society, *History of Medicine and Surgery*, 95–97.

[91] Nathan S. Davis, Jr., "The Later History of the Medical School," in Wilde, ed., *Northwestern University*, 3:320.

[92] Northwestern University Medical School, Minutes of Faculty Meetings, April 17, 1888.

[93] Daniel A. K. Steele and William E. Quine, "History of the College of Physicians and Surgeons," in Cutler, ed., *Medical and Dental Colleges of the West*, 341–346.

[94] Truman W. Miller, "History of the Chicago Policlinic," in *ibid.*, 453–456.

[95] W. Franklin Coleman, "History of the Post-Graduate Medical School and Hospital," in *ibid.*, 459–463.

[96] *Weekly Medical Review*, 7:52 (February 3, 1883); *Chicago Medical Register*, 1876–1877, 1886–1887.

CHAPTER V: PROFESSIONAL SOCIETIES AND PUBLICATIONS

[1] *Western Medical and Physical Journal, Original and Eclectic*, 1:xii (April, 1827).

[2] Higley, *Historical Sketch of the Academy*, 5.

³ Ralph S. Bates, *Scientific Societies in the United States* (Cambridge, Massachusetts, 1945), 65.

⁴ Charles B. Reed, "A Centennial Summary of Medicine," in *Illinois Medical Journal*, 77:442 (May, 1940).

⁵ "Semi-Centennial of the Illinois State Medical Society," in *Medical Standard*, 23:357 (June, 1900).

⁶ *North-western Medical and Surgical Journal*, N. S., 1:34 (May, 1852).

⁷ *Daily Chicago American*, June 29, 1840.

⁸ *Proceedings of the Medical Convention for the Purpose of Organizing the Illinois State Medical Society*, 4–5, 31. Though the present society claims an organic connection with the earlier body, there is no evidence that the members present at the convention of 1850 considered themselves to be reorganizing the defunct Medical Society of Illinois. No mention was made of any earlier organization and the delegates proceeded to draw up constitution, by-laws, and code of ethics exactly as if none existed. The only connecting link between the two bodies was the person of Dr. C. F. Hughes, secretary of the earlier society, who was the only man who was present at both conventions. See W. O. Ensign, "Medical Organization and the North Central Illinois Medical Association," in *Illinois Medical Journal*, 13:273–274 (March, 1908).

⁹ The Rock River Valley Society was formed in 1846 at Rockford and overlapped territory of Wisconsin and Indiana; the Aesculapian Society of the Wabash Valley was organized in 1847; Morgan and Peoria counties had short-lived societies in 1846 and 1847, respectively; and at Ottawa in 1847 the Medical Society of La Salle and Adjoining Counties was brought into being. *Illinois and Indiana Medical and Surgical Journal*, N. S., 1:252–259 (August, 1846); W. O. Ensign, "Medical Organization and the North Central Illinois Medical Association," in *Illinois Medical Journal*, 13:274 (March, 1908).

¹⁰ See the *Chicago American*, October 1, 1836, for Boone's announcement.

¹¹ Zeuch, "Early Medical Legislation and Organization in the Illinois Country," in *Bulletin of the Society of Medical History of Chicago*, 4:208 (July, 1930).

¹² *Biographical Sketches of the Leading Men of Chicago* (Wilson & St. Clair, Publishers, Chicago, 1868), 273–281; Zeuch, comp., *History of Medical Practice*, 1:208–209.

¹³ The only authoritative information on the history of the first two years of the Chicago Medical Society is found in a number of short sketches by Nathan S. Davis. After 1852 the minutes of the Society provide a reliable source of historical data. The sketches by Davis are located in the manuscript minutes of the Society, volumes 2 and 6, in the Chicago Historical Society. Much of the same ground is gone over in his published "A Brief History of the Chicago Medical Society from Its Origins to the End of Its First Half Century of Progress," in *Chicago Medical Recorder*, 21:199–204 (October, 1901). More published reminiscences are found in *ibid.*, 22:365–369 (May, 1902).

¹⁴ See the *Chicago Medical Journal*, N. S., 6:425 (September, 1863).

¹⁵ Chicago Medical Society, Minutes, April 5, 1852, August 3, 1858, February 4, 1903.

¹⁶ *Chicago Medical Journal*, N. S., 2:255–256 (April, 1859); N. S., 4:45 (January, 1861).

[17] Philip Van Ingen, *The New York Academy of Medicine: Its First Hundred Years* (New York, 1949), *passim*.

[18] Nathan S. Davis, Brief History of Medical Societies in Chicago, bound in volume 2 of the minutes of the Chicago Medical Society.

[19] Chicago Medical Society, Minutes, November 10, 1865, June 7, 1875, May 15, 1901. It is not certain that Simms actually attended, though plans for a joint reception with the Society of Physicians and Surgeons are mentioned in the minutes.

[20] *Ibid.*, April 24, 1863.

[21] *Ibid.*, June 18, July 2, 1877.

[22] *Chicago Medical Journal*, N. S., 1:101–113 (March, 1858). The endoscope, too, was swiftly adopted in Chicago; Desormeaux's lectures were reprinted in one of the Chicago journals. *Ibid.*, 24:177ff. (April, 1867); Chicago Medical Society, Minutes, May 21, 1883.

[23] *Ibid.*, October 3, 1881.

[24] *Ibid.*, April 1, 1889, April 2, 1894.

[25] "The Illinois State Medical Society: Archives Era," in *Illinois Medical Journal*, 77:396–397, 400 (May, 1940).

[26] Chicago Medical Society, Minutes, July 14, 1873.

[27] *Ibid.*, March 18, 1878. For an account of the Chicago Society of Physicians and Surgeons, see George H. Weaver, "The Chicago Society of Physicians and Surgeons," in *Bulletin of the Society of Medical History of Chicago*, 4:317–321 (January, 1933).

[28] Ludvig Hektoen, "Phases of the History of the Chicago Pathological Society," in Chicago Pathological Society, *Transactions*, 5:91 (May 12, 1902).

[29] Chicago Medical Society, Minutes, December 15, 1879.

[30] *Ibid.*, May 16, 1854.

[31] *Ibid.*, May 13, 1856.

[32] *Ibid.*, November 18, 1864.

[33] *Ibid.*, October 16, 1863, December 8, 1865, December 28, 1866, February 28, 1870.

[34] *Ibid.*, July 20, 1891.

[35] Bates, *Scientific Societies in the United States*, 85.

[36] Ludvig Hektoen, "Early Pathology in Chicago and Christian Fenger," in Institute of Medicine of Chicago, *Proceedings*, 11:263–272 (April 15, 1937).

[37] Edwin F. Hirsch, History of the Chicago Pathological Society, manuscript (1949), in Chicago Medical Society.

[38] Chicago Laryngological and Otological Society, *Constitution, By-Laws and Membership Roster* (n. p., [1948]), 2–3.

[39] James B. Herrick, "The Chicago Society of Internal Medicine," in Institute of Medicine of Chicago, *Proceedings*, 8:93–98 (June 15, 1930). See also his manuscript sketch, covering the earlier Society of Internal Medicine, in the files of the Chicago Medical Society.

[40] See the unpublished accounts in the files of the Chicago Medical Society.

[41] Harry A. Paskind, History of the Chicago Neurological Society, manuscript (1941), in Chicago Medical Society.

[42] Practitioners' Club, Minutes and Programs 1891–95, in Society of Medical History of Chicago Collection, John Crerar Library.

43 King, ed., *History of Homeopathy*, 1:349.

44 *Illinois Medical Journal*, N. S., 2:327–328 (December, 1900). This list includes only the regular organizations.

45 "Report of the Committee on Medical Literature," in American Medical Association, *Transactions*, 1:249–288 (1848).

46 *North-western Medical and Surgical Journal*, N. S., 3:335 (November, 1850).

47 "Report of the Committee on Medical Literature," in American Medical Association, *Transactions*, 6:99–130 (1953).

48 *Illinois Medical and Surgical Journal*, 1:1–3 (April, 1844).

49 Nathan S. Davis, "A Brief History of Medical Journalism in Chicago to the End of the Nineteenth Century," in *The Clinical Review*, 16:469 (Chicago, September, 1902).

50 *Chicago Medical Journal*, N. S., 1:192 (April, 1858).

51 *Ibid.*, 2:184 (March, 1859).

52 Davis, "A Brief History of Medical Journalism," in *The Clinical Review*, 16:470–472.

53 *Ibid.*, 472–476. After the turn of the century the movement for increased publications continued, with the establishment of such important journals as the A.M.A. *Archives*, more than a dozen journals for as many specialties, and the American Medical Association's *Today's Health* for lay readers.

54 G. Frank Lydston, "How to Write a Medical Article: A Plea for Plagiarism," in *Journal of the American Medical Association*, 41:1346 (November 28, 1903).

55 *Proceedings of the Testimonial Banquet Given in Honor of Prof. Christian Fenger, on November 3d, 1900, by the Medical Profession* (Chicago, 1900), 39; Holmes, "Medical Education in Chicago," in *Medical Life*, N. S., 18:574.

56 J. M. Toner to Nathan S. Davis, December 27, 1878, in Nathan Smith Davis papers, Northwestern University Medical School.

57 Same to same, January 4, 1879.

58 Board of Trustees, Newberry Library, to Nathan S. Davis, December 26, 1889, in Medical Library Association of Chicago Papers, Chicago Historical Society.

59 Chicago Medical Society, Minutes, April 2, 1894.

60 *Ibid.*, April 7, 1890.

61 Lewis and Smith, *Chicago*, 174.

62 Chicago Medical Society, Minutes, June 20, 1906.

CHAPTER VI: EMERGENCE OF CHICAGO AS A FORCE

1 Chicago Medical Society, Minutes, September 21, 1885, June 7, 1886.

2 Malcolm T. MacEachern, "Progress of Surgery in the State of Illinois," in *Illinois Medical Journal*, 77:453–454 (May, 1940).

3 E. R. Le Count, "Christian Fenger as Pathologist," in Chicago Pathological Society, *Transactions*, 6:2–9 (October 12, 1903); McArthur, "Christian Fenger as I Knew Him," in *Bulletin of the Society of Medical History of Chicago*, 3:54 (January, 1923); Ludvig Hektoen, "Early Pathology in Chicago and Chris-

tian Fenger," in Institute of Medicine of Chicago, *Proceedings*, 11:260 (April 15, 1937).

⁴ Christian Fenger, "Autobiography," in Ludvig Hektoen and Coleman G. Buford, eds., *The Collected Works of Christian Fenger, M.D., 1840–1902* (2 vols., Philadelphia, 1912), 1:4.

⁵ Frank Billings, "Christian Fenger," in *Surgery, Gynecology and Obstetrics*, 35:367 (September, 1922).

⁶ James B. Herrick, "Christian Fenger as I Knew Him, 1885 to 1902: A Study of Personality," in Institute of Medicine of Chicago, *Proceedings*, 13:323. The local medical bard, G. Frank Lydston, composed the following suggestive lines for a great testimonial banquet in Fenger's honor in 1900, *Proceedings of the Testimonial Banquet Given in Honor of Prof. Christian Fenger on November 3d, 1900, by the Medical Profession*, 42:

Oh, how things hev went an' changed, till now the world's all upside down.
Thar's no comfort now in practicin' in ole Chicago town.
We early settlers air a-kickin' hard; we're feelin' mighty sore,
Fer the game that wuz so easy isn't easy enny more.
We can't give satisfacshun, no matter what, er how we do,
In enny kind o' sickness from chills ter doloreux,
Onless we kin pacify 'em with some high-falutin' name—
Which the same it wuz onheard of 'fore
    That durned Chris Fenger came.

⁷ Ludvig Hektoen, "Notes on the History of Bacteriology in Chicago Prior to the Organization of Bacteriologic Teaching (about 1890)," in *Bulletin of the Society of Medical History of Chicago*, 5:4–5 (January, 1937).

⁸ Chicago Medical Society, Minutes, November 7, 1881.

⁹ Drs. Channing W. Barrett, Charles J. Kurtz, and William P. Schoen to J. P. Simonds, 1949–1950, Chicago Medical Society. See, too, Fenger and Holmes, "Antisepsis in Abdominal Operations," in *Journal of the American Medical Association*, 9:444 (October 1, 1887).

¹⁰ William G. Allen to J. P. Simonds, April 15, 1949, Chicago Medical Society.

¹¹ Byron Robinson, "Dr. Christian Fenger," in *Medical Review*, 36:257 (St. Louis, October 9, 1897).

¹² Coleman G. Buford, "Christian Fenger: A Biographical Sketch," in *Bulletin of the Society of Medical History of Chicago*, 1:196–202 (March, 1913).

¹³ Billings, "Christian Fenger," in *Surgery, Gynecology and Obstetrics*, 35:368.

¹⁴ William J. Mayo, "Murphy, John Benjamin," in Howard A. Kelly and Walter L. Burrage, eds., *American Medical Biographies* (Baltimore, 1920), 839.

¹⁵ Rupert M. Parker and Channing W. Barrett to J. P. Simonds, 1949–1950, Chicago Medical Society.

¹⁶ J. B. Murphy to N. S. Davis, Jr., February 20, 1907, in Nathan Smith Davis Papers, Northwestern University Medical School.

¹⁷ Others from Wisconsin who achieved fame were Frank Billings, Albert I. Bouffleur, Frank Cary, Archibald Church, David J. Davis, John M. Dodson, Henry B. Favill, James C. Gill, Ludvig Hektoen, Oscar A. King, E. R. Le Count, Franklin H. Martin, Albert J. Ochsner, Henry Palmer, Fred B. Robinson, Nicholas Senn, Bertram W. Sippy, and Frederick Tice. This information was made

available through the generosity of William S. Middleton, dean of the medical school at the University of Wisconsin, who lent the author his unpublished manuscript on "Wisconsin Men in Chicago Medicine."

[18] Loyal Davis, *J. B. Murphy, Stormy Petrel of Surgery* (New York, 1938), *passim.*

[19] G. W. C[rile], "Dr. John B. Murphy," in *Cleveland Medical Journal,* 15:532 (1916).

[20] Davis, *J. B. Murphy,* 282.

[21] Walter L. Bierring, "Biographies of the Presidents of the American Medical Association," in Fishbein, *History of the American Medical Association,* 718–719, quoting Sir Berkeley Moynihan.

[22] Davis, *J. B. Murphy,* 245–272.

[23] *Bulletin of the Chicago Medical Society,* 16:16–20 (October 14, 1916).

[24] Sir Berkeley Moynihan, "John B. Murphy—Surgeon," in *Addresses on Surgical Subjects* (Philadelphia, 1928), 107–108.

[25] Morris Fishbein, "Ludvig Hektoen: A Biography and an Appreciation," in *Archives of Pathology,* 26:3–18 (Chicago, 1938). A partial list of "Hektoen men" who have been important in Chicago medicine is the following: Peter Bassoe, D. J. Davis, George and Gladys Dick, Martin Fisher, Evarts A. Graham, Alice Hamilton, Howard T. Ricketts, E. C. Rosenow, James P. Simonds, Theodore Teakin, Ruth Tunnicliff, William B. Wherry, and Rollin Woodyat. See William Allen Pusey, "High Lights in the History of Chicago Medicine," in *Bulletin of the Society of Medical History of Chicago,* 5:190 (May, 1940).

[26] Herrick, *Memories of Eighty Years, passim.*

[27] Addresses by James B. Herrick and Dallas B. Phemister, in Billings Medical Club of Chicago, *A Service in Memory of Frank Billings* (Chicago, 1932).

[28] Frank Billings, "Chronic Focal Infections and Their Etiologic Relations to Arthritis and Nephritis," in *Archives of Internal Medicine,* 9:484–498 (Chicago, 1912).

[29] Ernest E. Irons, "The Theory of Focal Infection: Its Influence on the Practice of Medicine," in Institute of Medicine of Chicago, *Proceedings,* 16:272–273 (December 15, 1946).

[30] Address by Dallas B. Phemister in *A Service in Memory of Frank Billings.*

[31] Article by Morris Fishbein in *Chicago Daily News,* September 21, 1932; Rush Medical College, Faculty Minutes, October 20, 1932, Rush Medical College Library, Presbyterian Hospital.

[32] James B. Herrick, "Frank Billings," in *Bulletin of the Alumni Association of Rush Medical College,* 18:12 (August, 1924).

[33] Cutler, ed., *Medical and Dental Colleges of the West,* 96–99.

[34] A. J. Ochsner, "Nicholas Senn the Surgeon," in *Bulletin of the Alumni Association of Rush Medical College,* 4:13 (February, 1908).

[35] Byron Robinson, "Professor Senn's Clinic," in *Medical Review,* 33:218–219 (March 28, 1896).

[36] William E. Quine, "Nicholas Senn as a Man," in *Bulletin of the Alumni Association of Rush Medical College,* 4:7–10 (February, 1908).

[37] Nicholas Senn, "A Plea for the International Study of Carcinoma," in *Journal of the American Medical Association,* 46:1255 (April 28, 1906). The experiment was performed in 1901.

38 Howard A. Kelly, "Senn, Nicholas," in Kelly and Burrage, eds., *American Medical Biographies*, 1034–1036.

39 Lawson Tait, The Medical Tramp, undated manuscript in Nathan Smith Davis Papers, Northwestern University Medical School.

40 Quine, "Nicholas Senn as a Man," in *Bulletin of the Alumni Association of Rush Medical College*, 4:8–9.

41 *Chicago Daily News*, July 13, 1910.

42 Franklin H. Martin, *The Joy of Living: An Autobiography* (2 vols., Garden City, New York, 1933), 1:397.

43 Frank J. Jirka, *American Doctors of Destiny* (Chicago, 1940), 254.

44 Martin, *Joy of Living*, 1:409–431.

45 Chicago Medical Society, Council Minutes, December 9, 1913.

46 *Illinois Medical Journal*, 24:365–366 (December, 1913).

47 *Ibid.*, 25:44 (January, 1914).

48 Martin, *Joy of Living*, 1:436.

49 *Ibid.*, 1:438.

50 Edwin F. Hirsch, History of the Chicago Pathological Society, manuscript (1949), in Chicago Medical Society; J. J. Moore, "A Century of Pathology," in *Illinois Medical Journal*, 77:435–439 (May, 1940). Ninety-two Illinois pathologists were certified by the American Board as of June, 1950. See *Directory of American Specialists* (5th ed., Chicago, 1951), 795–799.

51 Chicago Medical Society, Minutes, November 2, 1874.

52 Danforth, *Life of Nathan Smith Davis*, 13.

53 William P. Schoen to J. P. Simonds, June 29, 1949, Chicago Medical Society.

54 Isaac A. Abt, "The Growth of Pediatrics in the Chicago Area," in *Medical Clinics of North America* (Philadelphia, January, 1946), 3–15, and "A Survey of Pediatrics during the Past 100 Years," in *Illinois Medical Journal*, 77:491–494 (May, 1940).

55 *Chicago Medical Journal and Examiner*, 42:17–21 (January, 1881); Joseph L. Baer, "A Century of Obstetrics and Gynecology," *Illinois Medical Journal*, 77:469–470 (May, 1940).

56 Chicago Medical Society, Minutes, November 19, 1883. The estimate was given by Oscar C. De Wolf, Chicago Health Commissioner, who was present at the meeting.

57 Morris Fishbein with Sol Theron De Lee, *Joseph Bolivar De Lee: Crusading Obstetrician* (New York, 1949), 45–46.

58 James E. Lebensohn, "Ophthalmology in Illinois 1840–1940," in *Illinois Medical Journal*, 77:480–485 (May, 1940). By June, 1950, there were approximately two thousand ophthalmologists certified by the American Board. *Directory of American Specialists* (5th ed.), 492–580.

59 Peter Bassoe, "The Early History of Neurology and Psychiatry in the Middle West," in *Bulletin of the Society of Medical History of Chicago*, 3:175 (October, 1923).

60 Chicago Medical Society, *History of Medicine and Surgery*, 107–108.

61 This is the same Bannister whose famous diary supplied William Seward with much of the knowledge on which he based his decision to purchase Alaska.

62 Peter Bassoe, "A Sketch of the Development of Psychiatry and Neurology

in Chicago," in Institute of Medicine of Chicago, *Proceedings*, 11:169–170 (December 15, 1936).

[63] William Allen Pusey, *The History of Dermatology* (Springfield, Illinois, 1933), 146–147.

[64] Erwin P. Zeisler, "Joseph Zeisler—Pioneer Chicago Dermatologist," in *Urologic and Cutaneous Review*, 51:187–190 (West Palm Beach, Florida, March, 1947); Emil H. Grubbé, *X-Ray Treatment: Its Origin, Birth and Early History* (St. Paul, Minnesota, 1949), *passim*.

[65] See Maximilian J. Hubeny and Percy J. Delano, "Progress in Radiology," in *Illinois Medical Journal*, 77:475–480 (May, 1940).

[66] Bernhard J. Stern, *American Medical Practice in the Perspectives of a Century* (New York, 1945), 49–50.

[67] Information supplied by Directory Department, American Medical Association, August, 1950.

[68] Henry E. Sigerist, *The Great Doctors: A Biographical History of Medicine* (rev. ed., New York, 1933). Approximately fifty biographies are included.

[69] See Richard H. Shryock, "Factors Affecting Medical Research in the United States, 1800–1900," in *Bulletin of the Society of Medical History of Chicago*, 5:1–18 (July, 1943).

[70] *Chicago Medical Journal and Examiner*, 47:156 (August, 1883).

[71] *Chicago Daily Tribune*, January 11, 1910.

[72] James P. Simonds, "Ludvig Hektoen: a Study in Changing Scientific Interests," in Institute of Medicine of Chicago, *Proceedings*, 14:286 (December 15, 1942).

[73] For a partial list of original medical research in Chicago, see Pusey, "High Lights in the History of Chicago Medicine," in *Bulletin of the Society of Medical History of Chicago*, 5:196–199.

[74] *Medical Standard*, 43:12–13 (December, 1920).

[75] *Bulletin of the Chicago Medical Society*, 21:22–23 (December 21, 1921).

[76] Illinois Medical Center District, *Fact Book: A Description of the Research, Healing and Teaching Institutions which Constitute the District . . . Their History . . . and a Glance at the Future* (Chicago, 1948), 24–25.

[77] *Chicago Sun-Times*, January 31, 1950.

[78] Chicago Medical Society, Council Minutes, June 8, 1943, April 12, 1949; *Chicago Sun-Times*, June 15, 1950.

[79] *Chicago Daily Tribune*, February 14, 1949.

[80] Illinois Medical Center District, *Fact Book*, 1–5.

CHAPTER VII: EXPANSION OF MEDICAL EDUCATION

[1] American Medical Association, Council on Medical Education and Hospitals, *Medical Education in the United States 1934–1939* (Chicago, 1940), 99, table 21.

[2] N. S. Davis, Jr., "The Later History of the Medical School," in Wilde, ed., *Northwestern University*, 3:321.

[3] Abt, *Baby Doctor*, 24.

[4] Northwestern University Medical School, *John Harper Long 1856–1918: A Tribute from His Colleagues* (n. p., [1918]), *passim*.

[5] John E. Rhodes, "The Making of a Modern Medical School: A Sketch of Rush Medical College," in *Medical News* (New York, November 16, 1901), 766–767.

[6] Bridge and Rhodes, "History of Rush Medical College," in Cutler, ed., *Medical and Dental Colleges of the West*, 34–37.

[7] Arthur E. Hertzler, *The Horse and Buggy Doctor* (New York, 1938), 42.

[8] Bridge and Rhodes, "History of Rush Medical College," in Cutler, ed., *Medical and Dental Colleges of the West*, 46.

[9] William E. Quine, "History of the College of Physicians and Surgeons of Chicago," in *Bulletin of the Society of Medical History of Chicago*, 1:64 (October, 1911).

[10] William A. Pusey, "The College of Physicians and Surgeons of Chicago," in *Adresses Delivered upon the Re-opening of the Medical Department of the University of Illinois, March 6, 1913* (n. p., [1913]), 39–41.

[11] Bayard Holmes to Jens Christian Bay, February 6, 1922, bound with the College of Physicians and Surgeons' *First Decennial Catalogue 1881–1891*, in the John Crerar Library.

[12] Holmes, "Medical Education in Chicago," in *Medical Life*, N. S., 39:32–41 (January, 1922).

[13] *Medical Standard*, 6:120 (October, 1889).

[14] Victor C. Vaughan, *A Doctor's Memories* (Indianapolis, 1926), 439.

[15] *Bulletin of the Alumni Association of Rush Medical College*, 7:24 (April, 1911).

[16] *Quarterly Bulletin of Northwestern University Medical School*, 10:57 (June, 1908).

[17] Winfred S. Hall, "Student Life at the Medical School," in Wilde, ed., *Northwestern University*, 3:428–430.

[18] *Medical Standard*, 38:457 (November, 1915).

[19] *Illinois Medical Journal*, N. S., 7:186–195 (February, 1905).

[20] Arthur D. Bevan, "Cooperation in Medical Education and Medical Service," in *Journal of the American Medical Association*, 90:1173–1175 (April 14, 1928). By 1950 the number of medical schools in America had declined under steady pressure to 79; there were the same year only five recognized schools in Illinois, all of them in Chicago.

[21] Victor Johnson, "The Council on Medical Education and Hospitals," in Fishbein, *History of the American Medical Association*, 896–898.

[22] Flexner listed the schools as the Chicago College of Medicine and Surgery, Hahnemann Medical College, Hering Medical College, Illinois Medical College, Bennett Medical College, Physio-Medical College of Medicine and Surgery, Jenner Medical College, National Medical University, Reliance Medical College, and Littlejohn College of Osteopathy. Abraham Flexner, *Medical Education in the United States and Canada: A Report to the Carnegie Foundation for the Advancement of Teaching* (New York, 1910), 216.

[23] *Ibid.*, 216–220.

[24] *Chicago Sunday Tribune*, May 21, 1911. For a reply to Egan's attack on Flexner's supporters in Illinois, see the long statement of Dr. J. F. Percy of Galesburg, Illinois, in *ibid.*, May 28, 1911.

[25] Chicago Medical Society, Council Minutes, April 9, 1912. The chairman

of the investigating committee spoke significantly of his aim "to collect facts by those of local residence instead of imported talent," thus making "haste unnecessary and the avoidance of superficial effort more certain."

[26] Northwestern University Medical School, *Annual Announcement*, 1911–1912.

[27] By 1939, only 657 of 3,226 applicants for admission to Chicago schools were found acceptable. The ratio between applicants and matriculants after World War II became even greater. Fred C. Zapffe, "Medical Education in Illinois during the Last One Hundred Years," in *Illinois Medical Journal*, 77:416 (May, 1940).

[28] Rush Medical College, *Annual Announcement*, 1914–1915; Rush Medical College, Faculty Meeting Minutes, February 7, 1918.

[29] *Bulletin of the Chicago Medical Society*, 20:26–27 (October 16, 1920).

[30] *Clinique*, 26:21–24 (Chicago, January, 1905).

[31] Bevan, "Cooperation in Medical Education and Medical Service," in *Journal of the American Medical Association*, 90:1175.

[32] Northwestern University Board of Trustees and Executive Committee, Minutes, June 22, 1891, Northwestern University.

[33] Pusey, "The College of Physicians and Surgeons," in *Addresses Delivered Upon the Re-opening of the Medical Department of the University of Illinois*, 47–50. For a full account of the background and course of the negotiations, see Quine, "History of the College of Physicians and Surgeons," *Bulletin of the Society of Medical History of Chicago*, 1:66–70 (October, 1911).

[34] Rush Medical College, *Annual Announcements*, 1898–1924.

[35] Northwestern University Medical School, *Annual Announcement*, announcements for the years 1910 through 1920.

[36] *Ibid.*, 1930–1950.

[37] J. Roscoe Miller, "Appreciations of Irving Samuel Cutter," in *Quarterly Bulletin of Northwestern University Medical School*, 19:66–68 (Spring, 1945).

[38] Barry J. Anson, "Northwestern University Medical School: Retrospect and Prospect," in *Quarterly Bulletin of Northwestern University Medical School*, 20:251 (Summer, 1946).

[39] Abraham Flexner, A Plan for the Development of Medical Education in Chicago, July, 1916, in University of Chicago Archives; Abstract of Minutes of Board of Trustees, University of Chicago, November 8, 1916.

[40] Franklin C. McLean and Nellie Gorgas, eds., "Medicine in the Division of Biological Sciences, University of Chicago," in *Methods and Problems of Medical Education* (Rockefeller Foundation, 19th series, 1931), 7–16.

[41] Emmet B. Bay, *The Quality of Care Rendered by the Universtiy of Chicago Clinics* (Chicago, 1932), 14–15.

[42] Mrs. Paul R. Cannon, clippings from *Inside Information*, a University Clinics Guild publication, Chicago Medical Society. The three institutions combining to form the orthopedic unit were the Gertrude Dunn Hicks Memorial Hospital, the Country Home for Convalescent Children. and the Home for Destitute Crippled Children.

[43] McLean and Gorgas, eds., "Medicine in the Division of Biological Sciences," in *Methods and Problems of Medical Education*, 2.

[44] Memorandum by Laird Bell, chairman of the Committee on Instruction

and Research, University of Chicago Board of Trustees, October 13, 1937. This memorandum was made available through the courtesy of Earl D. Hostetter, present secretary of the Rush Board of Trustees.

[45] *Ibid.*

[46] William Rainey Harper to John M. Dodson, December 18, 1900, in University of Chicago Archives.

[47] William Rainey Harper to F. M. Sperry, August 8, 1902, and E. Fletcher Ingals to William Rainey Harper, May 11, 1892, in University of Chicago Archives.

[48] Abstract of Minutes of the Board of Trustees, University of Chicago, May 3, 1898.

[49] Rush Medical College, Faculty Meeting Minutes, February 14, 1941; *Trustees of the Rush Medical College . . . vs. the University of Chicago, Complaint* Cook County Circuit Court, Case no. 41C 4423 (Chicago, 1941), 1–19.

[50] The information concerning Rush's recent activities derives from an interview with Earl D. Hostetter, secretary of the Rush Board of Trustees, May 4, 1950.

[51] *Chicago Daily News*, August 30, 1946.

CHAPTER VIII: THE CHICAGO MEDICAL SOCIETY

[1] Chicago Medical Society, Minutes, June 29, 1898, in Chicago Historical Society.

[2] *Ibid.*, February 25, 1903. For information on organization of the branch societies, see *ibid.*, June 15, 1904, June 20, 1906; Council Minutes, December 12, 1905, March 10, 1908, November 18, 1913; Trustee Minutes, January 19, 1909. The general minutes of the Society to 1912 and the trustee minutes to 1910 are located in the Chicago Historical Society. All council and trustee minutes since these dates are filed in the offices of the Society.

[3] Chicago Medical Society, Minutes, November 19, 1902, June 15, 1904.

[4] *Illinois Medical Journal*, 11:170 (February, 1907); Chicago Medical Society, Council Minutes, November 9, 1937.

[5] Chicago Medical Society, Minutes, June 21, 1905.

[6] *Ibid.*, 1862 (Appendix), June 21, 1905, February 12, 1943, March 12, 1946.

[7] *Ibid.*, 1903–1910; Chicago Medical Society, Elections and Campaign Literature, 1909–1918, Society of Medical History Collection, in John Crerar Library.

[8] William A. Evans, Historical Material Furnished by Dr. William A. Evans, undated manuscript in Chicago Medical Society.

[9] Chicago Medical Society, Minutes, June 17, 1908.

[10] Chicago Medical Society, Council Minutes, March 8, 1910.

[11] Chicago Medical Society, Elections and Campaign Literature, 1909–1918.

[12] Chicago Medical Society, Council Minutes, October 11, 1910.

[13] *Ibid.*, October 9, 1906.

[14] Chicago Medical Society, Minutes, June 19, 1907.

[15] Chicago Medical Society, Council Minutes, January 14, 1908.

[16] Fishbein, *History of the American Medical Association*, 235.

[17] Chicago Medical Society, Minutes, June 19, 1907.

[18] Chicago Medical Society, Council Minutes, November 8, 1910.
[19] *Chicago Daily News*, October 28, 1914.
[20] Michael M. Davis, *America Organizes Medicine* (New York, 1941), 174.
[21] Chicago Medical Society, Council Minutes, March 30, 1909.
[22] *Bulletin of the Chicago Medical Society*, 16:16 (June 2, 1917).
[23] Chicago Medical Society, Council Minutes, March 10, 1942, April 13, 1948.
[24] *Ibid.*, March 11, 1947.
[25] Chicago Medical Society, Minutes, June 21, 1905; Council Minutes, December 11, 1906.
[26] *Bulletin of the Chicago Medical Society*, 16:15 (May 5, 1917).
[27] The question of medical economics is discussed at length in Chapter XII.
[28] Bayard Holmes, The Duty of the Reader to the Medical Writer, undated manuscript in John Crerar Library.
[29] Chicago Medical Society, Council Minutes, November 27, 1906.
[30] *Ibid.*, February 8, 1910.
[31] See, for example, *ibid.*, January 9, 1923.
[32] *Ibid.*, February 11, 1913.
[33] *Ibid.*, April 12, 1932.
[34] *Ibid.*, November 14, 1933.
[35] See, for example, *ibid.*, May 1, 1945.
[36] *Ibid.*, March 10, 1942.
[37] *Ibid.*, March 12, November 12, 1946.
[38] J. B. Herrick, "The Chicago Society of Internal Medicine," in Institute of Medicine of Chicago, *Proceedings*, 8:94–95 (June 15, 1930).
[39] Frank P. Hammon, History [of] Chicago Society of Industrial Medicine and Surgery, manuscript (1949), in Chicago Medical Society. The Chicago Society of Anesthesiology was also inaugurated in 1920. For a summary of its history, see the short sketch in the History file of the Chicago Medical Society.
[40] Theron G. Randolph, History of Chicago Society of Allergy, manuscript (1950), in Chicago Medical Society.
[41] George H. Coleman, The Institute of Medicine of Chicago, manuscript (1950), in Chicago Medical Society.
[42] Chicago Institute for Psychoanalysis, *Report of the Five Year Period 1942–1947* [Chicago, 1947], 7ff.

CHAPTER IX: SOME SOCIO-MEDICAL PROBLEMS

[1] Edgar Sydenstricker, "Economic Status and the Incidence of Illness," in United States Public Health Service, *Public Health Reports*, 44:1833 (July 26, 1929); G. St. J. Perrott and Selwyn D. Collins, "Relation of Sickness to Income and Income Change in 10 Surveyed Communities," in *ibid.*, 50:621 (May 3, 1935); Rollo H. Britten, "Mortality Rates by Occupational Class in the United States," in *ibid.*, 49:1101 (September 21, 1934); Stern, *American Medical Practice*, 117.
[2] Edgar Sydenstricker, *Health and Environment* (New York, 1933), 84–132. This is the conclusion, too, of Gunnar Myrdal, *An American Dilemma* (New York, 1944), 142.

[3] Chicago Medical Society, Minutes, February 28, 1870.

[4] "Report on Topography, Climatology, and Epidemic Diseases of the State of Illinois," in American Medical Association, *Transactions*, 21:344–347 (1870).

[5] Chicago Board of Health, *Report*, 1893, p. 86. The paragraphs have been put into chronological order.

[6] Chicago Health Statistics Survey, Work Projects Administration, *Health Data Book for the 75 Local Community Areas of the City of Chicago* (Chicago, 1939), 49–130.

[7] Robert E. Lee Faris and H. Warren Dunham, *Mental Disorders in Urban Areas . . .* (Chicago, 1939), ix–x. Another important article dealing with the effect of economic change on health in Chicago is Lolagene C. Coombs, "Economic Differentials in Causes of Death," in *Medical Care*, 1:246–255 (Summer, 1941). See, too, Stern, *American Medical Practice*, 110–121.

[8] Abbott, *Tenements of Chicago*, x.

[9] Morris Fishbein, "Medicine as a World Problem," in *Hygeia*, 26:469 (July, 1948).

[10] Frederick Tice, "A Century of Tuberculosis in Illinois," in *Illinois Medical Journal*, 77:455 (May, 1940).

[11] City Homes Association, *A Study of Tuberculosis in Chicago* (Chicago, 1905), 3.

[12] "Theodore B. Sachs," in Institute of Medicine of Chicago, *Proceedings*, 1:16–18 (1916–1917).

[13] Jane Addams, *The Second Twenty Years at Hull-House . . .* (New York, 1930), 13–15.

[14] Tice, "A Century of Tuberculosis in Illinois," in *Illinois Medical Journal*, 47:458.

[15] Jirka, *American Doctors of Destiny*, 314–316.

[16] Irmengarde Eberle, *Modern Medical Discoveries* (New York, 1948), 131; *Chicago Sun-Times*, February 19, July 18, 1950.

[17] United States Public Health Service and National Tuberculosis Association, *Tuberculosis in the United States: Graphic Presentation*, 3 (1945): chart I.

[18] Chicago Medical Society, Council Minutes, January 14, 1947.

[19] United States Public Health Service, *The Chicago-Cook County Health Survey* (New York, 1949), 527–530; American Public Health Association, *Public Health in Illinois: Full Report of a Study Completed in June, 1942* (New York, 1942), 106.

[20] United States Public Health Service, *Chicago-Cook County Health Survey*, 502.

[21] Coombs, "Economic Differentials in Causes of Death," in *Medical Care*, 1:249–250.

[22] Chicago Medical Society, Council Minutes, March 14, 1939; United States Public Health Service, *Chicago-Cook County Health Survey*, 504. For additional background information on this problem see Marion Nelson, *The Negro Tuberculosis Problem in Chicago* (Chicago Tuberculosis Institute, 1936).

[23] Howard W. Haggard, *Devils, Drugs, and Doctors . . .* (New York, 1929), 5.

[24] Sydenstricker, *Health and Environment*, 99; Abt, *Baby Doctor*, 50.

[25] Chicago Medical Society, Council Minutes, March 30, 1909; J. C. Perry, *Public Health Administration in Chicago, Ill.: A Study of the Organization and*

Administration of the City Health Department (Washington, 1915), 48–50; Chicago Department of Health, *Report*, 1926–1930, p. 3.

[26] Bernhard J. Stern, *Medical Services by Government: Local, State, and Federal* (New York, 1946), 123.

[27] Charles J. Whalen, "The Future of Medicine," in *Illinois Medical Journal*, 65:27 (January, 1934).

[28] Mrs. Paul Cannon, clippings from *Inside Information*, a University of Chicago Clinics Guild publication, History file, Chicago Medical Society.

[29] Abt, *Baby Doctor*, 107; William C. Van Benschoten to J. P. Simonds, August 31, 1949, and clippings from *Inside Information*, Chicago Medical Society.

[30] Illinois Department of Public Health, *Report*, 1924–1925, p. 207.

[31] Fishbein with Sol T. De Lee, *Joseph Bolivar De Lee*, 232–234.

[32] Chicago Medical Society, Council Minutes, May 2, 1938, March 10, 1942.

[33] Malcolm T. MacEachern, *Manual on Obstetric Practice in Hospitals* (American Hospital Association, *Official Bulletin No. 209*, Chicago, 1940), 7–9.

[34] See Fishbein with Sol T. De Lee, *Joseph B. De Lee*, 55.

[35] *Chicago Sun-Times*, November 8, 1949.

[36] Haagensen and Lloyd, *A Hundred Years of Medicine*, 368–369; Warren S. Thompson and P. K. Whelpton, *Population Trends in the United States* (New York, 1933), table 31, p. 109; P. K. Whelpton, *Forecasts of the Population of the United States 1945–1975* (Washington, 1947), table 33, p. 49.

[37] *Chicago Sun-Times*, June 23, 1950.

[38] Haagensen and Lloyd, *A Hundred Years of Medicine*, 369–371.

[39] United States Public Health Service, *Chicago-Cook County Health Survey*, fig. VII, p. 467.

[40] Ernst P. Boas, *The Unseen Plague: Chronic Disease* (New York, 1940), 14–15.

[41] United States Public Health Service, *Chicago-Cook County Health Survey*, table 173, p. 1213.

[42] Institute of Medicine of Chicago, *Proceedings*, 12:332 (April 15, 1939).

[43] Chicago Medical Society, Council Minutes, June 8, 1948.

[44] *Illinois Cancer Bulletin* (Chicago, 1946–1950), *passim*.

[45] United States Public Health Service, *Chicago-Cook County Health Survey*, 1231–1233, 1241.

CHAPTER X: ORIGIN AND DEVELOPMENT OF HOSPITALS

[1] Haagensen and Lloyd, *A Hundred Years of Medicine*, 21–26.

[2] *Weekly Chicago Democrat*, December 28, 1847; *Chicago Daily Journal*, September 26, 1850.

[3] *North-western Medical and Surgical Journal*, N. S., 3:263, 492–493 (1850–1851).

[4] Sister Mary Therese, Administrator of Mercy Hospital, to J. P. Simonds, April 27, 1949, Chicago Medical Society.

[5] John B. Murphy, "The History of Mercy Hospital," in Wilde, ed., *Northwestern University*, 3:368–384.

[6] Packard, *History of Medicine in the United States*, 2:874.

[7] *Presbyterian Hospital of the City of Chicago: A Factual Account of Its History and Accomplishments* (reprinted from Illinois Medical Center District, *Fact Book*, Chicago, 1948).

[8] Note by Henry M. Lyman, assistant secretary, on pp. 2–3 of Minutes of the Board of Trustees of Rush Medical College 1872–1920, bound in two volumes in office of E. D. Hostetter, present secretary of Rush trustees. See, too, *Presbyterian Hospital of the City of Chicago: Sixtieth Anniversary 1883–1943*, a pamphlet published by the hospital.

[9] "The Story of Wesley," in Wesley Memorial Hospital, *Annual Report*, 1948, pp. 1–12 (Chicago, 1948).

[10] Edith B. Farnsworth, "Passavant Memorial Hospital—Some Phases of Its History," in *Quarterly Bulletin of Northwestern University Medical School*, 22:1–4 (Spring, 1948).

[11] Stern, *Society and Medical Progress*, xiv.

[12] Brother Ludolph Sattler, administrator, Alexian Brothers Hospital, to James P. Simonds, August 16, 1949, Chicago Medical Society.

[13] Sister M. Therese, superintendent, St. Mary of Nazareth Hospital, to J. P. Simonds, April 20, 1949.

[14] Sister M. Rosanna Peters, *The History of the Poor Sisters of St. Francis, Seraph of the Perpetual Adoration 1875–1940* (St. Francis Community Press, Lafayette, Indiana, 1944), 126–130; *Lewis Memorial Maternity Hospital* [Chicago, n. d.], pamphlet; Loretto Hospital, *Strategic Alaska* [Chicago, n. d.], pamphlet; Mother M. Dunstan, superintendent, Little Company of Mary Hospital, to J. P. Simonds, April 20, 1949.

[15] *St. Luke's Hospital: Eightieth Anniversary, 1865–1945* (n. p., 1945), pamphlet.

[16] Grant H. Adams, public relations director, Michael Reese Hospital, to J. P. Simonds, March 21, 1949.

[17] Margarete K. Burlin, director of publicity, Grant Hospital, to J. P. Simonds, March 28, 1949.

[18] Nicolay A. Grevstad, *The Norwegian-American Hospital, Chicago* (Chicago, 1930); N. N. Ronning, *Fiftieth Anniversary of the Lutheran Deaconess Home and Hospital* (n. p., 1947); both pamphlets.

[19] Clare Louise Smith, *The Evanston Hospital School of Nursing 1898–1948* (Chicago, 1948), 3–11.

[20] Clara D. Schafer, superintendent, South Chicago Community Hospital, to J. P. Simonds, April 30, 1949.

[21] Henrotin Hospital, *Fifty-fourth Annual Report*, 1940, pp. 1–3.

[22] Theresita E. Norris, An Historical Review of Provident Hospital, manuscript (1944), in Chicago Medical Society.

[23] M. O. Bousfield, "An Account of Physicians of Color in the United States," in *Bulletin of the History of Medicine*, 17:73–75 (January, 1945).

[24] *Ibid.*, 76–77; T. E. Norris, An Historical Review of Provident Hospital.

[25] Chicago Hospital for Women and Children, *Annual Report*, 1865–1866, pp. 1–2; 1866–1867, p. 6; 1877–1878, pp. 5–6; 1883–1884, pp. 6–8.

[26] Edna H. Nelson, "Women and Children's Hospital," in *Hospital Council Bulletin*, 4:9–10 (January, 1941). This was also issued as a separate publication, Chicago, 1941.

[27] Chicago Medical Society, Minutes, April 2, 1883.

[28] *Ibid.*, August 18, 1884.

[29] Neola Nortbaum, director of public relations, Children's Memorial Hospital, to J. P. Simonds, May 26, 1949.

[30] La Rabida Jackson Park Sanitarium, *Annual Report*, 1946.

[31] Council on Medical Education and Hospitals, American Medical Association, "Hospital Service in the United States," in *Journal of the American Medical Association*, 143:28–32 (May 6, 1950).

[32] Edward H. L. Corwin, *The American Hospital* (New York, 1946), 37.

[33] K. A. Carroll, manager, Veterans Administration Hospital, Hines, Illinois, to J. P. Simonds, March 21, 1949.

[34] Max Thorek, director, American Hospital of Chicago, to J. P. Simonds, May 30, 1949; *MacNeal Memorial Hospital* (1948); Charles Newberger, "Mount Sinai Hospital of Chicago," in *Bulletin of the Mount Sinai Hospital*, 1:3–11 (January, 1949).

[35] Belmont Hospital, 1950, manuscript, in Chicago Medical Society. For brief historical accounts of some of the other voluntary hospitals in Chicago, see the section on hospitals in Chicago Medical Society, *History of Medicine and Surgery*. For statistical information on all Chicago and Illinois hospitals, see *Journal of the American Medical Association*, 146:134–137 (May 12, 1951).

[36] *Chicago Daily American*, September 28, 1839.

[37] *Illinois and Indiana Medical and Surgical Journal*, N. S., 2:85–87 (April, 1847); James N. Hyde, *Early Medical Chicago* (Chicago, 1879), 42.

[38] Enid R. Rich, The Cook County Hospital, master's thesis, University of Chicago, 1927, pp. 18–31.

[39] *Chicago Daily Democratic Press*, January 25, April 20, August 25, 1855.

[40] Rich, Cook County Hospital, 13ff.

[41] *Chicago Medical Journal*, N. S., 2:452 (July, 1859).

[42] William E. Quine, "Early History of the Cook County Hospital to 1870," in Chicago Medical Society, *History of Medicine and Surgery*, 257–259.

[43] *Chicago Medical Journal*, 23:91–93 (February, 1866).

[44] Quine, "Early History of the Cook County Hospital," in Chicago Medical Society, *History of Medicine and Surgery*, 261–262.

[45] Henry M. Lyman, "A Bit of the History of the Cook County Hospital," in *Bulletin of the Society of Medical History of Chicago*, 1:27–28 (October, 1911).

[46] *Chicago Tribune*, January 17, 1870.

[47] *Chicago Medical Journal*, 27:62 (January, 1870).

[48] Frank Billings, "History of the Cook County Hospital from 1876 to the Present Time," in Chicago Medical Society, *History of Medicine and Surgery*, 264–265.

[49] Illinois Medical Center District, *Fact Book*, 25.

[50] Chicago Medical Society, Minutes, June 17, 1878.

[51] Billings, "History of Cook County Hospital," in Chicago Medical Society, *History of Medicine and Surgery*, 266–267.

[52] L. L. McArthur, "Christian Fenger as I Knew Him," in *Bulletin of the Society of Medical History of Chicago*, 3:53 (January, 1923); *Chicago Medical Recorder*, 35:194 (April, 1913); Herrick, *Memories of Eighty Years*, 77.

[53] "Warden's Annual Report of Cook County Hospital," in *Annual Reports of the Cook County Agent, Warden Insane Asylum and Poor House, Medical Sup't Cook County Insane Asylum, Warden Cook County Hospital, Cook County Physician, and Coroner* (Chicago, 1876), 85–88.

[54] *Weekly Medical Review*, 8:221 (September 22, 1883); *Medical Standard*, 6:183 (December, 1889); State Board of Charities, *Annual Report*, 1890, p. 316; Billings, "History of Cook County Hospital," in Chicago Medical Society, *History of Medicine and Surgery*, 265; Chicago Medical Society, Council Minutes, January 11, 1905.

[55] Chicago Medical Society, Minutes, April 20, August 3, 1874.

[56] Cook County Hospital, Obstetrical Records, 1883–1888, in John Crerar Library.

[57] *Chicago Daily News*, September 3, 1946.

[58] Sophonisba P. Breckinridge, *The Illinois Poor Law and Its Administration* (Chicago, 1939), 93–95. See also William W. Burke, The Supervision of the Care of the Mentally Diseased by the Illinois State Board of Charities, 1869–1909, doctor's dissertation, University of Chicago, 1934.

[59] Peter Bassoe, "The Early History of Neurology and Psychiatry in the Middle West," in *Bulletin of the Society of Medical History of Chicago*, 3:181–182 (October, 1923); George H. Weaver, "Edward Mead, M.D.: The Pioneer Neuropsychiatrist of Illinois," in *ibid.*, 3:282 (December, 1924); Peter Bassoe, "A Sketch of the Development of Psychiatry and Neurology in Chicago," in Institute of Medicine of Chicago, *Proceedings*, 11:165–166 (December 15, 1936); *Chicago Daily Journal*, February 18, 1852.

[60] Carl E. Black, "Origin of Our State Charitable Institutions," in *Journal of the Illinois State Historical Society*, 18:186–191 (Springfield, April, 1925). Parts of Dorothea Dix's memorable speech before the Illinois legislature may be found in the *Illinois and Indiana Medical and Surgical Journal*, N. S., 2:45–46 (April, 1847). The community of Jacksonville contained an unusually high percentage of educated and enlightened settlers, resulting in her leadership in the establishment of institutions, charitable and otherwise. In Jacksonville were founded the first college, the first medical school, the first insane asylum, and the first institution for the deaf and dumb in the state.

[61] Evans, John. Statement regarding his life given by Mrs. Evans and others. Photostatic copies in the Deering Library, Northwestern University, of manuscripts in the Bancroft Library, University of California, Berkeley.

[62] Bassoe, "Early History of Neurology and Psychiatry," *Bulletin of the Society of Medical History of Chicago*, 3:176–177.

[63] J. Wesley Whicker, "Dr. John Evans," in *Indiana Magazine of History*, 19:239 (September, 1923).

[64] Mrs. E. P. W. Packard, *The Prisoners' Hidden Life, or Insane Asylums Unveiled* (Chicago, 1868).

[65] Albert Deutsch, *The Mentally Ill in America: A History of Their Care and Treatment from Colonial Times* (rev. ed., New York, 1949), 306–307.

[66] *Ibid.*, 426.

[67] *Ibid.*, 242–243.

[68] Henry M. Hurd and others, *The Institutional Care of the Insane in the United States and Canada* (4 vols., Baltimore, 1916–1917), 2:280; *Chicago*

Tribune, May 25, 1870; Chicago Medical Society, Minutes, October 15, 1883; Brown, *History of Public Assistance in Chicago*, table 12, p. 128.

[69] "Annual Report of the Medical Superintendent of Cook County Insane Asylum," in Cook County Board of Supervisors, *Proceedings*, 1877, pp. 44–47.

[70] "Warden's Annual Report of the Cook County Insane Asylum and Poor House," in Cook County Board of Supervisors, *Proceedings*, 1877, pp. 25–26.

[71] *Chicago Times*, March 19, 1876.

[72] Victor Robinson, *The Don Quixote of Psychiatry* (New York, 1919), 59–60; see also Shobal V. Clevenger, *Fun in a Doctor's Life* (Atlantic City, 1909), 102–103.

[73] Shobal V. Clevenger, "Treatment of the Insane," in *Journal of the American Medical Association*, 27:900 (October 24, 1896).

[74] Clevenger, *Fun in a Doctor's Life*, 205–209; *Chicago Medical Journal and Examiner*, 49:502–507 (December, 1884).

[75] See, for example, Chicago Medical Society, Minutes, November 10, 1884, October 19, November 2, 1885; Board of State Commissioners of Public Charities, *Ninth Biennial Report*, 1886 (Springfeld, 1887), 118–119.

[76] Julia C. Lathrop, "The Cook County Charities," in *Hull-House Maps and Papers* (New York, 1895), 150–154.

[77] Chicago Medical Society, *History of Medicine and Surgery*, 243.

[78] E. F. Dombrowski, superintendent, Chicago State Hospital, to J. P. Simonds, April 3, 1949. Rising public confidence in the state's mental hospitals is reflected in the increasing number of voluntary admissions; see Stuart K. Jaffary, *The Mentally Ill and Public Provision for Their Care in Illinois* (Chicago, 1942), table 6, p. 96.

[79] Harry R. Hoffman, Sketch of History of the Illinois Neuropsychiatric Institute, manuscript (1945), Chicago Medical Society.

[80] United States Public Health Service, *Chicago–Cook County Health Survey*, 556.

[81] The Institute for Juvenile Research was founded in 1909 by Dr. William Healy to service the Chicago Juvenile Court and to undertake psychological studies on the problems of the adolescent. After the Institute has been in operation for half a dozen years, Dr. Healy published many of his findings in a book, *The Individual Delinquent* (Boston, 1915). The Institute has served as a model for similar organizations in a number of other cities. George S. Stevenson and Geddes Smith, *Child Guidance Clinics: A Quarter Century of Development* (New York, 1934), 15–18.

[82] United States Health Service, *Chicago–Cook County Health Survey*, 602–605.

[83] Louis S. Reed, *Blue Cross and Medical Service Plans* (Washington, 1947), 253, appendix C; H. Kenneth Scatliff, medical director, Chicago Hospital Service Corporation, to author, January 16, 1952.

[84] Reed, *Blue Cross and Medical Service Plans*, 241–242; Alexander Ropchan, *Chicago Hospital and Clinic Survey* (Chicago Council of Social Agencies, 1935), 4–7.

[85] United States Public Health Service, *Chicago–Cook County Health Survey*, 1081–1083.

CHAPTER XI: PUBLIC HEALTH WORK IN CHICAGO

[1] Shryock, *Development of Modern Medicine*, 79.

[2] *Chicago Daily News*, August 15, 1950.

[3] Rauch, *Sanitary History of Chicago*, 11–12.

[4] *Ibid.*, 14.

[5] Herman N. Bundesen, "One Hundred Years of Public Health in Chicago 1840–1940," in *Illinois Medical Journal*, 77:425 (May, 1940); *Chicago Daily Journal*, August 27, 1849.

[6] Rauch, *Sanitary History of Chicago*, 54–120; Bundesen, "One Hundred Years of Public Health," in *Illinois Medical Journal*, 77:425–426.

[7] Rauch, *Sanitary History of Chicago*, 26.

[8] Chicago Medical Society, Minutes, August 7, September 11, 1863, January 22, 29, April 1, 1864.

[9] Samuel A. Levinson, "History and Progress of the Scientific Work of the Cook County Coroner's Office," in Institute of Medicine of Chicago, *Proceedings*, 12:468–471 (November 15, 1939).

[10] Davis, "On the Intimate Relation of Medical Science to the Whole Field of Natural Sciences," in Illinois State Medical Society, *Transactions* (1853), 22.

[11] Chicago Medical Society, Minutes, May 16, 1854.

[12] *Ibid.*, July 6, 1858.

[13] Lewis and Smith, *Chicago*, 96–97. But after a decade or so, criticism was renewed. The *Chicago Medical Journal and Examiner*, for example, satirized the two-mile inlet in 1884 (vol. 49:128): "I put my trust, not in disinfection, not in combustion, not in antisepsis, not in agents capable of destroying bacteria, but in two miles of lake water! That is the safe limit! Whether agitated by a boisterous storm, or as placid as a mountain-girt basin, these two miles shall stretch between me and all my sanitary sins! I will micturate, defecate, eject excreta, at one end of these two miles, and drink my water at the other, and I shall be safe! No wonder they come to see my Water-works! With these shall I not be cholera-proof?"

[14] J. H. Rauch, *A Report to the Board of Health of the City of Chicago on the Necessity of an Extension of the Sewerage of the City* (Chicago, 1873), 3–4.

[15] *Chicago Medical Examiner*, 6:705–712 (December, 1865).

[16] Rauch, *Sanitary History of Chicago*, 118–120; John M. Toner, "Boards of Health in the United States," in American Public Health Association, *Reports and Papers*, 1:502–513 (1873); Rauch, *Sanitary History of Chicago*, 125.

[17] H. N. Bundesen, "One Hundred Years of Public Health," in *Illinois Medical Journal*, 77:426 (May, 1940); Chicago Relief and Aid Society, *Report of the Committee on Sick, Hospital, and Sanitary Measures* (Chicago, 1874), 3–12.

[18] Rauch, John H., *Public Parks: Their Effects upon the Moral, Physical and Sanitary Condition of the Inhabitants of Large Cities* (Chicago, 1869), 6.

[19] Rawlings and others, *Rise and Fall of Disease in Illinois*, 1:153–154. Mention should be made at least of Rauch's valuable compilation of information on medical colleges in connection with his work in medical education: *Report on Medical Education, Medical Colleges and the Regulation of the Practice of Medicine in the United States and Canada, 1765–1890* (Springfield, Illinois, 1890).

[20] Arthur R. Reynolds, "Three Chicago and Illinois Public Health Officers: John H. Rauch, Oscar C. De Wolf and Frank W. Reilly," in *Bulletin of the Society of Medical History of Chicago*, 1:89–108 (August, 1912).

[21] Charles-Edward A. Winslow, *The Conquest of Epidemic Disease; a Chapter in the History of Ideas* (Princeton, 1943), 12.

[22] Rawlings and others, *Rise and Fall of Disease in Illinois*, 2:328–342.

[23] Rauch, *A Report to the Board of Health of the City of Chicago on the Necessity of an Extension of the Sewerage of the City*, 7.

[24] Winslow, *Conquest of Epidemic Disease*, xi. The clauses in this quotation are reversed.

[25] Reynolds, "Three Chicago and Illinois Public Health Officers," in *Bulletin of the Society of Medical History of Chicago*, 1:110.

[26] Chicago Medical Society, *History of Medicine and Surgery*, 100.

[27] Chicago Medical Society, Minutes, April 15, 1889.

[28] *Chicago Medical Journal*, 28:567 (September, 1871). The editor of this journal called the Common Council the "hydra-headed monster of ignorance and obstinacy" for refusing the appropriation.

[29] *Chicago Times*, March 26, 1876.

[30] *Chicago Medical Journal*, 30:190–191 (March, 1873).

[31] *Chicago Medical Journal and Examiner*, 33:1107 (December, 1876).

[32] Winslow, *Conquest of Epidemic Disease*, ix–xi.

[33] Charles-Edward A. Winslow, *The Evolution and Significance of the Modern Public Health Campaign* (New Haven, 1923), 34–35, and *The Road to Health* (New York, 1929), 15.

[34] The Department of Health had opened a chemical laboratory in 1880, with R. S. G. Paton as chemist. Paton examined and reported on samples of vinegar, baking powder, milk, tea, sugar, candy, and syrup. Chicago Board of Health, *Report*, 1879–1880, p. 24.

[35] Fred O. Tonney, "The Introduction of Bacteriology into the Service of Public Health in Chicago," in *Bulletin of the Society of Medical History of Chicago*, 5:22–24 (January, 1937).

[36] Rawlings and others, *Rise and Fall of Disease in Illinois*, 2:342–356.

[37] Abt, *Baby Doctor*, 50.

[38] Ernest Hart, "Health Conditions of Chicago," in *Chicago Medical Recorder*, 5:10 (July, 1893).

[39] *Chicago Medical Recorder*, 5:371–379 (December, 1893).

[40] Harrison P. Eddy, "Historic Review of the Development of Sanitary Engineering in the United States: Sewerage and Drainage of Towns," in *American Society of Civil Engineers, Transactions*, 92:1229–1230 (1928).

[41] Frederic P. Gorham, "The History of Bacteriology and Its Contribution to Public Health Work," in Mazÿck P. Ravenel, ed., *A Half Century of Public Health* (New York, 1921), 80–81.

[42] *Medical Review*, 40:404–405 (St. Louis, November 25, 1899).

[43] Rawlings and others, *Rise and Fall of Disease in Illinois*, 2:349–350.

[44] George W. Fuller, "Historic Review of the Development of Sanitary Engineering in the United States: Water-Works," in *American Society of Civil Engineers, Transactions*, 92:1220–1221, table 2 (1928).

[45] Hart, "Health Conditions in Chicago," in *Chicago Medical Recorder*, 5:1–3.

[46] Chicago Medical Society, Minutes, May 2, 1892; Chicago Board of Health, *Report*, 1892, p. 6; *Chicago Medical Recorder*, 27:72–74 (January 15, 1905).

[47] Chicago Board of Health, *Report*, 1877, pp. 22–23; *ibid.*, 1904–1905, xiii–xv; *Medical Standard*, 32:63–64 (February, 1909); Chicago Medical Society, Council Minutes, March 30, 1909.

[48] United States Public Health Service, *Chicago–Cook County Health Survey*, 237, 244–246, 267.

[49] Chicago Medical Society, Council Minutes, June 12, 1934; Bundesen, "One Hundred Years of Public Health," in *Illinois Medical Journal*, 77:427.

[50] A. C. Baxter, "Development of Public Health Service in Illinois," in *ibid.*, 77:420–424 (May, 1940).

[51] S. B. Grubbs, "Public Health Administration in Illinois," in United States Public Health Service, *Public Health Reports*, 30:1479–1545 (May 21, 1915).

[52] Rawlings and others, *Rise and Fall of Disease in Illinois*, 1:182–186.

[53] Chicago Board of Health, *Report*, 1894, xvi–xix; Rawlings and others, *Rise and Fall of Disease in Illinois*, 2:360–365; John Dill Robertson, *A Report on an Epidemic of Influenza in the City of Chicago in the Fall of 1918* (Chicago, Department of Health, 1918).

[54] A. W. Hagenbach, "Practice at the County Infirmary," in *Chicago Medical Journal and Examiner*, 48:3 (January, 1884). Before the operation of the immunization process was clearly understood, suggestions were occasionally made that syphilis might be prevented through inoculation. Dr. G. C. Paoli told the Chicago Medical Society in 1870 that he had "no doubt, that syphilis can be inoculated by using matter taken from children whose parents had been affected by syphilis." Other doctors present concurred in his views. Chicago Medical Society, Minutes, January 3, 1870.

[55] *Chicago Medical Recorder*, 44:392 (October, 1922); *Medical Standard*, 45:9 (October, 1922).

[56] Chicago School of Sanitary Science, *Bulletin*, 16:141–143 (August 26, 1922).

[57] Chicago Board of Health, *Report*, 1926–1930, p. 3.

[58] Paul De Kruif, in collaboration with Rhea De Kruif, *Life among the Doctors* (New York, 1949), 147.

[59] *American Journal of Public Health*, 18:69–70 (January, 1928).

[60] Robert F. Steadman, *Public Health Organization in the Chicago Region* (Chicago, 1930), 200n.

[61] Bundesen, "One Hundred Years of Public Health in Chicago," *Illinois Medical Journal*, 77:429; Chicago Medical Society, Council Minutes, February 13, 1934.

[62] Chicago Medical Society, Council Minutes, July 28, 1937; O. C. Wenger, "An Evaluation of the Chicago Syphilis Control Program after One Year" (multigraphed, Chicago, 1938), 17–26, 35–36.

[63] Chicago Venereal Disease Control Program, *Progress Report, July 1, 1943 to October 31, 1947* (Chicago, 1947), 1–3.

[64] *Newsweek*, August 18, 1947, pp. 48–51. The dramatic decline in venereal disease rates in Chicago continued after 1947 as evidenced by the following table:

Year	Syphilis	Gonorrhea
1947	3.6	7.2
1948	2.9	7.2
1949	2.2	6.3
1950	1.8	4.7

[65] *Chicago Daily Tribune*, May 25, 1949.

[66] *Chicago Sun-Times*, February 19, July 18, 1950.

[67] *Chicago Daily News*, August 15, 16, 1950; *Journal of the American Medical Association*, 144:1261 (December, 1950).

[68] *A Summary of the Chicago–Cook County Health Survey Conducted by the United States Public Health Service* (Chicago, 1947), 1–6; United States Public Health Service, *Chicago–Cook County Health Survey*, 39, 45, 95–97, 215, 265–268, 628–629.

[69] Chicago Board of Health, *Report*, 1932, p. 3.

[70] Chicago Medical Society, Council Minutes, January 11, April 12, 1938.

[71] United States Public Health Service, *Chicago–Cook County Health Survey*, 969–971.

CHAPTER XII: SOCIAL AND POLITICAL ATTITUDES OF CHICAGO PHYSICIANS

This chapter originally appeared as "The Social and Political Attitudes of Midwestern Physicians, 1840–1940: Chicago as a Case History," in *Journal of the History of Medicine and Allied Sciences*, 8:133–164 (1953).

[1] *Western Journal of the Medical and Physical Sciences*, 1:ix–xii (1827).

[2] Rush Medical College, *Annual Announcement*, 1844, 7.

[3] *Chicago Medical Journal*, N. S. 2:48–49 (1848).

[4] *North-western Medical and Surgical Journal*, N. S., 1:133–142 (1848).

[5] E. Fletcher Ingals, "The Life and Work of Dr. Daniel Brainard," in *Bulletin of the Alumni Association of Rush Medical College*, 8:8 (1912).

[6] David Riesman, "American Contributions to Nosography," in *New England Journal of Medicine*, 219:592 (1938).

[7] James Eckman, "Anglo-American Hostility in American Medical Literature of the Nineteenth Century," in *Bulletin of the History of Medicine*, 9:34–36 (1941).

[8] Richard H. Shryock, "Public Relations of the Medical Profession in Great Britain and the United States: 1600–1871," in *Annals of Medical History*, N. S., 2:327 (1930).

[9] *Northwestern University Record*, June 1893, 33–34.

[10] *North-western Medical and Surgical Journal*, N. S., 5:184–192 (1856).

[11] *Ibid.*, N. S., 1:131–134 (1852).

[12] Charles N. Andrews, "Valedictory Address . . . on Retiring from the Presidency of the Illinois State Medical Society," in *Transactions of the Illinois Medical Society* (1855), 81.

[13] *Chicago Medical Journal*, 25:219–230 (1868). The triumph of the Americans was even greater, gloated the reporter, "when we remember that it was gained on European ground and that judges in this great international contest were Europeans."

[14] *Ibid.*, 32:340–341 (1875).

[15] For an example of continued sensitivity to English criticism, see the *Chicago Medical Journal and Examiner*, 45:620–625 (1882).

[16] Quoted in *Chicago Medical Times*, 14:155–156 (1882).

[17] M. Fishbein, *History of the American Medical Association, 1847 to 1947* (Chicago, 1947), 118.

[18] *Chicago Medical Journal and Examiner*, 41:504 (1880).

[19] *Weekly Medical Review*, 14:323–324 (1886).

[20] J. E. Lebensohn, "Ophthalmology in Illinois," in *Illinois Medical Journal*, 77:484 (1940).

[21] *Chicago Medical Journal and Examiner*, 48:193 (1884).

[22] *Weekly Medical Review*, 22:354 (1890).

[23] *Chicago Medical Recorder*, 10:267 (1896).

[24] *Medical Standard*, 22:453 (1899).

[25] *Medical Era*, 7:193–194 (1889).

[26] *Ibid.*, 6:97–98 (1888).

[27] Chicago Medical Society, Minutes, October 6, 1879.

[28] Chicago Department of Health, *Annual Report*, 1889, 83–114.

[29] *Ibid.*, 1894, 217.

[30] "Bayard Taylor Holmes," in *Dictionary of American Biography*, 9:161. For a more complete sketch of Holmes' life and work, see T. N. Bonner, "A Forgotten Figure in Chicago's Medical History," in *Journal of the Illinois State Historical Society*, 45:212–219 (1952).

[31] B. Holmes, "The Origin of the Economic Conscience: A Country-bred Boy's Education in Economics," in *Medical Life*, 31:260–263 (1924). Editor Victor Robinson devoted the entire July 1924 issue of *Medical Life* to tributes to Holmes and the printing of two of his last essays.

[32] B. Holmes, The Confession of a Socialist, undated manuscript in John Crerar Library.

[33] Scrapbook of clippings on Bayard Holmes, medical papers and typewritten manuscripts, John Crerar Library.

[34] "A Letter from Graham Taylor," in *Medical Life*, 31:253 (1924).

[35] *Chicago Medical Journal*, 29:5–7 (1872).

[36] *Ibid.*, 27:567 (1870).

[37] Chicago Medical Society, Minutes, January 19, 1874.

[38] Harold N. Moyer, "James Stewart Jewell," in *Bulletin of the Society of Medical History, Chicago*, 3:491 (1925).

[39] Bayard Holmes, "Faith, Evolution and Evolution Clubs," in *Chicago Medical Recorder*, 44:118–120 (1922).

[40] *Chicago Medical Journal*, 31:199–202 (1874).

[41] *Weekly Medical Review*, 10:403–406 (1894).

[42] B. Holmes, "Faith, Evolution and Evolution Clubs," in *Chicago Medical Recorder*, 44:120 (1922). For further examples of anti-evolutionism among Chicago physicians in the 1880's, see S. V. Clevenger, *Fun in a Doctor's Life*, 194–195; *Chicago Medical Journal and Examiner*, 45:615–616 (1882); and *Chicago Medical Times*, 22:500–501 (1890).

[43] Chicago Medical Society, Minutes, October 6, 1879.

[44] *Chicago Medical Journal and Examiner*, 39:319 (1879).

[45] George Rosen, "Disease and Social Criticism: A Contribution to a Theory of

Medical History," in *Bulletin of the History of Medicine*, 10:10 (1941).

[46] Henry Gradle, "The Germ Theory of Disease," in *Popular Science Monthly*, 23:578 (1883).

[47] *Medical Review*, 39:244–245 (1899).

[48] Henry B. Favill, "Speech Delivered at the University of Chicago, June, 1905," in *Henry Baird Favill: A Memorial Volume*, compiled by John Favill (Chicago, 1917), 178–196.

[49] *Medical Standard*, 30:116–117 (1907).

[50] William Allen Pusey, "Some of the Social Problems of Medicine," in *Journal of the American Medical Association*, 83:1905 (1924).

[51] See, for example, C.-E. A. Winslow, *The Road to Health* (New York, 1929), 130–131.

[52] Chicago Medical Society, Minutes, October 8, 1912.

[53] *Chicago Medical Recorder*, 1901–1910 *passim*, especially 31:648–49 (1909). Among the members of the twenty-one-man editorial board at this time were Archibald Church, E. Doering, Junius C. Hoag, Franklin H. Martin, S. C. Plummer, Arthur R. Reynolds, and Edmund Andrews.

[54] *Medical Standard*, 20:75 (1898); *Clinique*, 29:247–249 (1908).

[55] *Medical Standard*, 36:388–389 (1913).

[56] Chicago Medical Society, Minutes, October 29, 1902.

[57] *Ibid.*, February 18, 1903.

[58] Chicago Medical Society, Council Minutes, May 27, 1910.

[59] *Medical Standard*, 32:4–5 (1909).

[60] Chicago Medical Standard, *History of Medicine and Surgery*, 175.

[61] Arthur D. Bevan, "Medicine a Function of the State," in *Journal of the American Medical Association*, 62:821–823 (1914).

[62] *Illinois Medical Journal*, 22:729–730 (1912).

[63] S. V. Clevenger, "Physicians and the Progressive Party," in *Dr. Clevenger's Comments*, no. 1, 1–8, 1912, Collected Papers, John Crerar Library.

[64] Chicago Medical Society, Minutes, 1903–1910 *passim*.

[65] Chicago Medical Society, Minutes, January 11, February 8, 1910.

[66] *Medical Standard*, 29:1–2 (1906).

[67] *Ibid.*, 32:625–626 (1909).

[68] *Chicago Medical Recorder*, 45:820–821 (1923).

[69] *Illinois Medical Journal*, 63:193–198 (1933).

[70] *Ibid.*, 38:47 (1920). Whalen complained that at "any moment, at any place, one may expect to be reformed or investigated."

[71] *Ibid.*, 47:88 (1925).

[72] *Ibid.*, 1921–1927 *passim*.

[73] *Ibid.*, 61:186 (1932).

[74] W. A. Pusey, "Some of the Social Problems of Medicine," in *Journal of the American Medical Association*, 83:1905–1908, 1960–1964 (1924).

[75] Charles B. Reed, "State Medicine Means Regimentation and Nullity," in *Illinois Medical Journal*, 56:248 (1929).

[76] *Clinique*, 41 (1920).

[77] "The Doctor Must Sell Himself," in *Medical Standard*, 48:9 (1925).

[78] J. Lewis Webb, "Economic Laws Governing the Worker's Income," in *Bulletin of the Chicago Medical Society*, 32:23–28 (1930).

[79] *Bulletin of the Chicago Medical Society*, 35:525 (1933).
[80] Chicago Medical Society, Council Minutes, October 9, 1934.
[81] *Ibid.*, March 10, 1936.
[82] *Illinois Medical Journal*, 65:25–28 (1934).
[83] *Ibid.*, 68:293 (1935).
[84] Chicago Medical Society, Council Minutes, May 1, 1937.
[85] Edward H. Ochsner, *Social Insurance and Economic Security* (Boston, 1934), *passim*.

CHAPTER XIII: THE PROFESSION AND THE PUBLIC

[1] John H. Hollister, *Memories of Eighty Years: Autosketches, Random Notes and Reminiscences* (Chicago, 1912), 54.
[2] Carl E. Black, "Medical Practice in Illinois before Hard Roads," in *Bulletin of the Society of Medical History of Chicago*, 5:418 (June, 1946).
[3] *Chicago Medical Journal*, 23:489 (October, 1866).
[4] *Chicago Medical Review*, 6:444 (October 1, 1882).
[5] *Illinois Medical Bulletin*, 3:690 (Chicago, 1903).
[6] Black, "Medical Practice in Illinois before Hard Roads," in *Bulletin of the Society of Medical History of Chicago*, 5:422–423 (June, 1946).
[7] See Chicago Medical Society, Minutes, July 2, 1883.
[8] Alvin V. Cole to J. P. Simonds, April 5, 1949.
[9] John F. Williams, "The Work of the Physicians during the Chicago Fire," in *Bulletin of the Society of Medical History of Chicago*, 2:339–342 (March, 1922).
[10] George H. Weaver, "The Chicago Medical Relief Committee," in *Bulletin of the Society of Medical History of Chicago*, 2:334–338 (March, 1922).
[11] *Chicago Daily Journal*, June 12, 1848.
[12] *Chicago Daily Democratic Press*, August 12, 1854.
[13] *Chicago Daily American*, April 30, 1842.
[14] Danforth, *Life of Nathan Smith Davis*, 56.
[15] Evans, John. Statement regarding his Life given by Mrs. Evans and others. Photostatic copies in the Deering Library, Northwestern University, of manuscripts in the Bancroft Library, University of California, Berkeley.
For a fuller treatment of the political and social views of Chicago physicians see Thomas N. Bonner, "The Social and Political Attitudes of Midwestern Physicians, 1840–1940," in *Journal of the History of Medicine and Allied Sciences*, 7:133–164 (April, 1953).
[16] Norman Bridge, *The Marching Years* (New York, 1920), 90–96.
[17] See *Chicago Weekly Democrat*, June 13, 1857.
[18] D. W. G[raham] to Mary E. Bates, August 15, 1883, in John Crerar Library. For a fuller treatment of the problem from the standpoint of medical schools, see above, chapter IV.
[19] *Illinois and Indiana Medical and Surgical Journal*, 1:30–31 (April, 1846); Chicago Medical Society, Minutes, March 5, 1869.
[20] *Chicago Medical Journal*, 25:168–169 (March 1, 1868).
[21] Harry H. Moore, *Public Health in the United States* . . . (New York, 1923), 202.

Notes to Pages 231–240

[22] Quoted in E. R. Booth, History of Osteopathy . . . (rev. ed., Cincinnati, 1924), 214.

[23] Chicago Tribune, 1860–1875, passim.

[24] Ibid., January 9, 1870.

[25] North-western Medical and Surgical Journal, N. S., 1:161–165 (August, 1852); Illinois Medical and Surgical Journal, 1:97–105 (October, 1844); Chicago Medical Society, Minutes, December 7, 1858.

[26] See North-western Medical and Surgical Journal, 5:86–88 (April–May, 1848), N. S., 2:230 (September, 1849).

[27] Chicago Medical Journal and Examiner, 39:312 (September, 1879).

[28] Ibid., 56:139–141 (March, 1888).

[29] Illinois State Board of Health, First Annual Report, 1878, pp. 5–18.

[30] H. A. Johnson, "The Influence of the Work of the Illinois Medical Practice Act upon Medical Education," in Chicago Medical Journal and Examiner, 57:326–330 (December, 1888); ibid., 56:142–143 (March, 1888).

[31] Francis W. Shephardson, A Report on the Administration of the Medical Practice Act (Springfield, Illinois, 1919), 4.

[32] George Rosen, Fees and Fee Bills: Some Economic Aspects of Medical Practice in Nineteenth Century America (supplements to the Bulletin of the History of Medicine, No. 6, Baltimore, 1946), 33–34.

[33] Chicago Medical Society, Minutes, April 10, 1855.

[34] Ibid., November 29, 1869; Shryock, Development of Modern Medicine, 381–384.

[35] "Archive Years," in Illinois Medical Journal, 70:396 (May, 1940).

[36] Medical Standard, 22:318–319 (August, 1899).

[37] Chicago Medical Society, Minutes, January 23, 1901; Chicago Daily Tribune, January 1, 1911.

[38] Garceau, Political Life of the American Medical Association, 103–108.

[39] Chicago Medical Society, Minutes, January 5, 1865, June 29, 1866.

[40] Chicago Daily Tribune, March 23, 1880; Chicago Medical Journal and Examiner, 40:528–533 (May, 1880).

[41] Weekly Medical Review, 16:60 (July 16, 1887).

[42] Chicago Medical Society, Minutes, June 19, 1907; Chicago Medical Society, Council Minutes, March 10, 1908, February 13, 1912, May 1, 1913.

[43] Public Health Institute, How Laymen Cut Medical Costs (Chicago, 1948), 3–4, 8–9, 18–19.

[44] Ibid., 21–23; Bulletin of the Chicago Medical Society, 31:29–30 (April 13, 1929); Herrick, Memories of Eighty Years, 231.

[45] Herman N. Bundesen, "The High Cost of Illness," in Forum, 82:112 (August, 1929). Dr. Bundesen was finally reinstated as a member of the Chicago Medical Society in 1948 after having his application rejected several times by the council. Chicago Medical Society, Minutes, April 13, 1948.

[46] Schmidt had wide popular support. President Walter Dill Scott of Northwestern University and Rabbi Louis Mann came to Schmidt's defense; the Chicago Association of Commerce instituted an inquiry; business groups in general criticized the action of the Society. Commissioner Bundesen and Dr. Frank Billings appeared before the Association of Commerce to attest to the high professional and personal standing of Dr. Schmidt; Dr. Charles Mayo wired from

Rochester, Minnesota, that Schmidt was "a great man" and that his expulsion was "unfortunate." *Chicago Daily Tribune*, April 10, 11, 13, 1929; *Chicago Daily News*, April 10, 11, 12, 13, 15, 16, 1929.

[47] *Bulletin of the Chicago Medical Society*, 33:16–18 (October 11, 1930).

[48] C. B. Reed, "State Medicine Means Regimentation and Nullity," in *Illinois Medical Journal*, 56:251 (October, 1929).

[49] Alexander Ropchan, *Chicago Hospital and Clinic Survey* (Chicago Council of Social Agencies, 1935), 8ff.

[50] Chicago Medical Society, Council Minutes, November 13, 1934, October 8, 1940.

[51] Fishbein, *History of the American Medical Association*, 407–408.

[52] Chicago Medical Society, Committee on Medical Economics, *Report of a Study of the Abuse of Free Medical Service in Out Patient Practice* (multigraphed, Chicago, 1935), 6. The budget varied from $45.03 per month for a working woman living alone to $121.57 for a five-person family; persons earning this much or more were considered capable of paying a private physician.

[53] Chicago Medical Society, Council Minutes, February 11, March 10, April 14, 1936, February 9, March 9, 1937, February, 1938. The council was particularly upset by the clinic admission policies of the University of Chicago, which refused to employ any "means test" in screening applicants. See Council Minutes, February 13, 1934, June 4, 1935.

[54] *Ibid.*, April 8, 1913.

[55] J. L. White, "Hygiene and Doctors' Fees," in *Illinois State Medical Society, Transactions* (1889), 382–393.

[56] Chicago Medical Society, Minutes, May 19, 1890.

[57] See Chicago Medical Society, Council Minutes, June 12, 1906, February 12, 1907.

[58] Chicago Medical Society, Minutes, June 19, 1907.

[59] Nathan Sinai, Odin W. Anderson, and Melvin L. Dollar, *Health Insurance in the United States* (New York, 1946), 7–11.

[60] *Bulletin of the Chicago Medical Society*, 16:13–20 (February 24, 1917).

[61] A. D. Bevan, "Medicine a Function of the State," in *Journal of the American Medical Association*, 42:823 (March 14, 1914).

[62] Fishbein, *History of the American Medical Association*, 313.

[63] *Illinois Medical Journal*, 77:401 (May, 1940).

[64] R. L. Duffus, "Shall Medicine Be Socialized?" in *The New York Times*, December 4, 1932.

[65] The Chicago laymen on the committee were Michael M. Davis, director for medical services, Julius Rosenwald Fund, William F. Ogburn, professor of sociology, University of Chicago, and Amelia Sears, member of the Board of Commissioners, Cook County.

[66] Committee on the Costs of Medical Care, *Medical Care for the American People: The Final Report of the Committee on the Costs of Medical Care* (Chicago, 1932), 104–144, 152–183.

[67] Sinai and others, *Health Insurance in the United States*, 14ff.; James Rorty, *American Medicine Mobilizes* (New York, 1939), 31–35, 80–83; Fishbein, *History of the American Medical Association*, 417.

[68] Chicago Medical Society, Council Minutes, December 10, 1935.

[69] *Ibid.*, November 24, 1936, January 12, February 9, October 12, 1937.

[70] Chicago Medical Society, Committee on Medical Economics, *The Medical Care Required and Available in Cook County* (Chicago, 1939), 16–21.

[71] *Chicago Daily Tribune*, November 20, 1945.

[72] Clarence A. Peters, ed., *Free Medical Care* (New York, 1946), 3, 36–37.

[73] *Illinois Medical Journal*, 88:225–227 (November, 1945).

[74] New York Academy of Medicine, Committee on Medicine and the Changing Order, *Medicine in the Changing Order* (New York, 1947), xii.

[75] The pressure increased after 1948, when Federal Security Administrator Oscar Ewing convened a National Health Assembly, composed of groups and individuals interested in public health problems. The assembly, in its report, called attention to inequities in the distribution of medical care and cited the need for more physicians, hospitals, and other medical resources. Regarding payment of physicians' fees, the assembly declared that the principle of contributory health insurance should be utilized to abolish the economic barrier to adequate service, to avoid the indignity of a "means test," and to remove the burden of unpredictable costs. Tax funds should be used to provide services not available under the prepayment plans. But the assembly split on the issue of whether a continued voluntary system of prepayment was preferable to a compulsory federal plan. National Health Assembly, *America's Health: A Report to the Nation* (New York, 1949), 221–222. In his report to the president, however, Ewing recommended without reservation a system of national health insurance. Oscar R. Ewing, *The Nation's Health: A Ten Year Program* (Washington, 1948), xi.

[76] B. J. Stern, *Medical Services by Government*, 34; Chicago Medical Society, Council Minutes, February 13, 1945, March 12, 1946.

[77] Chicago Medical Society, Trustee Minutes, August 1, 1947; Chicago Medical Society, Council Minutes, November 9, 1948; and information supplied by Illinois Medical Service.

[78] Hertzler, *Horse and Buggy Doctor*, 9.

A Note on the Bibliography

The list of bibliographical sources that follows this note is still the most extensive yet published on Chicago medicine. In the intervening years, however, a number of additional books and articles have been written that discuss the history of medicine in the city. Scholars will find helpful the *Annotated Bibliography of Chicago History* (Chicago: Chicago Historical Society, 1979) by Frank Jewell, which is a careful compilation of works dealing with all phases of the city's life. Of histories of the city itself, the two most useful among more recent studies are Bessie Pierce's solid, three-volume *History of Chicago* (Chicago: University of Chicago Press, 1937–57, 1975), and Harold M. Mayer and Richard C. Wade's *Chicago: Growth of a Metropolis* (Chicago: University of Chicago Press, 1969). The latter is a ground-breaking study in urban history.

A number of books that have appeared since 1957 treat the major medical schools and universities of the Chicago area. Especially relevant are Leslie B. Arey, *Northwestern University Medical School, 1859–1959: A Pioneer in Educational Reform*, rev. ed. (Evanston: Northwestern University Medical School, 1979); Jim Bowman, *Good Medicine: The First 150 Years of Rush-Presbyterian-St. Luke's Medical Center* (Chicago: Chicago Review Press, 1987); and Edward P. Cohen, ed., *Medicine in Transition: The Centennial of the University of Illinois College of Medicine* (Urbana: University of Illinois Press, 1981). Other university histories that include sections on medical education are Harold F. Williamson and Payson S. Wild, *Northwestern University: A History, 1850–1975* (Evanston: Northwestern University Press, 1976); Richard Storr, *Harper's University* (Chicago: University of Chicago Press, 1966); and Wynton U. Solberg, *The University of Illinois, 1867–1894* (Urbana: University of Illinois Press, 1968). Ilza Veith wrote *The University of Chicago Clinics and Clinical Departments, 1927–1952: A Brief History of the Origins, the Formative Years, and the Present State of Medicine at the University of Chicago* (Chicago: University of Chicago Press, 1952). A full treatment of Abraham Flexner's visits in Chicago can be found in Patricia Spain Ward, "The Other Abraham: Flexner in Illinois," *Caduceus* 2 (Spring 1986): 1–66. For a thorough description and analysis of medical education in the late 1960s see Illinois Board of Higher Education, *Education in the Health Fields for the*

298 A Note on the Bibliography

State of Illinois, 2 vols. (Springfield: Illinois Board of Higher Education, 1968).

Newer biographical and autobiographical writings that illuminate phases of Chicago's medical history include Edwin F. Hirsch, *Frank Billings: The Architect of Medical Education, an Apostle of Excellence in Clinical Practice, a Leader in Chicago Medicine* [Chicago, 1966]; George Rosen, "Christian Fenger, Medical Immigrant," *Bulletin of the History of Medicine* 48 (Spring 1974): 129–45; Morris Fishbein, *Morris Fishbein, M.D.: An Autobiography* (Garden City, N.Y.: Doubleday, 1969); and Barbara Sicherman, *Alice Hamilton: A Life in Letters* (Cambridge: Harvard University Press, 1984), especially pp. 108–236. For a somewhat different view of Joseph B. De Lee's work as an obstetrician in Chicago, see Judith W. Leavitt, *Brought to Bed: Childbearing in America, 1750 to 1950* (New York: Oxford University Press, 1986), especially pp. 179–89.

Other books and articles of recent vintage that are worthy of mention include Thomas Philpott's *The Slum and the Ghetto* (New York: Oxford University Press, 1978), a revisionist history of housing policy in Chicago from 1880 to 1930; Michael Millman's *Politics and the Expanding Physician Supply* (Montclair, N.J.: Allenheld, Osmun, 1980), which includes much on recent medical policy in Illinois; Conrad Seipp's "Organized Medicine and the Public Health Institute of Chicago," *Bulletin of the History of Medicine* 62 (Fall 1988): 429–49, an account of a controversy that was still hot when the first edition of this book appeared; and Vanessa N. Gamble's "The Negro Hospital Renaissance: The Black Hospital Movement, 1920–1945," in *The American General Hospital: Communities and Social Context*, Diana E. Long and Janet Golden, eds. (Ithaca: Cornell University Press, 1989), an important article on black hospital development that includes new material on Provident Hospital.

Excellent photographic collections that include some pictures of Chicago medical practice in the Depression and World War II years are Robert L. Reid and Larry A. Viskochil, eds., *Chicago and Downstate: Illinois as Seen by the Farm Security Administration Photographers, 1936–43* (Urbana: University of Illinois Press, 1989), and John Stoeckle and George A. White, *Plain Pictures of Plain Doctoring* (Cambridge: MIT Press, 1985).

Bibliographical Sources

MANUSCRIPTS AND
OTHER COLLECTED MATERIALS

ANDREWS, EDMUND, Papers, in the Chicago Historical Society.

CHICAGO LARYNGOLOGICAL AND OTOLOGICAL SOCIETY, Proceedings 1899–1938, in the John Crerar Library.

CHICAGO MEDICAL SOCIETY, Historical Collection. Includes letters from older Chicago doctors and from hospital and specialty society directors sent in reply to a questionnaire from James P. Simonds, chairman of the Committee on Medical History of the Chicago Medical Society.

CHICAGO MEDICAL SOCIETY, Minutes:
General Meetings, 1852–1909, in the Chicago Historical Society;
Council Meetings, 1903–1912, in the Chicago Historical Society;
Council Meetings, 1912–1950, in the Chicago Medical Society;
Trustee Meetings, 1898–1910, in the Chicago Historical Society;
Trustee Meetings, 1910–1950, in the Chicago Medical Society.

DAVIS, NATHAN SMITH, Papers, in the Northwestern University Medical School.

EVANS, JOHN. Statement regarding his life and notes given by Mrs. Evans, Mrs. Dickinson, and Governor Sheldon of Colorado. Photostatic copies in the Deering Library, Northwestern University, of manuscripts in the Bancroft Library, University of California, Berkeley.

HOLLISTER, JOHN H., Papers, in the Chicago Historical Society.

HOLMES, BAYARD, Papers, in the John Crerar Library.

JOHN CRERAR LIBRARY, Medical Reprints. Include works of Isaac A. Abt, Edmund Andrews, Henry M. Bannister, William T. Belfield, Frank Billings, Norman Bridge, William H. Byford, Shobal V. Clevenger, Nathan Smith Davis, Sr., Nathan Smith Davis, Jr., William A. Evans, Joseph B. De Lee, Christian Fenger, Austin Flint, Malcolm L. Harris, Ludvig Hektoen, James B. Herrick, Bayard Holmes, James N. Hyde, Hosmer A. Johnson, G. Frank Lydston, Lewis L. McArthur, Franklin H. Martin, John B. Murphy, Albert H. Ochsner, Edward Ochsner, Robert B. Preble, William A. Pusey, Nicholas Senn, Max Thorek, Frederick Tice, Frank Waxham, and George H. Weaver.

KIMBERLY, EDMUND S., Papers, in the Chicago Historical Society.

MEDICAL LIBRARY ASSOCIATION OF CHICAGO, Papers, in the Chicago Historical Society.

NORTHWESTERN UNIVERSITY ARCHIVES, Correspondence concerning the relationship of the Medical School to the University.

NORTHWESTERN UNIVERSITY MEDICAL SCHOOL, Faculty Minutes, 1859–1891.

PRACTITIONERS' CLUB, Minutes and Programs. Society of Medical History of Chicago Collection, John Crerar Library.

RUSH MEDICAL COLLEGE, Minutes:

Board of Trustees, 1872–1920, in the possession of Earl D. Hostetter, Chicago;

Faculty, 1875–1941, in the Rush Medical Library, Presbyterian Hospital, Chicago.

SOCIETY OF MEDICAL HISTORY OF CHICAGO, Collections. Includes pamphlets, reprints, students' notebooks, diplomas, photographs, college announcements, catalogues, letters to Dr. John McLean from other Rush faculty members, 1843–1849; letters to Nicholas Senn 1888–1906; Chicago Medical Relief Committee records, 1871–1873; election and campaign literature of the Chicago Medical Society, 1909–1918; Cook County Hospital obstetrical records, 1883–1888; and some materials belonging to Dr. Mary E. Bates, first female intern at the Cook County Hospital. Uncatalogued manuscripts, John Crerar Library.

UNIVERSITY OF CHICAGO ARCHIVES, Correspondence concerning the relationship of Rush Medical School to the University.

PERIODICALS

American Journal of Public Health. New York, 1911–.

AMERICAN MEDICAL ASSOCIATION, *Journal*. Chicago, 1883–.

———, *Transactions*. 33 vols. Philadelphia, 1848–1882.

American Practitioner. 49 vols. Louisville, Kentucky, 1886–1905.

AMERICAN PUBLIC HEALTH ASSOCIATION, *Public Health Papers and Reports*. 37 vols. New York, 1873–1912.

American Review of Tuberculosis. Baltimore, 1917–.
AMERICAN SOCIETY OF CIVIL ENGINEERS, *Transactions.* New York, 1867–.
Annals of Medical History. 24 vols. New York, 1917–1942.
Archives of Internal Medicine. Chicago, 1908.
Archives of Pathology. Chicago, 1926–.
Bacteriological Review. Baltimore, 1937–.
Bulletin of the History of Medicine. Baltimore, 1933–. (Vols. 1-6, 1933–1938 as *Bulletin of the Institute of the History of Medicine.*)
Bulletin of the Johns Hopkins Hospital. Baltimore, 1889–.
CHICAGO GYNECOLOGICAL SOCIETY, *Transactions.* 12 vols. New York, 1891–1904.
CHICAGO HOMEOPATHIC MEDICAL SOCIETY, *Bulletin.* 10 vols. Chicago, 1917–1926.
Chicago Medical Examiner. 16 vols. Chicago, 1860–1875. (After 1871 as *Chicago Examiner.* In 1875 it was united with *Chicago Medical Journal* as *Chicago Medical Journal and Examiner*).
Chicago Medical Journal. 18 vols. Chicago, 1858–1875. (In 1875 became *Chicago Medical Journal and Examiner* when it absorbed the *Chicago Medical Examiner.*)
Chicago Medical Journal and Examiner. 58 vols. Chicago, 1844–1889. (Vols. 1–2 as *Illinois Medical and Surgical Journal;* vols. 3–4 as *Illinois and Indiana Medical and Surgical Journal;* vols. 5–14 as *Northwestern Medical and Surgical Journal;* vols. 15–32 as *Chicago Medical Journal.*)
Chicago Medical Recorder. Chicago, 1891–. (It became the *Radiological Review* in 1927 and the *Radiological Review and Mississippi Valley Medical Journal* in 1939.)
Chicago Medical Review. 63 vols. Chicago and St. Louis, 1880–1914. (Title varies: *Weekly Medical Review, Medical Review.*)
CHICAGO MEDICAL SOCIETY, *Bulletin.* Chicago, 1902–.
The Chicago Medical Times. 42 vols. Chicago, 1869–1910.
CHICAGO PATHOLOGICAL SOCIETY, *Transactions.* 15 vols. Chicago, 1894–1937.
Cleveland Medical Journal. 17 vols. Cleveland, 1902–1918.
The Clinical Review. 25 vols. Chicago, 1892–1907.
The Clinique. 47 vols. Chicago, 1880–1926.
The Homeopathic Student. 5 vols. Chicago, 1895–1900.
Illinois and Indiana Medical and Surgical Journal. 2 vols. Chicago

and Indianapolis, 1846–1848. (In 1848 it became the *North-western Medical and Surgical Journal.*)

Illinois Cancer Bulletin. Chicago, 1946–.

Illinois Medical and Surgical Journal. 2 vols. Chicago, 1844–1846. (In 1846 the name was changed to *Illinois and Indiana Medical and Surgical Journal.*)

Illinois Medical Bulletin. 8 vols. Chicago, 1900–1908.

Illinois Medical Journal. Springfield, 1899–.

ILLINOIS STATE HISTORICAL SOCIETY, *Journal.* Springfield, 1908–.

——, *Transactions.* Springfield, 1900–1936.

ILLINOIS STATE MEDICAL SOCIETY, *Transactions.* 48 vols. Springfield, 1850–1898.

INSTITUTE OF MEDICINE OF CHICAGO, *Proceedings.* Chicago, 1917–.

Journal of the History of Medicine and Allied Sciences. New Haven, Connecticut, 1946–.

The Medical Current. 12 vols. Chicago, 1885–1896.

Magazine of Western History. 14 vols. Cleveland and New York, 1884–1891. (Became the *National Magazine.*)

Medical Era. 21 vols. Chicago, 1883–1903.

Medical Freedom. 6 vols. New York, 1911–1916.

Medical Life. 45 vols. New York, 1894–1938.

Medical Mirror. 18 vols. St. Louis, 1890–1907.

Medical News. 87 vols. Philadelphia and New York, 1843–1905.

The Medical Standard. 54 vols. Chicago, 1887–1931. (Title varies.)

The Medical Visitor. 21 vols. Chicago, 1885–1905.

New England Journal of Medicine. Boston, 1828–.

Northwestern Journal of Homeopathy. 4 vols. Cedar Rapids, Iowa, 1889–1892.

Northwestern Journal of Homœopathia. 4 vols. Chicago, 1848–1852.

North-western Medical and Surgical Journal. 10 vols. Chicago and Indianapolis, 1848–1857. (In 1858 it became the *Chicago Medical Journal*; in 1852 a new series was commenced.)

NORTHWESTERN UNIVERSITY MEDICAL SCHOOL, *Bulletin.* Chicago, 1899–. (Suspended 1913–1939.)

RUSH MEDICAL COLLEGE, *Bulletin of the Alumni.* 18 vols. Chicago, 1904–1924.

SOCIETY OF MEDICAL HISTORY OF CHICAGO, *Bulletin.* Chicago, 1911–.

Surgery, Gynecology and Obstetrics. Chicago, 1905–.

Texas Medical Journal. 8 vols. Galveston, 1873–1879.
United States Medical and Surgical Journal.
Urologic and Cutaneous Review. St. Louis, 1897–. (1897–1912 as *American Journal of Dermatology and Genito-Urinary Diseases.*)
Western Journal of Medical and Physical Sciences. 12 vols. Cincinnati, 1827–1838. (Title varies: *Western Journal of the Medical and Physical Sciences.*)

NEWSPAPERS

Chicago Daily American (established 1839; discontinued 1842; published as *Daily Chicago American* 1839–1841).
Chicago Morning Democrat (daily; established 1840; title changed to *Chicago Democrat* 1846, and to *Chicago Daily Democrat* 1849; absorbed by *Chicago Daily Tribune* 1861).
Chicago Democrat (weekly; established 1833; title continues as *Weekly Chicago Democrat* 1846; and as *Chicago Weekly Democrat* 1857; absorbed by *Chicago Daily Tribune* 1861).
Chicago Examiner (established 1900; 1918 united with *Chicago Record-Herald* to form *Chicago Herald and Examiner*).
Chicago Express (daily; established 1842; discontinued 1844).
(Chicago) *Gem of the Prairie* (weekly; established 1844; merged with *Chicago Tribune* 1852).
Chicago Herald (established 1881; followed *Chicago Daily Telegraph* 1878–1881; published as *Chicago Herald* 1881–1895; as *Chicago Times-Herald* 1895–1901; as *Chicago Record-Herald* 1901–1914; as *Chicago Record-Herald & Inter Ocean* 1914; as *Chicago Record-Herald* 1914–1918. In 1918 combined with *Chicago Examiner* to form *Chicago Herald and Examiner.*)
(Chicago) *The Inter Ocean* (established 1872; became *Daily Inter Ocean* 1879; 1914 united with *Chicago Record-Herald* to form *Chicago Record-Herald & Inter Ocean*; 1914 name shortened to *Record-Herald.*)
Chicago Journal (daily; established 1844; followed *Chicago Express* 1842–1844; continued as *Daily Chicago Journal* 1853; and as *Chicago Evening Journal* 1861; absorbed by *Chicago Daily News* 1929).
Chicago Journal (weekly; established 1844; discontinued 1896?).
Chicago (Daily) News (established 1876).
Chicago Times (daily; established 1854; published as *Chicago Daily Times* 1854–1860; as *Daily Times and Herald* 1860; as *Daily Chicago*

Times 1860–1861; 1895 united with *Chicago Herald* to form *Chicago Times-Herald,* later *Chicago Herald and Examiner*).

Chicago Times (weekly; established 1854; name changed to *Times and Herald* 1860 after absorbing the *Herald;* 1861–95 as *Chicago Times;* discontinued 1895).

Chicago Tribune (established 1847; united with *Chicago Daily Press* 1858 as *Chicago Daily Press and Tribune;* 1859 as *Press and Tribune;* and 1860 as *Chicago Daily Tribune*).

BIOGRAPHICAL REFERENCE WORKS

AMERICAN COLLEGE OF SURGEONS, 1950–1952 *Year Book.* Chicago, 1950.

AMERICAN MEDICAL ASSOCIATION, *American Medical Directory.* 18th ed. Chicago, 1950.

ATKINSON, WILLIAM B., ed., *The Physicians and Surgeons of the United States.* Philadelphia, 1878.

Biographies of Physicians and Surgeons. Chicago, 1904.

Chicago Medical Blue Book. Chicago, 1895–.

Chicago Medical Register. 9 vols. Chicago, 1876–1887.

The Chicago Medical Register and Directory. Chicago, 1872–.

CHICAGO MEDICAL SOCIETY, *History of Medicine and Surgery and Physicians and Surgeons of Chicago.* Chicago, 1922.

CUTLER, H. G., ed., *Physicians and Surgeons of the West: Illinois Edition.* Chicago, 1900.

GROSS, SAMUEL D., ed., *Lives of Eminent American Physicians and Surgeons of the Nineteenth Century.* Philadelphia, 1861.

KELLY, HOWARD A., ed., *Cyclopedia of American Medical Biographies.* 2 vols. Philadelphia, 1912.

——, and BURRAGE, WALTER L., eds., *American Medical Biographies.* 3 vols. Baltimore, 1920.

——, *Dictionary of American Medical Biography.* New York, 1928.

MOSHER, CHARLES D., *Mosher's Centennial Historical Album Containing Photographs, Autographs and Biographies of Chicago Physicians.* Chicago, 1876.

Prominent Physicians, Surgeons, and Medical Institutions of Cook County in the Closing Year of the Nineteenth Century. Chicago, [1899].

SPERRY, F. M., ed., *A Group of Distinguished Physicians and Surgeons of Chicago.* Chicago, 1904.

STONE, R. FRENCH, ed., *Biography of Eminent American Physicians and Surgeons.* Indianapolis, 1894.

WATERMAN, ARBA NELSON, *Historical Review of Chicago and Cook County.* . . . 3 vols. Chicago, 1908.

WATSON, IRVING A., ed., *Physicians and Surgeons of America.* Concord, New Hampshire, 1896.

WILLIAMS, STEPHEN W., *American Medical Biography.* Greenfield, Massachusetts, 1845.

HISTORY OF MEDICINE

ALLEN, RAYMOND B., *Medical Education and the Changing Order.* New York, 1946.

BONNER, THOMAS N., "The Social and Political Attitudes of Midwestern Physicians, 1840–1940," in *Journal of the History of Medicine and Allied Sciences,* 7:133–164 (April, 1953).

BURR, C. B., *Medical History of Michigan.* 2 vols. Minneapolis, 1930.

BULLOCK, WILLIAM, *The History of Bacteriology.* New York, 1938.

CASTIGLIONI, ARTURO, *A History of Medicine.* 2d ed. New York, 1947.

CORWIN, EDWARD H. L., *The American Hospital.* New York, 1946.

DEUTSCH, ALBERT, *The Mentally Ill in America: A History of Their Care and Treatment from Colonial Times.* . . . Rev. ed. New York, 1949.

EBERLE, IRMENGARDE, *Modern Medical Discoveries.* New York, 1948.

FAIRCHILD, DAVID S., *History of Medicine in Iowa.* N. p., 1927.

FISHBEIN, MORRIS, *Frontiers of Medicine.* New York, 1933.

FRANK, LOUIS F., *The Medical History of Milwaukee 1834–1914.* Milwaukee, 1915.

GALDSTON, IAGO, *Progress in Medicine: A Critical Review of the Last Hundred Years.* . . . New York, 1940.

GARRISON, FIELDING H., *An Introduction to the History of Medicine.* . . . 4th ed. Philadelphia, 1929.

——, *Lectures on the History of Medicine, a Series of Lectures at the Mayo Foundation.* . . . Philadelphia, 1933.

GOODWIN, E. J., *A History of Medicine in Missouri.* St. Louis, 1905.

GUTHRIE, DOUGLAS, *A History of Medicine.* . . . Philadelphia, 1946.

HAAGENSEN, CUSHMAN, and LLOYD, WYNDHAM E. B., *A Hundred Years of Medicine.* New York, 1943.

HAGGARD, HOWARD W., *Devils, Drugs, and Doctors: The Story of the*

Science of Healing from Medicine-Man to Doctor. . . . New York, 1929.
——, *The Doctor in History.* New Haven, Connecticut, 1934.
JORDAN, PHILIP D., "Some Bibliographical and Research Aids to American Medical History," in *Ohio State Archaeological and Historical Quarterly,* 50:305–325 (December, 1941).
KEMPER, WILLIAM H., *A Medical History of the State of Indiana.* Chicago, 1911.
LEONARDO, RICHARD A., *History of Surgery.* New York, 1943.
MAJOR, RALPH H., *Disease and Destiny.* . . . New York, 1936.
METTLER, CECILIA A., *History of Medicine.* . . . Philadelphia, 1947.
MUMFORD, JAMES G., *A Narrative of Medicine in America.* Philadelphia, 1903.
NEWSHOLME, SIR ARTHUR, *The Story of Modern Preventive Medicine.* . . . Baltimore, 1929.
NEW YORK ACADEMY OF MEDICINE, *Medicine in the Changing Order.* New York, 1947.
OHIO STATE UNIVERSITY MEDICAL SCHOOL, *A Collection of Source Material Covering a Century of Medical Progress 1834–1934.* Blanchester, Ohio, 1934.
OSLER, WILLIAM, *The Evolution of Modern Medicine.* . . . New Haven, Connecticut, 1921.
PACKARD, FRANCIS R., *History of Medicine in the United States.* . . . 2 vols. New York, 1931.
PUSEY, WILLIAM ALLEN, *The History of Dermatology.* Springfield, Illinois, 1933.
RIESMAN, DAVID, *Medicine in Modern Society.* Princeton, 1938.
SHRYOCK, RICHARD H., *American Medical Research, Past and Present.* New York, 1947.
——, *The Development of Modern Medicine: An Interpretation of the Social and Scientific Factors Involved.* 2d ed. New York, 1947.
——, "Medical Sources and the Social Historian," in *American Historical Review,* 41:458–473 (April, 1936).
SIGERIST, HENRY E., *American Medicine.* New York, 1934.
——, *Civilization and Disease.* Ithaca, New York, 1943.
——, *The Great Doctors: A Biographical History of Medicine.* . . . Rev. ed. New York, 1933.
——, *A History of Medicine.* . . . vol. 1. New York, 1951.
SINGER, CHARLES JOSEPH, *A Short History of Medicine.* . . . New York, 1928.

SORSBY, ARNOLD, *A Short History of Ophthalmology.* . . . London, 1933.

STERN, BERNHARD J., *American Medical Practice in the Perspectives of a Century.* New York, 1945.

——, *Society and Medical Progress.* Princeton, New Jersey, 1941.

ZEUCH, LUCIUS H., comp., *History of Medical Practice in Illinois.* Vol. 1, *Preceding 1850.* Chicago, 1927.

ZILBOORG, GREGORY, in collaboration with GEORGE W. HENRY, *A History of Medical Psychology.* New York, 1941.

HISTORY OF CHICAGO

ADDAMS, JANE, *Twenty Years at Hull-House.* New York, 1910.

——, *The Second Twenty Years at Hull-House.* New York, 1930.

ALVORD, CLARENCE W., ed., *The Centennial History of Illinois.* 6 vols. Springfield, 1917–1920.

ANDREAS, ALFRED T., *History of Chicago: From the Earliest Period to the Present Time.* 3 vols. Chicago, 1884–1886.

——, *History of Cook County, Illinois: From the Earliest Period to the Present Time.* Chicago, 1884.

BERNERT, ELEANOR H., see WIRTH, LOUIS.

BURGESS, ERNEST W., and NEWCOMB, CHARLES, eds., *Census Data of the City of Chicago, 1920, 1930.* Chicago, 1931, 1933.

CURREY, JOSIAH SEYMOUR, *Chicago: Its History and Its Builders.* . . . 5 vols. Chicago, 1912.

DOLLAR, MELVIN L., Vital Statistics for Cook County and Chicago. 3 vols. Multigraphed. Chicago, 1942.

FEDERAL WRITERS' PROJECT, *Selected Bibliography: Illinois, Chicago and Its Environs.* American Guide Series. Chicago, 1937.

GOODSPEED, WESTON A., and HEALY, DANIEL D., eds., *History of Cook County, Illinois.* . . . 2 vols. Chicago, 1909.

KIRKLAND, JOSEPH, see MOSES, JOHN.

LEWIS, LLOYD, *Chicago: The History of Its Reputation.* Introduction and Part II by Henry Justin Smith. New York, 1929.

McILVAINE, MABEL, comp., *Reminiscences of Early Chicago (The Lakeside Classics).* Chicago, 1912.

——, *Reminiscences of Chicago during the Forties and Fifties (The Lakeside Classics).* Chicago, 1913.

——, *Reminiscences of Chicago during the Civil War (The Lakeside Classics).* Chicago, 1914.

——, *Reminiscences of Chicago during the Great Fire* (*The Lakeside Classics*). Chicago, 1915.

MOSES, JOHN, *Illinois, Historical and Statistical.* . . . 2 vols. Chicago, 1889–1892.

——, and KIRKLAND, JOSEPH, comps., *History of Chicago, Illinois,* 2 vols. Chicago, 1895.

NEWCOMB, CHARLES, *see* BURGESS, ERNEST W.

PEASE, THEODORE C., *The Story of Illinois.* 2d ed. Chicago, 1949.

PIERCE, BESSIE L., *A History of Chicago.* vol. 1. New York, 1937.

QUAIFE, MILO M., *Chicago and the Old Northwest 1673–1835.* . . . Chicago, 1913.

WIRTH, LOUIS, AND BERNERT, ELEANOR H., eds., *Local Community Fact Book of Chicago.* Chicago, 1949.

BOOKS AND PAMPHLETS

ABBOTT, EDITH, *The Tenements of Chicago 1908–1935.* Chicago, 1936.

ABT, ISAAC, *Baby Doctor.* New York, 1944.

ACKERKNECHT, ERWIN H., *Malaria in the Upper Mississippi Valley 1760–1900.* (Supplements to the *Bulletin of the History of Medicine,* No. 4). Baltimore, 1945.

Addresses Delivered upon the Reopening of the Medical Department of the University of Illinois. N. p., [1913].

AMERICAN FOUNDATION STUDIES IN GOVERNMENT, *American Medicine; Expert Testimony out of Court.* 2 vols. N. p. 1937.

AMERICAN MEDICAL ASSOCIATION, *Proceedings of the National Medical Convention Held in New York, May, 1846, and in Philadelphia, May, 1947.* N. p., n. d.

——, Council on Medical Education and Hospitals, *Medical Education in the United States 1934–1939.* Chicago, 1940.

AMERICAN PUBLIC HEALTH ASSOCIATION, "Public Health in Illinois: Free Report of a Study Completed in June, 1942." Mimeographed.

AMERICAN PUBLIC WELFARE ASSOCIATION, *Medical Care for the Unemployed and Their Families under the Plan of the Federal Emergency Relief Administration.* . . . [Chicago? 1934?].

ANDERSON, ODIN W., *see* SINAI, NATHAN.

AUGUSTIN, GEORGE, *History of Yellow Fever.* New Orleans, 1909.

BACHMAN, GEORGE W., and MERIAM, LEWIS, *The Issue of Compulsory Health Insurance.* Washington, D. C., 1948.

BARKER, LEWELLYS F., *Time and the Physician*. New York, 1942.

BATES, RALPH S., *Scientific Societies in the United States*. Cambridge, Massachusetts, 1945.

BAY, EMMET B., *The Quality of Care Rendered by the University of Chicago Clinics*. Chicago, 1932.

BAY, JENS CHRISTIAN, *Dr. Christian Fenger: The Man and His Work*. [Chicago?], 1940.

BEARD, CHARLES A., ed., *Whither Mankind?* New York, 1928.

BELFIELD, WILLIAM T., *On the Relations of Micro-organisms to Disease. . . .* New York, 1883.

BILLINGS MEDICAL CLUB OF CHICAGO, *A Service in Memory of Frank Billings*. Chicago, 1932.

BLACK, CARL E., and BESSIE M., *From Pioneer to Scientist: The Life Story of Greene Vardiman Black, "Father of Modern Dentistry," and His Son, Arthur Davenport Black. . . .* St. Paul, Minnesota, 1940.

BOAS, ERNST P., *The Unseen Plague: Chronic Disease*. New York, 1940.

BOOTH, E. R., *History of Osteopathy, and Twentieth-Century Medical Practice*. Memorial ed. Cincinnati, 1924.

BRECKINRIDGE, SOPHONISBA P., *The Illinois Poor Law and Its Administration*. Chicago, 1939.

BRIDGE, NORMAN, *The Marching Years*. New York, 1920.

BROWN, JAMES, *The History of Public Assistance in Chicago 1883–1893*. Chicago, 1941.

BUFORD, COLEMAN G., *see* Hektoen, Ludvig.

BULEY, R. CARLYLE, *see* PICKARD, MADGE E.

BUSHNELL, CHARLES J., *The Social Problem at the Chicago Stock Yards*. Chicago, 1902.

CABOT, HUGH, *The Patient's Dilemma: The Quest for Medical Security in America*. New York, 1940.

CHAMBERLAIN, CLAUDE W., comp., *General Information and Illinois Laws Relating to the Public Health*. State of Illinois, Department of Public Health, 1940.

CHASE, THOMAS N., ed., *Mortality among Negroes in Cities*. Atlanta, Georgia, 1903.

CHESBROUGH, ELLIS S., *Chicago Sewerage*. Chicago, 1858.

CHICAGO, CITY OF, *Report of the Board of Health*, 1867–.

——, City Council, *Sanitary Code*, 1911, *City of Chicago, with*

Amendments and Additions up to and including July 10, 1916. Chicago, 1916.

——, City Council, *Sanitary Code, 1922. . . .* Chicago, 1923.

——, Department of Health, *Report and Handbook for the Years 1911 to 1918 Inclusive*. Chicago, 1919.

——, Department of Health, *Report of Streams Examination, Chemic and Bacteriologic, of the Waters between Lake Michigan at Chicago and the Mississippi River at St. Louis. . . .* Chicago, 1902.

——, Department of Welfare, *Chicago Cares: A Decade of Service. Decennial Report of the Department of Welfare 1936–1946*. Chicago, 1946.

——, Municipal Reference Library, *Index to Municipal Legislation*. Chicago, 1937.

——, Sanitary District, *The Sanitary District of Chicago*. [Chicago], 1919.

(CHICAGO) CITY HOMES ASSOCIATION, *A Study of Tuberculosis in Chicago*. Chicago, 1905.

——, *Tenement Conditions in Chicago. . . .* Chicago, 1901.

CHICAGO HEALTH STATISTICS SURVEY, WORKS PROGRESS ADMINISTRATION, *Health Data Book for the 75 Local Community Areas of the City of Chicago*. Chicago, 1939.

CHICAGO HOSPITAL FOR WOMEN AND CHILDREN, *Annual Report, 1865–1891*.

CHICAGO INSTITUTE FOR PSYCHOANALYSIS, *Report of the Five Year Period 1942–1947*. [Chicago, 1947].

CHICAGO LARYNGOLOGICAL AND OTOLOGICAL SOCIETY, *Constitution, and By-Laws and Membership Roster*. [Chicago, 1948].

CHICAGO MATERNITY CENTER, *Annual Report, 1932–*.

CHICAGO MEDICAL SOCIETY, Committee on Medical Economics, *Report of a Study of the Abuse of Free Medical Service in Out Patient Practice*." Multigraphed. Chicago, 1935.

——, *The Medical Care Required and Available in Cook County*. Chicago, 1939.

CHICAGO RELIEF ADMINISTRATION, *Official Bulletin*. Nos. 361-540. Multigraphed. Chicago, May-November, 1937.

CHICAGO RELIEF AND AID SOCIETY, *Chicago Relief: First Special Report of the Chicago Relief and Aid Society*. Chicago, 1871.

——, *Report of the Committee on Sick, Hospital, and Sanitary Measures*. Chicago, 1874.

CHICAGO SOCIETY OF INDUSTRIAL MEDICINE AND SURGERY, *Constitution and By-Laws.* [N. d., n. p.].

CHICAGO VENEREAL DISEASE CONTROL PROGRAM, *Progress Report, July 1, 1943 to October 31, 1947.* Chicago, 1947.

CLEVENGER, SHOBAL V., *Address to the Chicago Academy of Medicine at the Organization Meeting, September 21, 1890.* Philadelphia, 1890.

——, *Fun in a Doctor's Life.* . . . Atlantic City, 1909.

——, *Treatment of the Insane.* Chicago, 1896.

COLE, ARTHUR C., *The Irrepressible Conflict 1850–1865.* New York, 1934.

COLLEGE OF PHYSICIANS AND SURGEONS, *First Decennial Catalogue 1881–1891, and the Announcement for 1892–1893.* Chicago, 1892.

COMMITTEE OF MEDICAL WOMEN, Council of National Defense, *Census of Women Physicians.* Rochester, New York, 1918.

COMMITTEE ON THE COSTS OF MEDICAL CARE. *Medical Care for the American People.* Chicago, 1932.

COOK COUNTY, Board of County Commissioners, *Annual Report of the Cook County Agent, Warden Insane Asylum and Poor House, Medical Sup't to Cook County Insane Asylum, Warden Cook County Hospital, Cook County Physician, and Coroner.* Chicago, 1876.

——, Board of County Commissioners, *Proceedings, 1876–1877.* Chicago, 1878.

——, Circuit Court, *Trustees of the Rush Medical College . . . vs. The University of Chicago. . . , Complaint.* Case no. 41C 4423. Chicago, 1941.

COUNCIL OF SOCIAL AGENCIES OF CHICAGO, Health Division, *Annual Report, 1937–1939.*

CUTLER, H. G., ed., *Medical and Dental Colleges of the West: Chicago.* Chicago, 1896.

DANFORTH, ISAAC N., *The Life of Nathan Smith Davis.* . . . Chicago, 1907.

DAVIS, LOYAL, *J. B. Murphy, Stormy Petrel of Surgery.* New York, 1938.

DAVIS, MICHAEL M., *America Organizes Medicine.* New York, 1941.

DAVIS, NATHAN SMITH, *The Basis of Scientific Medicine and the Proper Methods of Investigation.* Chicago, 1891.

——, *History of Medical Education and Institutions in the United States.* . . . Chicago, 1851.

——, *History of Medicine, with Code of Medical Ethics.* Chicago, 1903.

——, *History of the American Medical Association from Its Organization up to January, 1855.* Philadelphia, 1855.

——, *The History, Present Status, and Future Progress of Practical Medicine.* Chicago, 1893.

——, *Inaugural Address Delivered at the Opening of the Medical Department of Lind University.* Chicago, 1859.

——, *Lecture Introductory to the Fifth Annual Course of Instruction in the Chicago Medical College.* Chicago, 1863.

——, *Lectures on the Principles and Practice of Medicine. . . .* Chicago, 1884.

——, *The Present Status of Bacteriologic Investigations and Their Relations to Etiology and Therapeutics.* Chicago, 1895.

——, *What Are the Most Efficient and Practical Means for Limiting the Prevalence and Fatality of Pulmonary Tuberculosis.* Chicago, 1899.

DEELMAN, HERMAN T., ed., *Surgery a Hundred Years Ago.* London, 1925.

DE KRUIF, PAUL, *Man Against Death.* New York, 1932.

——, in collaboration with Rhea De Kruif, *Life among the Doctors.* New York, 1949.

DE LEE, JOSEPH B., *The Chicago Lying-in Hospital and Dispensary, and the Chicago Maternity Center.* Chicago, 1934.

Directory of American Specialists. 5th ed. Chicago, 1951.

DOLLAR, MELVIN L., *see* Sinai, Nathan.

DOWNING, CARTER H., *Principles and Practice of Osteopathy.* Kansas City, 1923.

DRAKE, DANIEL, *A Systematic Treatise, Historical, Etiological, and Practical, on the Principal Diseases of the Interior Valley of North America. . . .* 2 vols. Vol. 1, Cincinnati, 1850; vol. 2, Philadelphia, 1854.

DUNHAM, WARREN H., *see* FARIS, ROBERT E. LEE.

EARLE, CHARLES W., *The Demand for a Woman's Medical College in the West. . . .* Waukegan, Illinois, 1879.

——, *Progress in the Study and Practice of Medicine by Women.* Chicago, 1891.

——, *Synopsis of Lectures on Obstetrics.* Chicago, 1885.

EMBREE, EDWIN R., *Julius Rosenwald Fund; Review of Two Decades 1917–1936.* Chicago, 1936.

EVANS, JOHN, *Memorial of Doctor John Evans Praying the Establishment of a System of Quarantine Regulations for the Prevention of the Spread of Cholera.* 39 Congress, 2 session, House Miscellaneous Document, no. 66. Washington, D. C., 1866.

EWING, OSCAR R., *The Nation's Health: A Ten Year Program.* Washington, D. C., 1948.

FARIS, ROBERT E. LEE, and DUNHAM, H. WARREN, *Mental Disorders in Urban Areas.* . . . Chicago, 1939.

FAVILL, JOHN B., ed., *Henry Baird Favill: A Memorial Volume.* Chicago, 1917.

FENGER, CHRISTIAN, *Proceedings of the Testimonial Banquet Given in Honor of Prof. Christian Fenger, on November 3rd, 1900, by the Medical Profession.* Chicago, 1900.

FIELD, DAVID D., *The Genealogy of the Brainerd Family in the United States.* . . . New York, 1857.

FISHBEIN, MORRIS, *A History of the American Medical Association 1847 to 1947.* Philadelphia, 1947.

———, with Sol Theron De Lee, *Joseph Bolivar De Lee, Crusading Obstetrician.* New York, 1949.

FLEXNER, ABRAHAM, *I Remember: The Autobiography of Abraham Flexner.* New York, 1940.

———, *Medical Education in the United States and Canada.* . . . New York, 1910.

GARCEAU, OLIVER, *The Political Life of the American Medical Association.* Chicago, 1941.

GERHARD, FRED., *Illinois as It Is.* . . . Chicago, 1857.

GORGAS, NELLIE, *see* McLEAN, FRANKLIN.

GRADLE, HENRY, *Bacteria and the Germ Theory of Disease: Eight Lectures Delivered at the Chicago Medical College.* Chicago, 1883.

GREVSTAD, NICOLAY A., *The Norwegian-American Hospital, Chicago.* [Chicago, 1930].

GROVE, ROBERT D., *see* Linder, Forest E.

GRUBBÉ, EMIL H., *X-Ray Treatment: Its Origin, Birth and Early History.* St. Paul, Minnesota, 1949.

GUNN, JANE A., *Memorial Sketches of Doctor Moses Gunn by His Wife.* . . . Chicago, 1889.

HAGGARD, HOWARD W., *The Science of Health and Disease; a Textbook of Physiology and Hygiene.* New York, 1927.

Hall & Smith's Chicago City Directory for 1853–'54. Chicago, 1853.

HARRISON, LEONARD V., *see* MAYERS, LEWIS.

HEALTH INSURANCE COUNCIL, Survey Committee, *A Survey of Accident and Health Coverage in the United States as of December 31, 1948*. N. p., 1949.

HEALY, WILLIAM, *The Individual Delinquent*. Boston, 1920.

HEITMAN, FRANCIS B., *Historical Register and Dictionary of the United States Army*. . . . 2 vols. Washington, D. C., 1903.

HEKTOEN, LUDVIG, and BUFORD, COLMAN G., eds., *The Collected Works of Christian Fenger, M.D., 1840–1902*. 2 vols. Philadelphia, 1912.

HENROTIN HOSPITAL, *Annual Report*, 1940, 1946. [Chicago? n. d.].

HERRICK, JAMES B., *Memories of Eighty Years*. Chicago, 1949.

HERTZLER, ARTHUR E., *The Horse and Buggy Doctor*. New York, 1938.

HIGLEY, WILLIAM K., *Historical Sketch of the Academy* (Chicago Academy of Sciences, *Special Publication No. 1*). Chicago, 1902.

HOLLISTER, JOHN H., *Memories of Eighty Years: Autosketches, Random Notes and Reminiscences*. Chicago, 1912.

Hull-House Maps and Papers. New York, 1895.

HURD, HENRY M., and others, *The Institutional Care of the Insane in the United States and Canada*. 4 vols. Baltimore, 1916–1917.

HYDE, JAMES N., *Early Medical Chicago*. . . . Fergus' Historical Series no. 11. Chicago, 1879.

ILLINOIS, STATE OF, Board of Commissioners of Public Charities, *Ninth Biennial Report, 1886*. Springfield, 1887.

——, Board of Health, *Annual Report, 1873–1913*. Springfield, 1879–1914.

——, Commission on Occupational Diseases, *Report of Commission on Occupational Diseases to His Excellency Governor Charles S. Deneen*. Chicago, 1911.

——, Department of Public Health, *Annual Report, 1917–*. Springfield, 1919.

ILLINOIS MEDICAL CENTER DISTRICT, *Fact Book: A Description of the Research, Healing and Teaching Institutions which Constitute the District . . . Their History . . . and a Glance at the Future*. Chicago, 1948.

ILLINOIS STATE MEDICAL SOCIETY, *Proceedings of the Medical Convention for the Purpose of Organizing the Illinois State Medical Society Held at Springfield, June 4, 1850*. . . . Chicago, 1850.

INFANT WELFARE SOCIETY OF CHICAGO, *Annual Report, 1911–*. [Chicago, 1911?].

JAFFARY, STUART K., *The Mentally Ill and Public Provision for Their Care in Illinois*. Chicago, 1942.

JERGER, JOSEPH A., *Doctor—Here's Your Hat! The Autobiography of a Family Doctor*. New York, 1939.

JIRKA, FRANK J., *American Doctors of Destiny*. . . . Chicago, 1940.

JOHNSON, CHARLES B., *Sixty Years in Medical Harness*. New York, 1926.

JOHNSON, GLENN H., *Relief and Health Problems of a Selected Group of Non-Family Men*. Chicago, 1937.

JOHNSON, H. A., *History of the Chicago Medical College: An Introductory Lecture to the College Session of 1870–71*. Chicago, 1870.

JUETTNER, OTTO, *Daniel Drake and His Followers: Historical and Biographical Sketches*. Cincinnati, 1909.

KING, WILLIAM H., ed., *History of Homeopathy and Its Institutions in America*. . . . 4 vols. Chicago, 1905.

KLEM, MARGARET C., *Prepayment Medical Care Organizations*. Washington, D. C., 1945.

KNOPF, S. ADOLPHUS, *A History of the National Tuberculosis Association*. . . . New York, 1922.

Lakeside Annual Directory of the City of Chicago, 1874–75. Chicago, 1875.

LA RABIDA JACKSON PARK SANITARIUM, *Annual Report*, 1946. [Chicago? n. d.].

LEIGH, ROBERT D., *Federal Health Administration in the United States*. New York, 1927.

Lewis Memorial Maternity Hospital. Chicago, n. d.

LEWIS, MIRIAM, see BACHMAN, GEORGE W.

LIND UNIVERSITY, Medical Department, *First Annual Announcement*. Chicago, 1859.

LINDER, FOREST E., and GROVE, ROBERT D., *Vital Statistics Rates in the United States 1900–1940*. Washington, D. C., 1943.

LORETTO HOSPITAL, *Strategic Alaska*. Chicago, n. d.

LYDSTON, G. FRANK, *How Simmons, "Our Peerless Leader," Became a Regular*. Chicago, [1909?].

——, *The Medical Frankenstein*. Chicago, 1909.

——, *Where Is the Spirit of '76?* [Chicago? 1909?]

——, *Why I Write for Independent Journals*. [Chicago?], 1908.

MACEACHERN, MALCOLM T., *Manual on Obstetric Practice in Hospitals* (American Hospital Association, *Official Bulletin no. 209*). Chicago, 1940.

McLEAN, FRANKLIN, and GORGAS, NELLIE, eds., "Medicine in the Division of Biological Sciences, University of Chicago," in *Methods and Problems of Medical Education* (Rockefeller Foundation, 19th series). New York, 1931.

McMECHEN, EDGAR C., *Life of Governor Evans*. Denver, Colorado, 1924.

MANHEIMER, STEPHEN, *An Historical Sketch of Mount Sinai Hospital*. [Chicago?], 1940.

MARTIN, FRANKLIN H., *The Joy of Living: An Autobiography*. 2 vols. New York, 1933.

MAURY, DABNEY H., *The Water Works System of the City of Chicago*. Chicago, 1911.

MAYERS, LEWIS, and HARRISON, LEONARD V., *The Distribution of Physicians in the United States*, New York, 1924.

MOORE, HARRY H., *Public Health in the United States*. . . . New York, 1923.

MOYNIHAN, SIR BERKELEY, *Addresses on Surgical Subjects*. Philadelphia, 1928.

MYRDAL, GUNNAR, *An American Dilemma*. New York, 1944.

NATIONAL HEALTH ASSEMBLY, *America's Health: A Report to the Nation*. New York, 1949.

NELSON, EDNA H., *The Women's and Children's Hospital*. [Chicago], 1941.

NELSON, MARION, *The Negro Tuberculosis Problem in Chicago*. Chicago, 1936.

NEWSHOLME, SIR ARTHUR, *Medicine and the State*. Baltimore, 1932.

The Northwestern Medical Almanac. N. p., 1870.

NORTHWESTERN UNIVERSITY, *Annual Catalogue of the Medical School*, 1910–50.

NORTHWESTERN UNIVERSITY MEDICAL SCHOOL, *John Harper Long 1856–1918: A Tribute from His Colleagues*. N. p., [1918].

NORWOOD, WILLIAM F., *Medical Education in the United States before the Civil War*. Philadelphia, 1944.

OCHSNER, EDWARD H., *Social Insurance and Economic Security*. Boston, 1934.

PACKARD, MRS. E. P. W., *The Prisoner's Hidden Life, or Insane Asylums Unveiled*. Chicago, 1868.

PERRY, JAMES C., *Public Health Administration in Chicago, Ill.: A Study of the Organization and Administration of the City Health Department*. Washington, D. C., 1915.

PETERS, CLARENCE A., ed., *Free Medical Care*. New York, 1946.

PETERS, M. ROSANNA, *The History of the Poor Sisters of St. Francis Seraph of the Perpetual Adoration 1875–1940*. Lafayette, Indiana, 1944.

PICKARD, MADGE E., and BULEY, R. CARLYLE, *The Midwest Pioneer: His Ills, Cures, & Doctors*. Crawfordsville, Indiana, 1945.

POOLEY, WILLIAM V., *The Settlement of Illinois from 1830 to 1850*. Madison, 1908.

The Presbyterian Hospital of the City of Chicago, Sixtieth Anniversary 1883–1943. [Chicago], 1943.

PUBLIC HEALTH INSTITUTE, *How Laymen Cut Medical Costs*. Chicago, 1948.

PUSEY, WILLIAM A., *A Doctor of the 1870's and 80's*. Springfield, 1932.

QUAIFE, MILO M., *Chicago as a Medical Center; The Surgeons of Fort Dearborn*. [Chicago? 1913].

QUINE, WILLIAM E., *Addresses Delivered at a Memorial Service at the College of Medicine of the University of Illinois*. Chicago, 1923.

RAPER, HOWARD R., *Man against Pain: The Epic of Anesthesia*. New York, 1945.

RAUCH, JOHN H., *Intramural Interments in Populous Cities and Their Influence upon Health and Epidemics*. Chicago, 1866.

——, *Public Parks: Their Effects upon the Moral, Physical and Sanitary Condition of the Inhabitants of Large Cities*. Chicago, 1869.

——, *Report on Medical Education, Medical Colleges in the Regulation of the Practice of Medicine in the United States and Canada, 1765–1890*. Springfield, Illinois, 1890.

——, *A Report to the Board of Health of the City of Chicago on the Necessity of an Extension of the Sewerage of the City*. Chicago, 1873.

——, *A Sanitary History of Chicago from 1833 to 1870*. Chicago, 1871.

RAVENEL, MAZŸCK P., ed., *A Half Century of Public Health*. New York, 1921.

RAWLINGS, ISAAC D., and collaborators, *The Rise and Fall of Disease in Illinois*. 2 vols. Springfield, 1927.

REED, LOUIS S., *Blue Cross and Medical Service Plans*. Washington, D. C., 1947.

REGENBURG, BERNARD, *Economic and Social Status of Patients of the Public Health Institute of Chicago.* Chicago, 1931.

REYNOLDS, JOHN, *My Own Times.* Belleville, Illinois, 1855.

RHODES, JOHN E., *The Making of a Modern Medical School: A Sketch of Rush Medical College.* [Chicago?], 1901.

RILEY, ELMER A., *The Development of Chicago and Vicinity as a Manufacturing Center Prior to 1880.* Chicago, 1911.

ROBERTSON, JOHN DILL, *A Report on an Epidemic of Influenza in the City of Chicago in the Fall of 1918.* Chicago, 1918.

ROBINSON, VICTOR, *The Don Quixote of Psychiatry.* New York, 1919.

——, *Victory over Pain.* New York, 1946.

RONNING, N. N., *Fiftieth Anniversary of the Lutheran Deaconess Home and Hospital.* [Chicago], 1947.

ROPCHAN, ALEXANDER, *Chicago Hospital and Clinic Survey.* Chicago, 1935.

ROREM, C. RUFUS, *Blue Cross Hospital Service Plans.* 2d ed. N. p., 1944.

——, *Private Group Clinics.* Washington, D. C., 1931.

——, *The Public Investment in Hospitals.* Chicago, 1930.

RORTY, JAMES, *American Medicine Mobilizes.* New York, 1939.

ROSEN, GEORGE, *Fees and Fee Bills: Some Economic Aspects of Medical Practice in Nineteenth Century America (Supplements to the Bulletin of the History of Medicine, No. 6).* Baltimore, 1946.

ROSS, ISHBEL, *Child of Destiny.* New York, 1949.

RUSH MEDICAL COLLEGE, *Annual Announcements*, 1844–1845, 1847–1853, 1855–1880, 1898–1924.

——, *Dedicatory Exercises of the New Building of Rush Medical College.* Chicago, 1876.

SCOTT, WALTER D., *John Evans 1814–1897: An Appreciation.* Evanston, Illinois, 1939.

SHAFER, HENRY B., *The American Medical Profession 1783 to 1850.* New York, 1936.

SHEPARDSON, FRANCIS W., *A Report on the Administration of the Medical Practice Act.* Springfield, 1919.

SHIPMAN, GEORGE E., *Homeopathy, Allopathy, and the City Hospital. . . .* Chicago, 1857.

SINAI, NATHAN, ANDERSON, ODIN W., and DOLLAR, MELVIN L., *Health Insurance in the United States.* New York, 1946.

St. Elizabeth's Hospital, Chicago. Chicago, 1930.

St. Luke's Hospital: Eightieth Anniversary 1865–1945. Chicago, 1945.

SMITH, CLARE LOUISE, *The Evanston Hospital School of Nursing 1898–1948.* Chicago, 1948.

SMITH, GEDDES, see STEVENSON, GEORGE S.

South Side Dispensary of Chicago, Report . . . for the Seven Years Ending Aug. 31st, 1887. Chicago, 1877.

SPIVAK, JOHN L., *The Medical Trust Unmasked.* New York, 1929.

STEADMAN, ROBERT F., *Public Health Organization in the Chicago Region.* Chicago, 1930.

STERN, BERNHARD J., *Medical Services by Government: Local, State and Federal.* New York, 1946.

——, *Medicine in Industry.* New York, 1946.

STEVENSON, GEORGE S., and SMITH, GEDDES, *Child Guidance Clinics: A Quarter Century of Development.* New York, 1934.

STIEGLITZ, EDWARD J., *A Future for Preventive Medicine.* New York, 1945.

A Summary of the Chicago-Cook County Health Survey Conducted by the United States Public Health Service. Chicago, 1947.

SWIFT, LOUIS F., *Yankee of the Yards.* Chicago, 1927.

SYDENSTRICKER, EDGAR, *Health and Environment.* New York, 1933.

THOMPSON, WARREN S., and WHELPTON, P. K., *Population Trends in the United States.* New York, 1933.

UNITED STATES PUBLIC HEALTH SERVICE, *The Chicago-Cook County Health Survey.* New York, 1949.

——, *Tuberculosis in the United States.* 3 vols. New York, 1943–1945.

UNIVERSITY OF ILLINOIS, *Addresses Delivered upon the Reopening of the Medical Department of the University of Illinois, March 6, 1913.* [Chicago, 1913].

VAN INGEN, PHILIP, *The New York Academy of Medicine: Its First Hundred Years.* New York, 1949.

VAUGHAN, VICTOR C., *A Doctor's Memories.* Indianapolis, 1926.

WEBB, CONSTANCE B., *A History of Contagious Disease Care in Chicago before the Great Fire.* Chicago, 1940.

WENGER, O. C., *An Evaluation of the Chicago Syphilis Control Program after One Year.* Chicago, 1938. Multigraphed.

WESLEY MEMORIAL HOSPITAL, *Annual Report,* 1948. [Chicago, 1948].

WHELPTON, P. K., *Forecasts of the Population of the United States, 1945–1975.* Washington, D. C., 1947.

——, *see also* Thompson, Warren S.

WILBUR, RAY L., *The March of Medicine: Selected Addresses and Articles on Medical Topics 1913–1937.* Stanford University, 1938.

WILDE, ARTHUR H., ed., *Northwestern University: A History 1855–1905.* 3 vols. New York, 1905.

WILLIAMS, ELMER L., ed., *"That Man Bundesen."* [Chicago], 1931.

WINSLOW, CHARLES-EDWARD A., *The Conquest of Epidemic Disease: A Chapter in the History of Ideas.* Princeton, 1943.

——, *The Evolution and Significance of the Modern Public Health Campaign.* New Haven, 1923.

——, *The Road to Health.* New York, 1929.

WOMAN'S HOSPITAL MEDICAL COLLEGE, *Annual Announcement,* 1870–1896.

WOODY, THOMAS, *A History of Women's Education in the United States.* 2 vols. New York, 1929.

Index

ACTH, discovery of, 104
Abbott, Edith, 136
Abt, Isaac, 66, 99, 141; his *System of Pediatrics*, 99
Academy of the Medical Sciences (Chicago), 73–74
Academy of Medicine (New York), 73, 249
Administrative Committee of the Central Service for the Chronically Ill, 132
Advertising, medical, 12–13, 76, 90, 126–127, 129–130, 236, 238–240, 243–244
Aged, the, as a medical problem, 20, 133, 143–145, 196, 198
Agassiz, Louis, 182
Alabama, 70
Albert Merritt Billings Memorial Hospital, 94, 119, 120, 150, 156
Alexian Brothers Hospital, 152, 153
Ambulance service, in Chicago, 128, 132; in New York, 128
Amerman, George K., 160
American Association of Industrial Physicians and Surgeons, 245
American Association for Labor Legislation, 215, 244
American Bar Association, 124, 248
American Board of Ophthalmology, 101
American Board of Pathology, 98
American College of Osteopathic Medicine and Surgery, 63
American College of Radiology, 105–106
American College of Surgeons, 96–98, 105
American Dental Association, 105
American Hospital, 158
American Hospital Association, 105, 245, 247, 248
American Medical Association, 10, founded 14, 17, 23, 37–38, 45, 46,

51, 52, 53, 56, 60, 61, 70, 78, 79, 85, 91, 97, 105, 111, 122, 127, 134, 203, 216–217; on insurance and cost of medical care, 248–249; Council on Medical Education and Hospitals, 113–114, 215; Council on Pharmacy and Chemistry, 196–197; Judicial Council, 239–240, 241
American Medical Temperance Society, 228
American Neurological Association, 102
American Public Health Association, 183, 194, 248
American Society of Anesthesiologists, 106
American Surgical Association, 103
Amoebic dysentery, outbreak in 1933, 194–195
Andrews, Edmund, 34, 35, 42–43, 53, 70, 74, 202
Andrews, Edward Wyllis, 85
Anesthesia, reception in Chicago, ix, 9, 16, 43, 104
Angell, James B., 92
Antibiotics, 143, 250
Antisepsis, development of, 33, 151; reception of in Chicago, ix, 34, 35, 37, 147, 148, 161
Appendicitis, 88, 90
Arlt, Ferdinand, 74
Armour, Phillip Danforth, 103
Armour Laboratories, 104
Arthritis, 93
Asepsis, 35, 37, 87, 92, 148, 153
Association of American Physicans and Surgeons, 106, 204
Association of Internes and Medical Students, 248
Atomic Energy Commission, 106
Attica, Indiana, 49
Axford, William L., 21